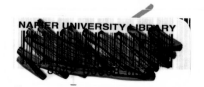

SUDDEN INFANT DEATH SYNDROME

Sudden Infant Death Syndrome

Medical Aspects and Psychological Management

edited by

JAN L. CULBERTSON, Ph.D.
Associate Professor of Pediatrics and Director of Neuropsychology,
Child Study Center, University of Oklahoma Health Sciences Center

HENRY F. KROUS, M.D.
Director of Pathology, Children's Hospital and Health Center, and
Clinical Professor of Pathology, University of California, San Diego

R. DEBRA BENDELL, Ph.D.
Psychological Director, High Risk Clinic, University of Miami
School of Medicine

Edward Arnold
A division of Hodder & Stoughton
LONDON   MELBOURNE   AUCKLAND

618.92026 CUL

The authors gratefully acknowledge the expertise and many contributions of
Ms. Sue Mullins in the preparation of this book.

First published in Great Britain, 1989
by Edward Arnold, the educational, academic
and medical division of Hodder and Stoughton
Limited, 41 Bedford Square, London WC1B 3DQ.

The paper used in this publication meets the minimum requirements of American National
Standard for Information Sciences—Permanence of Paper for Printed Library Materials,
ANSI Z39.48-1984.

British Library Cataloguing in Publication Data

Sudden infant death syndrome.

1. Babies. Sudden infant death syndrome
I. Culbertson, Jan L. II. Krous, Henry F.   III. Bendell, R. Debra
618.92'01

ISBN 0-340-49381-6

Whilst the advice and information in this book is believed to be true and accurate at the date
of going to press, neither the author nor the publisher can accept any legal responsibility or
liability for any errors or omissions that may be made.

Contents

Contributors

J. Bruce Beckwith, M.D., is Chairman of Pathology at the Children's Hospital, Denver, Colorado. He was formerly Director of Laboratories at the Children's Orthopedic Hospital and Medical Center in Seattle, Washington, Professor of Pathology and Pediatrics at the University of Washington School of Medicine, and Director of the SIDS research project at the Children's Orthopedic Hospital and Medical Center.

R. Debra Bendell, Ph.D., Psychological Director, High Risk Clinic, at the University of Miami School of Medicine, is author of the articles "The Impact of the Apneic Infant on Family Life," "Prematurity and the Family," and "Longitudinal Follow-Up of SIDS Families."

Abraham B. Bergman, M.D., Director of Pediatrics at Harborview Medical Center and Professor of Pediatrics at the University of Washington in Seattle, served as President of the National SIDS Foundation from 1972–1977. He is the author of *The "Discovery" of SIDS: Lessons in the Practice of Political Medicine,* as well as twenty-six other publications on SIDS.

Jan L. Culbertson, Ph.D., is Associate Professor of Pediatrics and Director of Neuropsychology at the Child Study Center, University of Oklahoma Health Sciences Center. She has co-authored numerous chapters and articles in the areas of pediatric and clinical child psychology and neuropsychology, including "Apneic Infants: Early Development, Temperament and Maternal Stress." She is editor of the *Division 37 Newsletter* and secretary of the Section on Clinical Child Psychology of the American Psychological Association.

Christian Guilleminault, M.D., Associate Director of the Sleep Disorders Clinic and Research Center and Professor of the Department of Psychiatry and Behavioral Sciences, Stanford University, received his neurologic and psychiatric training in Paris and Geneva. Devoted to human sleep pathology, he initiated the concept of "internal medicine during sleep."

Dorothy H. Kelly, M.D., Assistant Professor of Pediatrics at Harvard Medical School and Associate Pediatrician and Coordinator of the Pediatric Pulmonary Laboratory at Massachusetts General Hospital, has conducted extensive research and is the author of many articles on apnea of infancy. She has served on the American Academy of Pediatrics Prolonged Infantile Apnea Task Force.

Henry F. Krous, M.D., Director of Pathology, Children's Hospital and Health Center, San Diego, and Clinical Professor of Pathology, University of California, San Diego, has authored contributions on SIDS, especially in the areas of human and experimental pathology. He is a member of the Medical Research Board and former member of the Board of Trustees of the National Sudden Infant Death Syndrome Foundation and is on the Editorial Board of *Pediatric Pathology.*

Frederick Mandell, M.D., Children's Doctor and Associate Clinical Professor of Pediatrics, Harvard Medical School; Senior Associate in Medicine, Children's Hospital, Boston, Massachusetts; Consulting Pediatrician; Vice Chairman, National SIDS Foundation; Director, Massachusetts SIDS Center; Editor, *Pediatric Alert;* Associate Editor, *Child Health Alert;* and unpublished poet, is the author of many writings on SIDS.

Donald R. Peterson, M.D., M.P.H., Professor of Epidemiology at the University of Washington in Seattle, has been engaged in research on SIDS for the past twenty years. In addition to articles published in scientific journals, he has written a review on the evolution of the epidemiology of SIDS and has contributed chapters in several books.

Peter J. Schwartz, M.D., is Associate Professor of Medicine at the University of Milan, Italy, and Professor of Physiology and Biophysics at the University of Oklahoma Health Sciences Center. His main area of expertise is the neural control of circulation, particularly the relationship between the autonomic nervous system and sudden cardiac death. He is the Editor of *Neural Mechanisms in Cardiac Arrhythmias,* and of *Clinical Aspects of Life-Threatening Arrhythmias.*

Daniel C. Shannon, M.D., is Director of the Pediatric Pulmonary Unit at Massachusetts General Hospital and Associate Professor of Pediatrics in the Harvard-MIT School of Health Sciences and Technology where he also directs the respiratory pathophysiology section. His research is focused on systems analysis of respiratory control. He is a member of the American Physiological Society, Society for Pediatric Research, American Pediatric Society, and American Thoracic Society.

Terri L. Shelton, Ph.D., Pediatric/Clinical Psychologist within the Department of Pediatrics, University of Iowa, provides outpatient services to the Infant and Young Child Clinic and consultative services to the Infant Apnea Clinic within the Pediatric Pulmonary Department, University of

Iowa. She has conducted several research projects relating to infantile apnea.

Lois Sims Slovik, M.D., Director of Family Therapy at the Massachusetts General Hospital and Clinical Instructor at the Harvard Medical School, has been clinically involved with monitoring parents since 1978. Her specific area of expertise is in working with parents who have been monitoring for more than twelve months (i.e., 1–9 years).

Bradley T. Thach, M.D., Professor of Pediatrics at Washington University School of Medicine and Neonatologist at St. Louis Children's Hospital, St. Louis, Missouri, has conducted research on pharyngeal and upper airway physiology, maturation of respiratory control, and infantile apneic spells. He is a member of the American Physiological Society, American Thoracic Society, and Society for Pediatric Research.

Diane J. Willis, Ph.D., Professor of Medical Psychology, Department of Pediatrics, and Director of Psychological Services, Child Study Center, University of Oklahoma Health Sciences Center, has authored or co-authored numerous chapters and articles in the area of exceptionality and pediatric psychology. She is past Editor of the *Journal of Clinical Child Psychology* and *Journal of Pediatric Psychology* and past President of the Society of Pediatric Psychology, Section on Clinical Child Psychology, and the Division of Children, Youth, and Family Services of the American Psychological Association.

Foreword

Before 1960 there was virtually no organized or systematic professional approach to what was then known as crib death. Young, healthy infants died suddenly and inexplicably. Coroners and the few medical examiners who existed duly noted those deaths; however, they did not know what to do about them or even how to interpret them. A few fortunate, usually rather well-to-do families received support and consolation from their family physicians or pediatricians, but the great majority had no one to whom to turn.

Twenty-five years later, that grievous situation has changed radically for the better. As we look back, it is difficult to imagine that so many people suffered so much in those relatively recent days. In the interim, two processes have occurred: (1) a realization by professionals that these survivors really need help, and (2) a conceptualization of the specific roles various health professionals might assume in helping families of SIDS infants, especially in the prevention of mental illness among the survivors.

The idea of providing help specifically for grieving parents who had lost their babies to Sudden Infant Death Syndrome (SIDS) emerged almost simultaneously about 1960, in at least three places: Baltimore, Seattle, and Greenwich, Connecticut. In each of those places, one pair of stricken, intelligent parents decided that something had to be done because there was no one to assist families like themselves. Each couple independently sought help from a physician. Mr. and Mrs. Saul Goldberg of Baltimore, Maryland, turned to the late Dr. Russell Fisher, then medical examiner for the state of Maryland. With his help they founded the Guild for Infant Survival. The efforts of Senator and Mrs. Fred Dore of Seattle, along with their pediatrician, Dr. Robert Polley, resulted in the initiation of several medical research projects as well as new state legislation requiring autopsies for all infants suspected of having died from SIDS. Mr. and Mrs. Jed Roe of Greenwich, Connecticut, were joined by their pediatrician in establishing the Mark Addison Roe Foundation in memory of their infant son. That organization later became the National Sudden Infant Death Syndrome Foundation.

Thus, pediatricians and pathologists were the first professionals who responded to the needs of those bereaved families. As the number of SIDS families increased, they were able to attract more and more members of the medical profession to their cause, and finally they influenced federal agencies as well. The passage of the SIDS Act of 1974 (Public Law 93-270) represented the ultimate victory of those parents and their physicians, as it provided funds for regional centers to perform autopsies and provide information and counseling to SIDS families.

At the National Institute for Child Health and Human Development (NICHD), Dr. Eileen Hasselmeyer, a nurse, responded to the wave of parental pressure to aid SIDS families; she had a profound influence on the growing movement. Not only did she interest unprecedented numbers of the world's leading scientists in the subject but also she took an active role in systematizing efforts to aid families. In 1972 she served as Project Officer for an institute grant to sponsor seminars on SIDS for nurses across the country, who, in turn, helped affected families. Two nurses from the National SIDS Foundation, Peg Pomeroy and Carolyn Szybist, managed those seminars.

In 1972 Dr. Abraham Bergman of Seattle, funded by an NICHD grant, led a massive research project in 150 U.S. communities in an attempt to learn how SIDS families were being served at the local level (Bergman, A. B. 1973. Final report of a study on the management of sudden infant death syndrome (SIDS) in the United States. NICHD Contract #NICHD-72-2738). Seventy-four countries were studied by teams of medical student investigators. Only 23 percent were judged to provide good or excellent service to families, 30 percent were judged fair, and 47 percent provided poor or no service.

In 1973, partly as a response to the results of the Bergman study, the National Institute of Mental Health provided a grant to mobilize community resources for professionals across the nation. Two nurses again did the work: Kathy Peterson in the western states and Barbara French in the east. Everywhere they went, they met with pathologists and county and state health officials in an attempt to establish professional programs for SIDS families. Their work was outstanding and served as a model for the subsequent Maternal and Child Health federally funded programs that emerged in the late 1970s.

When the first federally funded projects took shape in 1975 and 1976, through the efforts of the Maternal and Child Health (MCH) Division of HEW, various professionals began to participate in learning about SIDS, teaching others about SIDS, and serving SIDS families. Included were psychologists, psychiatrists, social workers, emergency medical technicians, and emergency room personnel. When the federally funded MCH projects reached their peak in 1979–81, about fifty areas across the country were receiving optimal assistance. Autopsies were provided routinely and without charge to families. Parents were notified promptly about the results of postmortem examinations. Public health nurses made home visits to all SIDS families to offer assistance and provide additional ancillary services, as deemed necessary. Public awareness and understanding of SIDS had been improved at all levels of the population through the educational services of project personnel, so that individual cases were managed appropriately by professionals in homes, emergency rooms, and even funeral homes.

Since the 1950s, health and mental health professionals have played an ever more prominent role in assisting the familes of SIDS victims. In the beginning, only the occasional pediatrician or family doctor felt compelled to hold out a hand to those stricken parents. Later pathologists, especially pediatric and forensic pathologists, began to serve in the same way. As the various federal projects became established across the nation, more and more professional workers joined the ranks. Included among them were social workers, public health nurses, psychologists, emergency room personnel, and emergency medical technicians.

The outreach is not yet perfect. There are still many parts of the country where unfortunate incidents occur, but the progress that has been made in this sphere in the last fifteen years is impressive to those of us who have witnessed it firsthand.

Ideally all of the health and mental health professionals who come into contact with the families of recent SIDS victims will one day be thoroughly acquainted with the problem and prepared to conduct themselves appropriately. One hopes that they will be supportive and gentle, helpful but not overbearing, and always sensitive to the shock and grief of these relatives who, in a sense, are victims themselves.

MARIE VALDES-DAPENA, M.D.
Pediatric Pathologist and Professor of Pathology
University of Miami School of Medicine

Introduction

Sudden Infant Death Syndrome (SIDS) has been occurring clinically for centuries, but it has been recognized as a relatively distinct entity for only a few decades. Since the 1940s there has been systematic research regarding the etiology, clinicopathologic correlations, and prevention of this syndrome, an overview of which is provided in this volume. The concept and definition of SIDS were not formalized until 1969 at the Second International Conference on Causes of SIDS, and SIDS was not specified as an official cause of death until 1979 when ICD-9 came into use. The past two decades have witnessed a virtual explosion of new information about SIDS from the medical field; however, study regarding the care of survivors of SIDS victims has received less attention. This still elusive syndrome continues to cause enormous grief for parents, siblings, and extended family. Even with recent improvement in diagnostic accuracy, some episodes of SIDS may be viewed with suspicion by child protection agencies, health care professionals, legal and judicial personnel, and even extended family members. Parents of SIDS victims have been and still can be needlessly subjected to intrusive, unnecessarily insensitive investigations of their caretaking. Their grieving is often compounded by unwarranted guilt and lack of needed support by family, friends, and society. It is clear that careful pathological studies must be conducted to delineate cases of SIDS from criminal neglect and infanticide. It is also clear that appropriate management of SIDS dictates not only a careful diagnostic process but also dictates that attention be given to the potentially devastating psychosocial aspects of SIDS for the survivors.

This volume grew out of the need for a comprehensive text that would aid both health and mental health professionals in the understanding and management of SIDS from a psychobiological perspective. Part I, Medical Aspects of Sudden Infant Death Syndrome and Infantile Apnea, provides a comprehensive review of the most recent data on SIDS, including an overview of its epidemiology and pathology as well as a review of the major theories of etiology and pathogenesis. These include theories relating to upper airway obstruction; cardiac dysfunction caused by sympathetic imbalance; infections, such as those resulting from respiratory syncytial virus; and hyperthermia. Many of the authors of this volume are themselves pioneers in the medical and psychological research on SIDS and have contributed to the explosion of new information about this syndrome. They have provided both a historical and current perspective on the many theories of causation and the associated clinical and medical research that support or nullify the theoretical positions adopted. No one theory is emphasized; our intent is to provide an overview of research underlying several aspects of SIDS. Despite the elusive nature and the lack of definitive clinical markers for SIDS, the burgeoning medical research has led to a proliferation of knowledge in developmental physiology, which in itself might provide the basis for a text. Part I provides health practitioners with a detailed medical review of SIDS.

This volume also attempts to integrate medical and psychological issues in the management of SIDS by focusing on the circumstances of the survivor-victims of SIDS and their special needs. Part II, The Psychological Impact and Management of Sudden Infant Death Syndrome, systematically explores family responses to either the loss of a child or the perceived risk of losing a child. The psychological impact of SIDS upon families is profound, due not only to the loss of the infant but also to the special nature of SIDS deaths. Death is sudden and unexpected, usually during sleep, oftentimes without identifiable antecedents or plausible explanations. The death therefore causes a severe grief reaction, which may be complicated by a high level of suspicion and a sense of guilt among surviving family members. Medical and mental health professionals are concerned with providing support to the family and preventing pathological grief reactions that may be disruptive not only to individual family members but also to marital and family functioning in general. The effects of the SIDS death on surviving siblings is explored in depth, with special attention given to a child's conceptualization of death and ways to facilitate normal mourning. Finally, the special circumstances of infants with prolonged interrupted infantile apnea are addressed, with attention to the psychological stresses arising in families because of the monitoring requirements of those afflicted infants. Throughout the psychological portion of the book, an attempt is made to provide an in-depth discussion of family reactions to either the loss or threatened loss of an infant, methods of assessing the reactions of family members, and identification of risk for psychopathology as well as methods of intervention. The mental health practitioner should find this text practical and clinically relevant in addressing the needs of clients affected by SIDS.

The fascinating history of political action responses from the lay and medical communities which led to the development of the National SIDS Foundation is described. This story of grass roots efforts by bereaved parents, pediatricians, and pathologists is important to understanding the growth of research and public information regarding SIDS over the past thirty years. During this time, SIDS has gone from a relatively unknown entity, both in the professional and public sector, to universal recognition as a clinicopathologic entity. The joint advocacy effort of both lay and professional persons has provided the major impetus for the growth and development of knowledge about SIDS.

It is hoped that this volume will have a wide range of professional relevance, applicable to pediatricians, pathologists, emergency room physicians, educational directors of pediatric residency training programs, pediatric nurses, pediatric psychologists, psychiatrists, social workers, clergy, and others who come into contact with the victim-survivors of SIDS. Although much of the manuscript relates to biological and clinical research, portions of it may also be appropriate to the public at large, particularly those nonmedical professionals who may be in caretaking roles with young children (e.g., day care centers).

Finally, it is hoped that this volume will contribute to the better understanding of SIDS and early infantile apnea and to improved care of the survivor-victims.

PART I

Medical Aspects of Sudden Infant Death Syndrome and Infantile Apnea

1

The Epidemiology of Sudden Infant Death Syndrome

DONALD R. PETERSON, M.D.

In the United States, the terms "crib death" and "sudden, unexpected, unexplained infant death (SUUID)" have been superseded to a large extent by the designation sudden infant death syndrome (SIDS) in both lay and scientific circles. The term "cot death" seems to be preferred in Great Britain. Coined in 1969, SIDS was defined as "the sudden death of any infant or young child, which is unexpected by history, and in which a thorough post mortem examination fails to demonstrate an adequate cause of death" [1]. Evaluating a history, conducting a thorough examination, and deciding what might be an adequate cause of death are highly subjective processes; diagnostic decisions based on such processes may vary, not only from one pathologist to the next but also from one time to the next for the same pathologist. Furthermore, the process of diagnosis by exclusion, which the definition prescribes, results in a conclusion based on negative evidence; this axiomatically engenders less confidence than one based on positive findings.

In assigning SIDS as a cause of death, a pathologist, either consciously or unconsciously, may take two other factors into account. One is that SIDS victims typically die while unattended, presumably while asleep, and are therefore found dead at various intervals after being put down for a nap or for the night. The other factor that influences the diagnosis of SIDS is the age of the infant. Even before the definition of SIDS was promulgated, the age distribution of sudden infant deaths had been described by several investigators [2]. Virtually no episodes occur among infants less than one week of age. SIDS episodes increase in frequency with each successive week until the twelfth week and then decrease gradually until the thirty–sixth week. This distribution distinguishes SIDS from other major causes of death during infancy (Table 1.1) and contributes to classifying a sudden infant death as SIDS. Figure 1.1 compares the age distribution of SIDS with that of all infant deaths combined.

The definition of SIDS is germane, indeed vital, to the study of its epidemiology. Epidemiology deals with the occurrence of diseases, disabili-

TABLE 1.1 Major Components of Infant Mortality, King County, Washington, 1969–1977, Age Distribution Percentages

Assigned Cause of Death	Number of Infants	Attained Age at Death (weeks)			
		≤1	2–4	5–26	27–51
		%	%	%	%
Hyaline membrane disease	77	91	9	—	—
Respiratory distress syndrome	308	84	15	—	1
Asphyxia of the newborn	178	93	4	2	1
Immaturity	141	98	2	—	—
Birth injury	239	92	7	1	—
Congenital malformation	359	50	20	21	9
Infection	142	32	25	30	13
Sudden infant death syndrome	322	—	8	85	7
All other	232	48	12	25	15

ties, and deaths in human populations. Accurate enumeration of SIDS occurrences requires a community-wide system of surveillance that identifies all possible SIDS victims. It also requires that every possible case be examined by means of diagnostic criteria that are both sensitive and specific. Sensitivity is a measure of the proportion of cases that are correctly classified by the criteria; cases that are incorrectly classified as noncases are falsely negative leading to underenumeration of cases. Specificity is a measure of the proportion of noncases correctly classified as such; noncases that are incorrectly classified as cases are falsely positive leading to overenumeration of cases. Neither of these two measures can be calculated for SIDS because of the obvious lack of a standard against which the prevailing criteria can be compared. An epidemiologist who elects to study SIDS faces a case definition dilemma analogous to measuring a worm in units of length marked on a rubber band; results will be approximate rather than precise.

In an attempt to improve precision in case definition, designers of one epidemiologic study had three pathologists independently assess morphologic material from both SIDS and non-SIDS victims. They were not informed which was which. When the three concurred, the diagnosis of SIDS was deemed appropriate. Later discussion among the three examiners resolved differences in the final classification to be used for analysis of the study material.

In accepting the less-than-ideal but best available definition of SIDS, epidemiologists have had to interpret their data circumspectly, allowing for greater variance than would be the case if a definite diagnostic marker, pathognomonic for SIDS, were available.

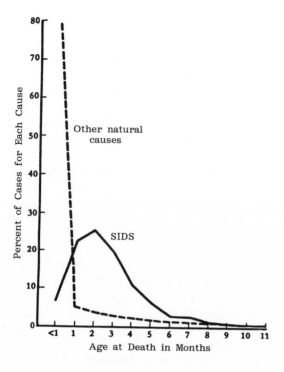

FIGURE 1.1. Age at death of SIDS occurrences versus all other natural causes of infant death. California, 1976–1978. *Source:* California SIDS Information and Counseling Project.

Is SIDS a New Syndrome?

According to Beckwith [3], the phenomenon that now is labeled SIDS has been described anecdotally since medieval and perhaps even biblical times. In 1834 Fearn [4] published a description of two sudden infant deaths that he investigated postmortem; his observations and speculation about their possible cause is comparable to contemporary accounts of SIDS. For centuries, suffocation as a result of overlaying by the mother or wet nurse was believed to be responsible for these events. During the nineteenth and early twentieth centuries, these episodes often were attributed to suffocation because of an enlarged thymus gland; suffocation by bedclothing or bedding and even cats sleeping with an infant and stealing its breath were thought to be causally related. The phenomenon of sudden infant death, which obviously has existed for centuries, has been the source of much grief and sorrow. In the early 1990s the noted Irish playwright and poet W. B. Yeats wrote "The Ballad of Moll Magee," which dramatically describes a mother's remorse at the sudden demise of her infant; in it she laments her fate and her possible shortcomings as a mother and endures the scorn of others [5]. These psychosocial consequences are no different today than at the turn of the century.

How Common is SIDS?

Epidemiologists did not become involved in research on SIDS until the mid 1960s [6]; since then, quantitative data on SIDS occurrence have been forthcoming from many parts of the world.

The incidence of SIDS usually is expressed as the proportion of live births that eventuate in SIDS in a calendar year. In the United States, this proportion generally ranges between two and three per thousand live births per annum (0.2 percent–0.3 percent) in various communities with intensive surveillance and resources for uniform diagnosis. These small proportions, when applied to all births in the United States in 1981, yield a putative estimate of 7,258 to 10,888 SIDS episodes each year.

In the eighth revision of the *International Classification of Diseases, Adapted* (ICDA), the rubric 795.0 was designated for SIDS. In the ninth revision (1978), nosological rules for identifying SIDS as a cause of death were made more comprehensive and the rubric was changed to 798.0. During 1981, the latest year for which United States infant mortality data are available, 5,295 deaths were officially recorded as due to SIDS. Because SIDS surveillance and adherence to diagnostic criteria vary from community to community, this number probably is somewhat less than the true value. Based on this figure, the 1981 incidence in the United States was 1.46 per 1,000 live births. Khoury and colleagues at the Centers for Disease Control, U.S. Public Health Service, published trends in post-neonatal mortality in the United States for the period 1962 through 1978 [7]. During this interval, SIDS rates first increased dramatically and then stabilized in 1975. The authors concluded that these results are partially explained by coding and reporting phenomena. Although the proportion of infants that become SIDS victims is small (a few tenths of one percent), the large number of births in the United States generates a sizeable number of families that experience the tragedy of SIDS each year.

SIDS occurrences also can be expressed as a proportion of all infant deaths. When infant deaths are extremely numerous, as in many developing countries, occurrences of SIDS are obscured by the multitude of other more obvious causes that compete for victims in early infancy; diarrheal diseases, malnutrition, and fulminant infections are examples. However, when the total infant death rate reaches a level of approximately fifteen per 1,000 live births, SIDS becomes a perceptibly significant proportion of the total (10 to 20 percent). As mentioned, SIDS occurs rarely, if at all, during the first week of life when most infant deaths occur; SIDS comprises from 40 to 60 percent of all deaths that occur after the first week of life and before the first birthday.

Relative to the number of live births each year, SIDS may be considered uncommon. On the other hand, in relation to infants dying after the first week of life, SIDS is the most common cause of death in infancy.

Where Does SIDS Occur?

Intuitively, one pictures SIDS episodes as domiciliary occurrences, and most are. However, SIDS also occurs in automobiles, in daycare facilities, in the homes of the parents' friends during visits, and while the infant is under the care of a babysitter (a particularly trying experience for both parents and sitter). A few infants have succumbed to SIDS while in the hospital for non-life-threatening conditions [8].

Whether the parents live in a city, suburb, or rural setting has no effect on the occurrence of SIDS; whether they live in the mountains or at sea level similarly makes little difference. The number of SIDS victims per 1,000 live births is somewhat higher in the Pacific Coast states than elsewhere in the United States for reasons that are not yet apparent.

SIDS occurs among Eskimos and Athabascan Indians in Alaska. SIDS incidents have been described among rural Guatemalan Indians, residents of Singapore and Malaysia, the Maoris living in New Zealand, and in Tasmania. Parallels of latitude obviously are no barrier to SIDS. The geographic distribution of the syndrome with respect to meridians of longitude also encompasses the earth with reports of SIDS from Europe, Africa, North America, Asia, and Australia.

For the reasons cited, comparison of rates of occurrence among countries must be made circumspectly. Statistically significant differences are not relevant; because the data are not derived from sampling and the data bases are generally huge, virtually all differences will be statistically significant. Occurrence rates for most countries range from 1.5 to 3.5 SIDS episodes per 1,000 live births. Northern European countries report rates below this range, with Sweden reporting a SIDS incidence of 0.5 per 1,000 live births; Sweden also has the lowest total infant mortality in the world.

When Does SIDS Occur?

SIDS occurs around the clock, with approximately two-thirds of its victims found dead between noon and midnight; the nature of SIDS precludes accurate assessment of the exact time of death. No consistent pattern of SIDS frequency by days of the week has been identified. SIDS usually occurs more often during the colder months of the year in either hemisphere.

Figure 1.2 depicts annual occurrence rates in King County, Washington, within a fifteen-year period during which a tight surveillance system and uniform diagnostic criteria were employed. The graph reveals annual variation between 1.5 and 3.0 per 1,000 live births, but no trend. In addition, there was a profound decrease in deaths during the first week of life with no counterpoint increase in either SIDS or postperinatal non-SIDS deaths. Non-SIDS deaths also decreased, particularly during the lat-

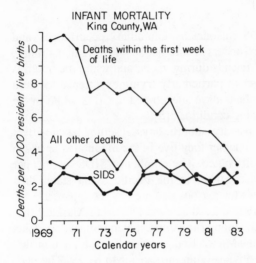

FIGURE 1.2. Secular trends of SIDS incidence compared with those for infants dying within the first week of life and all other infant deaths.

ter half of the 1969–1983 period. A virtually flat SIDS occurrence pattern also has been noted in St. Louis, Missouri (L. Hillman, personal communication, 1984) and Auckland, New Zealand (S. Tonkin, personal communication, 1984).

Review of Major Developments and Pertinent Literature

In epidemiologic circles, the terms *risk factor* and *association* are used more or less interchangeably. The terms have a statistical connotation signifying an excess proportion of cases in certain population subsets. These population subsets serve as epidemiologic descriptors that may or may not be links of consequence in the chain of causation. Unfortunately, some investigators assume that all so-called risk factors have positive predictive value and therefore are causally associated when, in fact, they may be only indirectly related to a causal variable or not related at all.

Whom Does SIDS Strike?

SIDS strikes all segments of society, but not equally. In the United States, rates of occurrence for blacks and Eskimos are two or three times higher than for whites [9]. Contrary to early studies [10, 11], a recent and much more extensive investigation suggested that the incidence of SIDS is not significantly higher among American Indians than among Caucasians [12]. In New Zealand a similar disparity in rates was shown between Polynesians and Caucasians [13]. Curiously, there is little or no male SIDS preponderance among these minority groups, which otherwise is on the order of 1.5:1.0.

SIDS occurrence rates are higher for babies weighing less than 2,500

TABLE 1.2 SIDS Occurrence Rates according to Maternal Age Groups and Birth Rank Categories, King County, Washington, 1969–1980

Maternal Age Group (years)	Birth Ranks					
	1		2		≥3	
	SIDS	SIDS/1,000 Live Births	SIDS	SIDS/1,000 Live Births	SIDS	SIDS/1,000 Live Births
14–19	65	3.6	30	11.3	8	7.0
20–25	45	1.1	78	2.5	74	6.2
26–31	24	1.0	34	1.3	44	3.7
32–37	5	1.4	7	1.2	16	1.5
All ages	139	1.6	149	2.3	142	4.0

grams at birth; most of these low-birth-weight SIDS infants weigh between 2,000 and 2,500 grams, after a gestation of more than thirty-seven weeks. This indicates that they are small for their gestational age and that growth *in utero* was retarded. Plural births usually result in low birth weight, and SIDS occurs about twice as often among plural as singleton births. Postnatal growth of babies who subsequently die of SIDS also has been shown to be retarded [14].

Infants of younger mothers succumb to SIDS proportionately more often than infants of older mothers, as shown in Table 1.2. The table also indicates that the pattern is the same for each of the three birth rank classifications (1, 2, and 3), and that increasing birth rank regularly results in higher incidence. Beyond maternal age 25 years, these trends tend to disappear. It has been shown that the maternal age trends are not an artifact produced by the calendar year of the mothers' births [15].

SIDS occurs relatively more often among infants of unmarried mothers, infants of mothers who have not completed high school, infants of mothers who have had inadequate prenatal care, and among infants from economically stressed families.

All of these factors interrelate to some degree. Moreover, these same factors also have been associated with most other causes of infant mortality, so they are nonspecific. More important, they account for only a portion of the families that experience SIDS. For these reasons, they do not qualify as SIDS predictors.

Similarly, cigarette smoking and drug abuse are associated with SIDS as well as with other causes of infant mortality. It is not known whether the prenatal growth retardation in SIDS is a result of smoking during pregnancy or of some other causal mechanism. Contrary to what one might expect, breast feeding does not protect against SIDS.

Several attempts have been made to identify a profile of factors that would permit detection of SIDS-susceptible infants prior to death but to no avail [16]. Adverse social circumstances of families clearly threaten the well-being of infants, but many SIDS episodes occur in families that ostensibly live under optimal social and economic circumstances.

The possibility that some genetic factor is responsible for SIDS has been explored in several ways. Froggatt's landmark case-control study in Northern Ireland in the 1960s revealed no evidence of sex chromatin abnormalities or consanguinity [17]. Studies of twins indicate that both members of a pair seldom are SIDS victims; between 4 percent and 8 percent of SIDS episodes in twins involve both babies. Like and unlike sex pairs do not differ in this respect. Full first cousins of SIDS probands have a SIDS incidence of approximately two per 1,000 live births, which is the expected rate for any birth cohort. In one study, parents of SIDS babies had significantly different frequency distributions of HLA (human leukocyte antigen) when compared with blood donors and healthy unrelated volunteers. The distribution of SIDS victims according to blood type has been reported differently in several studies, usually unstratified by race, and further confused by methodology with some investigators reporting blood type of the mother and others that of the infant. SIDS does occur in subsequent siblings of a SIDS proband [18], but estimates of the probability of a repetition in a family vary considerably, as shown in Table 1.3. The 95 percent limits of the estimates overlap, which may be construed as evidence that the true value lies somewhere within the range of reported rates. Additional research is needed to establish a credible value so that SIDS parents can be counseled about the risk of SIDS in a subsequent sibling. No pedigree studies of SIDS in extended families have been published; the many diagnostic labels previously appended to infant deaths that are now classified SIDS preclude confidence in results of pedigree analysis beyond the immediate generation.

There are repeated reports that about one-half of SIDS parents indicate their infant had symptoms suggestive of a mild, antecedent respiratory infection within two weeks prior to demise. Because none of these reports included a non-SIDS group for comparison, it is not known whether this association is distinctive of SIDS.

Current Understanding

Fortunately, SIDS occurs relatively rarely, ranging from 0.5 to 3.0 per 1,000 live births in different countries of the world. As infant deaths from other causes decline, SIDS accounts for an increasing proportion of the total infant mortality. The evidence suggests that the phenomenon of sudden infant deaths probably has occurred for centuries throughout the world at a relatively constant rate.

The age-at-death distribution of SIDS is the single, most consistent, unique, and provocative characteristic yet identified. SIDS very rarely occurs during the first week of life when infants are most vulnerable. The

TABLE 1.3 Comparison of Estimates of Risk of SIDS among Siblings

Author	Country	SIDS/ 1,000 Siblings	95 Percent Confidence Limits*
Froggatt	Northern Ireland	16.7	6.1–36.4
Peterson	United States	19.0	9.5–34.7
Beal	South Australia	20.0	9.3–43.4
Irgens	Norway	4.8	1.5–11.2

*"Confidence limits for the expected value of a Poisson distribution." 1966. In *Handbook of Tables of Probability and Statistics*, ed. by W.H. Beyer. Cleveland: Chemical Rubber Company, p. 191.

SIDS age range subsumes the period when profound maturational changes and adaptations take place. The rate of growth is greater than it will ever be again, which requires both efficient anabolic processes and adequate energy sources. Circadian rhythm and sleep cycles become established. The content of the diet changes frequently with concomitant changes in the intestinal flora. The infant is exposed to a host of antigens while the immunologic legacy from its mother is diminishing exponentially, and it is increasingly exposed to an ever expanding array of pathogenic agents. Neuronal circuits proliferate and integrate with rapid development of both motor and sensory function.

As a result of these considerations, research in SIDS has become the province of pediatric pathologists, physiologists, physiological chemists, psychologists, microbiologists, and immunologists—to mention some of the scientific disciplines that have been brought to bear. Results of this enterprise have been inconclusive, at least partly because of the lack of appropriate study subjects. By necessity, siblings of SIDS babies, their parents, and infants with periodic apnea have been used as SIDS surrogates. Whether these groups are valid surrogates is debatable, except in instances in which a trait or attribute under study can be considered a phenotypic expression of some gene that renders an infant susceptible to SIDS.

The unique age distribution pattern of SIDS has been identified wherever it has been adequately studied. Because of such consistency, one can argue that SIDS probably stems from a single underlying cause. Alternatively, one can postulate a mix of etiologic factors, which in the aggregate results in the age distribution pattern observed. This explanation, though less likely than the former, has its advocates. Arnon [19] championed the view that some babies with infant botulism die suddenly and unexpectedly, and therefore comprise a small proportion (perhaps 5 percent) of SIDS episodes as currently defined. He based his view, in part, on the similarity of the distribution of age at onset of infant botulism to that of SIDS. The peak age for infant botulism occurs about thirty days earlier than for SIDS, and the range in ages is compressed. Arnon also presented evidence suggesting that other clostridial species may be implicated in SIDS as well.

Denborough et al. [20] reported that the father of a child who had died of SIDS had a myopathy, which predisposes to malignant hyperthermia, an often fatal, but rare complication of anesthesia. Denborough questioned parents of fifty SIDS victims about anesthetic deaths or serious reactions to anesthetic agents, myopathy, or SIDS among family members. Skeletal muscle biopsy specimens taken during elective surgery were obtained from fifteen parents (representing thirteen SIDS victims) with a family medical history of any one of the three conditions. The specimens were tested in vitro for sensitivity to caffeine and halothane. Five of the fifteen exhibited increased contractility indicative of susceptibility to malignant hyperthermia. Denborough concluded, "This observation raises the possibility that an acute disorder of myoplasmic calcium metabolism may be implicated in some sudden infant deaths." Some SIDS infants reportedly have been wet with sweat or unexpectedly warm to the touch when found, and have had lesions in the intestinal mucosa that also occur in cases of heat stroke [21].

Postmortem serum concentration of triiodothyronine (T_3) and free thiamine (vitamin B_1) have been found elevated to a greater extent in SIDS victims than in specimens from babies dying of other causes [22–26]. Both of these compounds are potent energy production catalysts; their increased concentration could be the result of hyperthermia during the process of dying; alternatively, they may be postmortem artifacts without etiologic significance.

It has been amply demonstrated that some infants with periodic apnea succumb to SIDS; such events have occurred even when the infant was attached to an apnea monitor and the parents were schooled in resuscitation techniques. These events have not been quantified accurately, but they probably comprise no more than 2 percent of all SIDS episodes. Infants with severe periodic apnea have been termed "near misses" (for SIDS) or "abortive SIDS." These terms tend to create parental anxiety and to generate semantic confusion in the scientific community, as well.

Collectively, infant botulism, malignant hyperthermia, and periodic apnea may account for as much as 10 percent of SIDS occurrences. Assuming this is so, the question remains, are the remaining 90 percent all of a kind? Until there is evidence to the contrary, epidemiologists will have to assume that the answer is affirmative in order to maintain a working hypothesis.

Figure 1.2 reveals that during a fifteen-year span in King County, Washington, SIDS occurrences did not increase or decrease significantly. Figure 1.3 indicates that three salient "risk factors" (parity ≥ 2, teenage mothers, and low birth weight babies) have decreased substantially during the same interval. These changes occurred of themselves and thus provide a natural experiment that tests the predictive power, or lack of it, of these

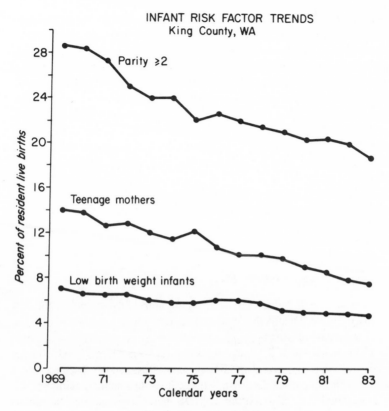

FIGURE 1.3. Secular trends of three salient infant risk factors.

factors. Brandt [27] showed that percentages of low-birth-weight infants in the entire United States have declined in a similar fashion. Thus, the trends shown in Figure 1.3 are not the result of some aspect of human reproduction unique to King County.

Why Does SIDS Occur?

"Why does SIDS occur?" is a question posed rhetorically to suggest that perhaps an answer couched in general terms is preferable to nonresponse, even though an explicit explanation is not possible at this time. It seems reasonable to infer from the global distribution of SIDS in both time and space that whatever the cause, it must be an inherent concomitant of the process of human reproduction. With occurrence rates generally confined to rather narrow limits of variation with respect to both time and place, the cause also must be a relatively constant force within birth cohorts. The age distribution pattern links SIDS to a window of vulnerability during which major development of vital biological functions takes place. The fact that postmortem tissue changes sufficient to cause death are absent in SIDS infants suggests that death comes as a result of some failure of function essential to life.

The fact that incidence among different ethnic groups varies consistently in the same direction suggests that different genetic pools may be involved with the genesis of SIDS. If this is so, heritability of SIDS must be multigenic, because previous studies provide no evidence to support a single gene explanation. The fact that non-white races do not exhibit a substantial male preponderance typical of whites may be a subtle clue that the fundamental flaw in SIDS originates with conception. Intrauterine growth retardation, which persists postnatally, is compatible with this concept.

With respect to thinking about SIDS causation, the phenomenon of twinning might be a useful biological model. All of the salient factors discussed (except the age-at-death distribution, of course) apply in general to both SIDS and twins.

Summary and Recommendations

The phenomenon of sudden infant death apparently has occurred for centuries, worldwide. Deaths that cannot be explained on the basis of circumstantial, clinical, or postmortem evidence comprise what is now termed SIDS. The incidence of SIDS averages about two per 1,000 live births per annum; the long-term trend in annual rates is essentially flat. As infant deaths from other causes diminish, SIDS constitutes an increasing proportion of the total. The distribution of SIDS in society is similar to that for other components that comprise the spectrum of infant mortality. The age distribution of SIDS is unique; most episodes occur during the second, third, and fourth months of life. SIDS has been studied from an epidemiologic point of view since the early 1960s. The goal of epidemiologists is to provide clues to causation that ultimately will result in prevention of death or disability; thus far, this goal has not been achieved with SIDS.

What if this goal is never realized? Should epidemiologists give up? The mystery surrounding SIDS devastates the parents of its victims; not knowing even a proximate cause of SIDS creates uncertainty and diminishes self assurance. Perhaps the burden of anxiety, guilt, shame, or blame would be dissipated by a knowledge of what went wrong, even though nothing could have been done in advance to prevent the occurrence. Thus, epidemiology has a role in the continuing search for clues as to why these infants die.

How Can Epidemiology Contribute in the Future?

Discovery of an objective diagnostic marker for SIDS would require epidemiologists to repeat the gamut of earlier studies to determine whether redefinition of SIDS altered our present comprehension, and in what way. Current concern and uncertainty about the precision of rates of occurrences would be dissipated. The issue of whether SIDS is a single entity or a collection of heterologous entities that appear similar but are fundamentally different could be resolved. Infant botulism, infant apnea, and genetic predisposition to malignant hyperthermia could be placed in proper perspective in relation to SIDS events without these stigmata.

In the meantime, the current definition will have to suffice. The association of infant apnea with SIDS needs to be studied systematically; an epidemiologic study of infant apnea would provide instructive comparisons. The thrust of most of the previous research has been directed at maternal attributes and circumstances at the expense of paternal ones. This avenue of investigation deserves further exploration. Although classic Mendelian inheritance clearly is not operative in SIDS, the role of polygenic inheritance remains an open question. Denborough's discovery of a possible link between the malignant hyperthermia trait and SIDS warrants more research. Studies are under way, not only to confirm Denborough's observation but also to expand the scope of factors in the family medical history that may be variants of malignant hyperthermia.

The National Sudden Infant Death Syndrome Foundation commissioned research to provide a better estimate of the likelihood of SIDS in a subsequent sibling. The results revealed that earlier estimates of risk of recurrence were inflated and that the risk in the United States is close to that shown for Norway in Table 1.3 [28].

The final chapter on SIDS epidemiology remains to be written. There is still work to be done; there is still reason to hope that the mystery that is SIDS will be solved.

References

1. Bergman, A.B., J.B. Beckwith, and C.G. Ray, eds. 1970. *Sudden Infant Death Syndrome—Proceedings of the Second International Conference on Causes of Sudden Death in Infants.* Seattle: University of Washington Press.
2. Wedgwood, R.J., and E.P. Benditt, eds. 1963. *Sudden Death in Infants—Proceedings of the Conference on Causes of Sudden Death in Infants.* U.S. Public Health Service Publication No. 1412.
3. Beckwith, J.B. 1973. The sudden infant death syndrome. *Current Problems in Pediatrics,* 3(8). Chicago: Year Book Medical Publishers.
4. Fearn, S.W. 1834. Sudden and unexplained death of children (letter to the editor). *Lancet* 1:246.
5. Yeats, W.B. 1906. *Collected Poems.* New York: Macmillan Publishing Company.
6. Peterson, D.R. 1980. Evolution of the epidemiology of the sudden infant death syndrome. *Epidemiologic Reviews* 2:97–112.

7. Khoury, M.J., J.D. Erickson, and M.J. Adams. 1984. Trends in postneonatal mortality in the United States, 1962 through 1978. *JAMA* 252:367–372.
8. Peterson, D.R., and J.B. Beckwith. 1974. The sudden infant death syndrome in hospitalized babies. *Pediatrics* 54:644–646.
9. Fleshman, J.K., and D.R. Peterson, 1977. The sudden infant death syndrome among Alaskan natives. *Am J Epidemiol* 105:555–558.
10. Kraus, J.F., and N.O. Borhani. 1972. Post-neonatal sudden unexplained death in California: A cohort study. *Am J Epidemiol* 95(6):497–510.
11. Blok, J.H. 1978. The incidence of sudden infant death syndrome in North Carolina's cities and counties: 1972–1974. *Am J Public Health* 68(4):367–372.
12. Kaplan, D.W., A.E. Bauman, and H.F. Krous. 1984. Epidemiology of sudden infant death syndrome in American Indians. *Pediatrics* 74(6):1041–1046.
13. Tonkin, S. 1974. "Epidemiology of SIDS in Auckland, New Zealand." In *SIDS, 1974—The Francis E. Camps International Symposium on Sudden and Unexpected Deaths in Infancy,* ed. R.R. Robinson. The Canadian Foundation for the Study of Infant Deaths.
14. Peterson, D.R. 1981. The sudden infant death syndrome: Reassessment of growth retardation in relation to maternal smoking and the hypoxia hypothesis. *Am J Epidemiol* 113:583–589.
15. Peterson, D.R., G. vanBelle, N.M. Chinn. 1982. Sudden infant death syndrome and maternal age. *JAMA* 247:2250–2252.
16. Murphy, J.F., R.G. Newcombe, and J.R. Sibert. 1982. The epidemiology of the sudden infant death syndrome. *J Epidemiol Community Health* 36:17–21.
17. Froggatt, P., M.A. Lynas, and G. MacKenzie. 1971. Epidemiology of sudden unexpected death in infants ('cot death') in Northern Ireland. *Br J Preventive and Social Med* 25:119–134.
18. Irgens, L.M., R. Skjaerven, and D.R. Peterson. 1984. Prospective assessment of recurrence risk in sudden infant death syndrome siblings. *J Pediatr* 104:349–351.
19. Arnon, S.S. 1984. Breast feeding and toxigenic intestinal infections—missing links in crib death? *Rev Infect Dis* 6:193–201 Supplement.
20. Denborough, M.A., G.J. Galloway, and K.C. Hopkinson. 1982. Malignant hyperpyrexia and sudden infant death. *Lancet* 2:1068–1069.
21. Stanton, A.N., D.J. Scott, and M.A.P.S. Downham. 1980. Is overheating a factor in some unexpected infant deaths? *Lancet* 1:1054–1057.
22. Chacon, M.A., and J.T. Tildon. 1981. Elevated values of triiodothyronine in victims of sudden infant death syndrome. *J Pediatr* 99:758–760.
23. Root, A.W., and W.K. Lee. 1983. Sudden infant death syndrome and triiodothyronine—clarification of a relationship (editorial). *J Pediatr* 102:251–252.
24. Davis, R.E., G.C. Icke, and J.M. Hilton. 1982. High serum thiamine and the sudden infant death syndrome. *Clin Chim Acta* 123:321–328.
25. Davis, R.E., G.C. Icke, and J.M. Hilton. 1983. "Sudden infant death and abnormal thiamine metabolism." In *Sudden Infant Death Syndrome,* ed. J.T. Tildon, L.M. Roeder, and A. Steinschneider. New York: Academic Press.

26. Wyatt, D.T., M.M. Erickson, R.E. Hillman, and L.S. Hillman. 1984. Elevated thiamine levels in SIDS, non-SIDS and adults—postmortem artifact. *J Pediatr* 104:585–588.
27. Brandt, E.N. 1984. Infant mortality—progress report. *Public Health Reports* 99:284–288.
28. Peterson, D.R., E.E. Sabotta, and J.R. Daling. 1986. Infant mortality among subsequent siblings of infants who died of sudden infant death syndrome. *J Pediatr* 108:911–914.

2

The Pathology of Sudden Infant Death Syndrome: An Overview

HENRY F. KROUS, M.D.

The last two decades have witnessed an exponential growth in the literature of sudden infant death syndrome (SIDS). To be sure, most of it has
focused upon clinical and pathophysiologic events prior to death of infants, many of whom have been considered at high risk for SIDS. However, pathologists have not been idle; in fact, their studies have provided
important hypotheses that have guided clinical research. The purpose of
this chapter is threefold: first, to provide a historical perspective; second,
to delineate our current understanding of the pathologic anatomy of SIDS;
and, third, to suggest future directions for investigation.

Historical Considerations

Stricken with grief at the sudden and unexpected death of their young infant, parents are desperate for an explanation yet are told by their physicians that no one knows why. However, this admission of ignorance belies
the fact that an enormous amount of information about SIDS and disorders
potentially related to or masquerading as SIDS continues to accumulate.
This encouraging situation can be appreciated most easily when placed in
historical perspective.

Review of the literature about sudden, unexpected death in infancy provides substance to the proposal that SIDS existed even before the birth of
Christ. The lack of earlier recognition of SIDS can be ascribed to its rarity
compared to infectious diseases, malnutrition, and other disorders that accounted for the vast majority of infant deaths. Overlaying and infanticide,
disorders of the thymus, and fulminant infections were given much attention as causes of the sudden, unexpected deaths of healthy infants.

Overlaying and Infanticide

Among Judeo-Christian cultures, overlaying is perhaps the earliest recorded cause of SIDS. The sagacity of King Solomon is prefaced in the
biblical quotation in I Kings 3:19–20, "and this woman's child died in the

night; because she overlaid it. And she arose at midnight, and took my son from beside me, while thine handmaiden slept, and laid it in her bosom, and laid her dead child in my bosom."

For centuries overlaying was considered a sin in the Catholic Church; however, judgments delivered by the Ecclesiastical courts upon the alleged perpetrators were less harsh than those for murder committed by other means. For example, the Cummean of the seventh century states that individuals guilty of overlaying "shall do penance for an entire year on bread and water and for two years more abstain from wine and flesh." [1] By the fourteenth century, overlaying had become a pardonable sin in the Catholic Church [2]. Two hundred years later, society's efforts to prevent overlaying were demonstrated by the manufacture of the arcuccio in Florence, Italy [3]. This cagelike device fit over the infant and prevented either bedclothes or the mother (or wet nurse) from lying directly on the baby; openings on either side of the arcuccio allowed breast feeding.

Overlaying was an accepted cause of infant death in Europe and the United States well toward the end of the nineteenth century. In 1841, an overseer of a Virginia plantation was of the opinion that the death of an infant slave was due to maternal overlaying [4]. Perhaps, the most heartless and misguided attitudes toward overlaying are those recorded in 1892 by Templeman, a forensic pathologist in Dundee, Scotland. His fascinating report on 258 infants records many features characteristic of SIDS including male predominance, higher wintertime incidence, and gross pathologic findings, which have not been substantially altered even today [5]. However, he noted that a majority of these infants died on Saturday night, when many of the parents allegedly had been drinking and, in their stuporous state, had overlain their infants upon retiring to bed. To the misfortune of the parents, he concluded these infants' deaths were a consequence of ignorance, drunkenness, and overcrowding; in some instances he postulated that the parents hoped to claim life insurance benefits. It was his recommendation that parents be forbidden from sleeping with their infants and that those parents who allegedly had overlain their infants be prosecuted. Whereas overlaying is a conceivable cause of infant death, it is important to note that the majority of cases of SIDS appear to occur when the infant is alone in the crib.

As recently as November 1984, a British Home Office pathologist was of the opinion that most cases of SIDS were caused by parents smothering their infants. The prestigious British medical journal *Lancet* editorialized that the epidemiologic profile of SIDS argues strongly against this assertion [6]. The journal noted that if SIDS were caused by smothering, "one would expect cot death to be most frequent in very young infants, who are most vulnerable, who have to be fed at night, and whose mothers are most likely to be suffering from fatigue and puerperal depression. The hypothesis does not seem to explain why cot deaths peak at 10 weeks of age when infants are beginning to sleep through the night, why the incidence rate is nearly three times higher in the winter than in the summer, why the incidence rate is higher for second than for first children, and why it diminishes as the age of the mother increases." Fortunately, such attitudes and conclusions have largely disappeared; in the vast majority of cases, the autopsy findings differentiate SIDS from infanticide.

Thymic Enlargement

As early as 1614, lethal tracheal compression by an enlarged thymus ("mors thymica" according to Plater) [7] was considered a cause of sudden, unexpected infant death. This theory apparently achieved wider popularity and greater validity with the description in 1830 of Kopp's "thymic asthma" (quoted by Lee) [8]. Kopp's thymic asthma occurred in apparently well infants who awakened during the night with a peculiar piping cry, whistling inspirations, and barely perceptible expirations, followed by sudden death. Necropsy revealed an "enlarged" thymus allegedly compressing the trachea.

Two subsequent papers, one in 1842 by Lee [8] and the other in 1858 by Friedleben [9], demonstrated that the thymuses of these infants were, in fact, no larger than those of healthy infants who died suddenly of other causes such as accidents; these authors concluded that the thymus rapidly shrinks in volume and weight in response to stress of any sort. Conversely, the earlier investigators had compared the size of the thymus glands of healthy infants dying suddenly with those of infants who had suffered subacute or chronic illnesses prior to their deaths, an obviously inappropriate control group against which to make comparisons.

It is worth remembering that quite massive lymphomatous neoplastic enlargement of the thymus must develop before respiratory embarrassment is seen. The cartilaginous rings of the trachea, even though quite compliant during early infancy, provide considerable resistance to extrinsic compression.

Status Thymicolymphaticus

Despite the earlier publications of Lee [8] and Friedleben [9], the thymus continued to play a role in the explanation of sudden, unexpected infant deaths into the early 1930s. In 1889, Dr. Arnold Paltauf, a Viennese physician, proposed a new condition, which he termed status thymicolymphaticus, to account for sudden infant death [10]. This "syndrome" was characterized by thymic and lymphoid hyperplasia, generalized arterial (especially aortic) hypoplasia, small adrenals, postadolescent hypogonadism, and sudden death. The mechanism of death was never clearly understood; thymic enlargement with tracheal compression, anaphylaxis, and nutritional and metabolic imbalance were suggested. The belief that lethal tracheal compression could be caused by an enlarged thymus achieved even wider recognition with its "validation" by the great American physician, Sir William Osler [11]. It was not until 1931 that status thymicolymphaticus was debunked following analysis of large amounts of data by a special committee, the results of which were reported by Young and Turnbull [12]. The committee concluded that there was "no evidence that so-called status thymicolymphaticus has any existence as a pathological entity."

Fulminant Infection

Because of the diversity of microbiologic organisms and their equally wide array of clinical manifestations, it is not surprising that infection has received substantial attention as a potential cause of sudden, unexpected infant death. In 1895, French physicians were of the opinion that the first attack of "suffocating catarrh of children" could cause severe pulmonary congestion and death in infants less than six months of age [13]. In 1934, Dr. Sidney Farber, a founding father of pediatric pathology, isolated streptococcal organisms from two infants whose sudden deaths initially had been ascribed to suffocation [14]. He concluded that the fulminant clinical course of these infants precluded the development of pathologic lesions that could be identified with either the naked eye or a microscope. In 1938, Goldbloom and Wigglesworth identified microscopic pulmonary inflammation at autopsy in nineteen of thirty cases of sudden, unexpected infant death [15].

The belief that fulminant infection played the primary role in SIDS appears to have reached its zenith in the landmark papers of Werne and Garrow published between 1942 and 1953 [16–19]. During meticulous postmortem examinations, these forensic pathologists from the New York City Borough of Queens found that 33 percent of infants who died suddenly and unexpectedly had suffered a recent upper respiratory infection, that pulmonary inflammation was commonly identified microscopically, and that bacteria were frequently grown from postmortem cultures. With the advantage of hindsight, it is now apparent that their positive postmortem cultures must be interpreted very cautiously.

Because the bodies of these infants typically remained for several hours in warm surroundings before discovery, postmortem bacterial migration allowed isolation of these organisms, especially coliforms, from the lungs. Therefore, their presence should not necessarily be considered pathogenic. In their classic paper in 1956, Adelson and Kinney found that "no single bacterial organism or group of organisms were cultured from any site with a degree of consistency sufficient to indicate that it had probable etiologic significance" [20]. Findings in 95 of 120 blood cultures, all cerebrospinal cultures, and 119 of 120 viral cultures obtained at necropsy were negative. The negative viral culture findings represent more the technology of the era than the infectious status of the host. In 1970, Ray and colleagues isolated viruses from 37.5 percent of SIDS cases compared with 16.2 percent of controls [21]. Because none of the viruses were isolated from the blood or tissues, these investigators concluded that the infants were not dying of fulminant infection, but that the virus was acting as a triggering mechanism to a catastrophe of cardiorespiratory control.

Nevertheless, respiratory infections may be a significant risk factor for SIDS. Both are more common during the winter months, occur more frequently in large families, and SIDS is frequently preceded by upper respiratory infection. Prospective studies showed microbiologic and/or histologic evidence of respiratory virus infection in approximately 25 percent of SIDS cases [22, 23]. Recently, increasing emphasis has been placed upon respiratory syncytial virus (RSV) infection because the RSV infection has been associated with sudden, unexpected death of infants [23–26]. Furthermore, apnea develops in 15 percent to 25 percent of infants infected with RSV [25, 27]; when associated with sleep, apnea also is considered by some investigators as a risk factor for SIDS [28]. Upper respiratory infections increase the duration and frequency of sleep apnea [29] and decrease pharyngeal muscle tone predisposing to collapse of the upper airway [30]. Finally, of course, the question here is: Should these deaths be considered SIDS or lethal viral RSV infection? The answer depends upon one's perspective and definition.

Arnon and colleagues published a series of papers in which they postulated that a small proportion of SIDS cases were a result of infant botulism [31–33]. In their original study, they identified either the organism and/or the toxin of *Clostridia botulinum* in 10 of 211 infants with SIDS and in none of the sixty-nine controls [31]. Subsequently, they demonstrated a similar age distribution in SIDS and infant botulism and the presence of a secretory IgA antibody capable of agglutinating *C. botulinum*, which may account for the higher incidence of SIDS in bottle-fed infants compared with breast-fed infants. They further showed that the toxins of *C. difficile* can cause the rapid death of infant rhesus monkeys whose findings at necropsy are similar to those of the SIDS infant [31–36]. A more recent paper again suggested an apparent link between *C. botulinum* infection and some cases of SIDS [37]. These are intriguing findings, but there remain significant questions such as the apparent contradiction between the hypotonia and constipation of infant botulism and evidence suggesting agonal autonomic nervous system discharge in some SIDS victims [38].

In summary, the temporal association between SIDS victims and infection is inescapable, yet other infants die of SIDS who have no clinical, microbiologic, or pathologic evidence of infection. Clearly, many questions remain to be answered.

Pathology

Gross Internal and External Findings

In 1892, Templeman provided a remarkably complete description of apparent SIDS victims that has not been substantially altered to this day. He wrote,

The external appearances presented by the body are chiefly of a negative character. There are no marks of violence to be observed. As a rule there is no flattening of the nose and face from pressure. Postmortem lividity comes on early, and is especially well marked on that side of the body on which the infant has been lying; the face is placid and calm; the eyes sometimes slightly congested, but not staring; the lips are livid, and the tongue not protruded. Frothy mucus, often tinged with blood, is generally seen about the mouth and nostrils. The hands are sometimes tightly clenched . . . a complete or partial examination presented the usual appearances found in cases of death by asphyxia, viz., a varying degree of congestion of the cerebral membranes—more or less engourgement of the internal organs, especially the lungs and kidneys, and the large thoracic veins, a fluid condition of the blood, which was dark in colour; and generally a distended condition of the right side of the heart, while the left was nearly or altogether empty and contracted . . . in about half the cases examined small punctiform haemorrhages were observed beneath the pleura and pericardium. The larynx, trachea, and bronchi as a rule are congested, and contained some frothy, often blood-stained mucus [5].

To his description, several other commonly observed features can be added. The infants appear normally nourished and hydrated. The diapers usually are wet and contain stool, and the bladder and rectum are typically empty [38]. In some cases, the hands clutch fibers apparently from the bedclothes. The lungs are congested and edematous, but gross evidence of pneumonia is not identified. The thymus is of normal size and shows little, if any, microscopic evidence of involution.

Intrathoracic Petechiae

Intrathoracic petechiae, seen in approximately 80 percent of cases, are the most common and visible pathologic findings in SIDS [38, 39]. They were first described by Fearn in 1834 in two five- and six-month-old infants who died during the night [40]. He attributed their deaths to a "violent action" of the heart. In 1843, Professor F. T. Berg of Sweden noted "alla var lungytan under pleura bespranged med sma flackar af capillar haemorrhagi" at autopsy of infants dying under similar circumstances [41].

Despite the frequent occurrence of intrathoracic petechiae in SIDS, their pathogenesis and significance remain to be clarified. It has been argued that their distribution is indicative of terminal upper airway obstruction. Templeman observed petechiae confined to the thoracic cavity of infants whom he suspected died because of overlaying [5]. Adelson and Kinney also remarked upon the presence of petechiae, yet did not find them helpful in differentiating SIDS from other causes of death [20]. However, careful analysis of their data reveals that the majority of the SIDS cases and eight of eleven of their controls who died of unequivocal upper airway obstruction (strangulation, neck compression, hanging, aspiration) had intrathoracic petechiae. Apparently none of the SIDS cases and only two of the controls who were victims of terminal airway occlusion had subdiaphragmatic petechiae.

In 1959, Handforth developed perhaps the first animal model to produce intrathoracic petechiae [42]. He killed rats by occluding their tracheas, observed intrathoracic petechiae at necropsy, and concluded that the agonal event in SIDS is laryngospasm. A decade later, Beckwith noted that posterior thymic petechiae were more numerous below than above the innominate vein in SIDS victims [43]. He hypothesized that this large vein acted as a dampening mechanism to changes in intrathoracic pressure occurring as a result of breathing against an occluded upper airway. Krous extended these observations by determining the microscopic distribution of intrathoracic petechiae in SIDS [39]. It was his hypothesis that if pressure changes within the chest were important in their pathogenesis, petechiae should occur more frequently near the surfaces of the thoracic viscera than in their central portions. This was true in the case of the thymus and heart. The distribution of pulmonary petechiae, on the other hand, suggested they were a result of left ventricular failure developing in response to breathing against an obstructed upper airway. In the same laboratory, Krous and colleagues observed pathophysiologic changes indicative of left heart failure in rabbits that were killed by repeated tracheal obstruction at end-expiration and that had pulmonary petechiae at necropsy [44]. The increases in pulmonary wedge pressure were similar to those observed by Buda et al. in adult men with obstructive sleep apnea syndrome [45]. Bromberger-Barnea elegantly described the cardiovascular pathophysiology that occurs when inspiring against a closed airway [46].

In an attempt to obtain indirect evidence of the pathogenesis of these hemorrhages, Krous and Jordan formally analyzed their visceral distribution following various modalities of death [47]. With few exceptions, they found that petechiae limited to the chest cavity occurred in SIDS and lethal upper airway obstruction; in contrast, visceral petechiae were seen on both sides of the diaphragm when the patient's terminal course was complicated by hypoxemia, hypercarbia, metabolic acidosis, coagulation defects, or infection.

On the presumption, yet unproven, that intrathoracic petechiae are the consequence of breathing against an occluded upper airway in SIDS, it is natural to ask where the obstruction occurs. The nose, larynx, and trachea are buttressed by cartilage, thus resisting collapse. The pharynx, on the other hand, is composed only of soft tissue and therefore constitutes the only collapsible segment of the upper airway. During inspiration, intra-pharyngeal pressure is less than atmospheric pressure, which tends to collapse the pharynx. Patency is maintained by delicately balanced neuro-muscular mechanisms [48].

There are several factors during infancy, not present during adulthood, that predispose to upper airway obstruction and may be important in SIDS. The upper airway of an infant is narrower than that of an older child or adult, because the cervical viscera occupy a relatively higher position in the neck [30, 49, 50]. In infants, the uvula nearly touches the epiglottis, whereas in adults these two structures are separated by a few centimeters. Furthermore, the immature development of the temporomandibular joints allows greater mobility and easy posterior displacement of the tongue and mandible, which narrows the airway.

Malformations of the mandible, such as in Pierre Robin syndrome [51], are associated with high mortality in early infancy [52, 53]. Guilleminault et al. demonstrated a small upper airway in some near miss SIDS infants who were siblings of SIDS victims, and in members of their families [54]. Upper respiratory infections also reduce pharyngeal muscle tone, which facilitates upper airway collapse [30, 54].

A large body of literature associates obstructive sleep apnea with SIDS, and this disorder may be another important factor. Guilleminault et al. noted frequent episodes of obstructive sleep apnea thirty hours prior to the sudden, unexpected death of a twenty-one-week-old female infant who was considered at autopsy to be a victim of SIDS [55]. Information regarding the presence of intrathoracic petechiae at autopsy was not provided.

Hypoxic Tissue Markers

In the 1970s, Naeye and colleagues reported subtle tissue changes, which have become known as the "hypoxic tissue markers," suggesting that many SIDS victims experience chronic or recurrent hypoxia and hypox-emia prior to death. The hypoxic tissue markers included increased pulmonary arteriolar muscle thickening, right ventricular hypertrophy, increased periadrenal brown fat, carotid body abnormalities, increased hepatic erythropoiesis, adrenal medullary hyperplasia or hypoplasia, and brainstem gliosis [56]. The latter marker is discussed in the Neuropathology section of this review. There have been numerous attempts to reproduce Naeye's provocative findings, the confirmation of which has important implications not only for treatment but also for prevention.

Pulmonary Arteriolar Muscle. In 1973, Naeye reported that nearly one-half of forty SIDS victims had increased pulmonary artery muscle mass compared with thirty-nine control infants [57]. Three-fourths of this increase was due to hypertrophy and one-fourth was due to hyperplasia of smooth muscle in the media. A point counting technique was used to evaluate twenty arteries between 30 and 100 microns in diameter in hematoxylin and eosin stained slides; it is not stated whether the arteries were chosen at random or how many points were counted. The latter issue is of particular importance because the relative standard error increases dramatically when only a small number of points are counted and the variable being analyzed comprises a small percentage of the whole [58]. In Naeye's study, endothelial nuclei were the reference point from which the volume of medial smooth muscle was calculated. Figures 1 and 2 in Naeye's paper are also cause for concern. The control cases show no decrement in pulmonary arteriolar smooth muscle between one and twelve months of age [57], yet following birth the amount of smooth muscle in small pulmonary arteries declines rapidly [59]. Since Naeye's article, several papers have addressed the same issue [60–66]. Only Mason et al. [60] and Weiler and deHaardt [65] found medial thickening. However, Mason did not provide important data about the controls, such as their ages and causes of death, and he ascribed to technical differences in his observation that the mean of some ratios in his SIDS cases were uniformly twice as large as those reported by Naeye [60]. Using electronic planimetry, Weiler and deHaardt measured ninety arteries between 50 and 500 microns in diameter and calculated a media index defined as the ratio of the medial thickness divided by the diameter of the artery [65]. They found the media index was higher in arteries of any size in SIDS than in controls. It is noteworthy that eight of sixteen controls were more than six months of age and twenty-seven of thirty-three SIDS cases were less than six months of age. Thus the difference between the SIDS and control cases may be due simply to the skewing of age in opposite directions. Using the same methods as Naeye, Valdes-Dapena et al. found neither abnormally thick medias nor medial hypertrophy in the pulmonary arterioles in SIDS [64]. Their statistical evidence of medial hyperplasia suggests less cytoplasm per smooth muscle cell in SIDS compared with controls, yet their Table 3 indicates no differences.

Using radial measurements, Williams et al. found that fifteen SIDS cases did not differ significantly from six controls with respect to mean percent wall thickness of small pulmonary arteries, but that medial smooth muscle extended more peripherally in SIDS [63]. The validity of these observations comes into question when one notes that the ages of only two controls are comparable to the time when most SIDS deaths occur and that the values for the controls differ from those previously reported by one of the authors [67].

Most recently, Singer and Tilly employed planimetric techniques augmented by computerized image analysis to compare the media of pulmonary arterioles ranging from 10 to 150 microns in diameter in SIDS cases and controls [66]. Compared to controls, there was neither significant thickening nor hypercellularity in SIDS. Since there were also no differences in arterioles between 10 and 30 microns in diameter, these investigators were unable to confirm the observation of Williams et al. [63] regarding greater peripheral extension of arteriolar smooth muscle in SIDS. In the study of Singer and Tilly, the expected decrement in medial muscle with advancing age was observed in controls and SIDS cases [66].

Right Ventricular Hypertrophy. Alveolar hypoxia produces pulmonary vasoconstriction, which leads to pulmonary hypertension and, if chronic or recurrent, thickening of the media of the small arteries of the lungs [68]. Over time, pulmonary hypertension causes right ventricular hypertrophy (RVH). In 1976, Naeye reported RVH in eighty-five SIDS victims compared to thirty controls [69]. RVH was expressed as the ratio of the weight of the right ventricular free wall x 1,000, divided by the body weight. Using the same method of measurement and calculation, Valdes-Dapena found no differences between 177 SIDS cases and 50 controls [70]. In both of these studies, the mean values for RVH in SIDS cases are nearly identical; the different conclusions rest solely upon lower mean values for Naeye's controls. In the remaining investigation into this issue, RVH was expressed as the ratio of the weight of the right ventricular free wall divided by the combined weight of the left ventricle and interventricular septum; RVH was not identified in six SIDS victims [63].

Carotid Body Abnormalities. In 1976, Naeye et al. reported that among fifty-six SIDS victims, 35 percent had a decreased volume and 14 percent had an increased volume of the chemoreceptor glomus cells in the carotid bodies compared to the controls [71]. Their observations, which were based upon carotid body glomus cell volume expressed as a function of body weight, can be questioned since the size of the carotid body can show a tenfold variability at any given crown–heel length [72]. Dinsdale concluded the carotid bodies of SIDS cases did not differ from those of the controls [72].

In a very poorly controlled study, Cole et al. observed fewer neurosecretory granules in the carotid bodies of SIDS victims than in those of controls and suggested this may be a pathognomonic marker of SIDS [73]. This unjustified conclusion is based upon electron micrographs that reveal considerable tissue autolysis and very inappropriate controls, including a man dying of a myocardial infarction.

In the most meticulous and carefully controlled study to date, Perrin et al. found that the carotid bodies in SIDS were normal and that they did not differ from controls with respect to the cross-sectional area of chemoreceptor cells or the frequency, distribution, or size of neurosecretory granules [74].

In a more recent paper, Perrin et al. demonstrated that despite the structural similarity, there was a tenfold increase in dopamine and a threefold increase in norepinephrine content of the carotid bodies of SIDS cases compared with controls [75]. This intriguing observation, which indicates a lack of correlation between morphology and biochemistry, deserves further investigation, especially since dopamine is known to inhibit respiratory responses to hypoxia [76], and there may be a relationship between these biochemical abnormalities and intrathoracic petechiae [77].

Perrin et al. developed a line of reasoning to show that the elevated catecholamine levels were not indicative of chronic hypoxia but rather may reflect an acute abnormality in neurotransmitter metabolism or release from the carotid bodies in SIDS [75]. Krous et al. showed that dopaminergic and beta adrenergic blockade inhibits the ability of norepinephrine to produce intrathoracic petechiae in rats killed by a single sustained occlusion of the trachea [77]. To date, the observations of Perrin et al. are unconfirmed and additional studies are necessary.

Periadrenal Brown Fat. A relationship between the "brownness" of fat and chronic hypoxemia has been suggested [78]. In 1974, Naeye compared the percentage of periadrenal brown fat cells in forty-eight non-hypoxemic controls, thirty hypoxemic controls and ninety-one SIDS victims, sixty-five of whom had no pulmonary inflammation [79]. He observed a significantly higher percentage of brown fat cells in SIDS victims between 2.5 and 5 months of age than in age-matched nonhypoxic controls; the values in the SIDS victims were similar to those in the hypoxemic controls. When he addressed this same subject two years later, he excluded all infants less than five months of age, thereby excluding most SIDS cases from analysis [69]. The adrenal sections were not standardized with respect to left or right side, or to adipose tissue around the head, body, or tail of the gland.

Using the same method, Valdes-Dapena et al. repeated this study in ninety-nine SIDS victims without pulmonary inflammation and two comparably aged control groups [80]. It does not appear the sections were standardized. One control group consisted of ninety-nine infants who died of cyanotic congenital heart disease and the other was composed of seventy-five healthy infants who died within minutes after an accident. Among infants less than five months of age, when most SIDS events occur, there was no difference in brown fat in SIDS victims compared with controls. Conversely, among infants between 5.1 and 12 months of age, more brown fat was observed in SIDS victims than in controls. In this age group, the ages of the SIDS cases and controls were skewed in opposite directions [81]; thus, the differences may be an expected finding [82, 83]. Emery and Dinsdale noted the fat around the same adrenal shows considerable variation in appearance [83]. Therefore, unlike previous investigators, they studied only the fat confined to the adrenal hilum. Because, in their opinion, the "simple division of fat into brown and non-brown is extremely subjective," they divided the fat cells into seven categories based on the degree of cytoplasmic loculation rather than on the presence of reticular cytoplasm as done by Naeye et al. [69, 79] and Valdes-Dapena et al. [80]. Among infants less than five months of age, Emery and Dinsdale found less brown fat in SIDS than in controls, but there were no differences between these groups after age five months [83]. These results are opposite those of Naeye [79].

Hepatic Erythropoiesis. Although the liver is not an important site of postnatal erythropoiesis, it is able to produce erythrocytes in response to chronic hypoxemia. In 1974, Naeye reported the presence of hepatic erythropoiesis in one-sixth of ninety-one SIDS victims, whether or not they had pulmonary inflammation [79]. In contrast, none of forty-eight nonhypoxemic controls revealed this finding. In SIDS cases, he found hepatic erythropoiesis correlated positively with the presence of thickened pulmonary arteries, right ventricular hypertrophy, and periadrenal brown fat retention [69, 79]. In an attempt to confirm these observations, Valdes-Dapena et al. studied 115 SIDS cases and 154 controls, 57 of whom were accident victims and 97 of whom died of cyanotic congenital heart disease [84]. With the exception of infants between birth and one month of age, the SIDS victims had a higher grade of hepatic erythropoiesis than either control group; however, the differences were not statistically significant. Furthermore, in each age group of SIDS cases and nearly all of the control groups, the standard deviation was larger than the mean, indicating wide variation from case to case and statistical heterogeneity. Neither of these investigations of hepatic erythropoiesis addressed the vital issues of standardization of microscopic sections, prematurity, postconceptional age, socioeconomic class, or anemia.

Postmortem biochemical evidence of accelerated erythropoiesis in SIDS has not been forthcoming. Kozakewich et al. did not find serum erythropoietin levels significantly different in SIDS victims compared with non-SIDS infants dying suddenly and unexpectedly [85]. Furthermore, age and hepatic erythropoiesis did not correlate with serum erythropoietin level in SIDS infants. In another study, erythrocyte glucose-6-phosphate dehydrogenase, ortidine monophosphate decarboxylase, and fetal hemoglobin levels were similar in SIDS infants and controls [86].

Adrenal Glands. Inconsistent observations have been made in comparisons of the adrenal glands of SIDS and controls. Both increased and decreased adrenal chromaffin mass [87, 88], increased fetal and decreased permanent cortex have been reported in SIDS cases [89]. In Suzuki's study, the weights of the adrenal glands did not differ between groups [89]. The use of available rather than standardized microscopic sections of the adrenals may explain these discordant results, especially when one recalls that the tissues in these glands are not evenly distributed. The adrenal chromaffin profile area of forty-one SIDS infants and eighteen controls was not different in the study by Patrick and Patrick, who utilized computerized image analysis of partially standardized sections of the adrenals [90].

Summary of Hypoxic Tissue Marker Literature. Despite the provocative observations of Naeye and colleagues, none of the hypoxic tissue markers have been confirmed unequivocally. There are at least three areas of difficulty with nearly all of the studies. The first is the relative unavailability of controls appropriately matched to the SIDS population [81]. Second, the tissue sections have not been standardized, and third, the analytical method may not have been optimal for comparison of the study groups [57, 64].

Neuropathology

Because SIDS is associated with sleep and substantial evidence suggests respiratory dysfunction, sleep apnea has evolved into a major area of investigation. An understanding of the maturation of neural control of respiration may not only explain mechanisms of death but also provide a means by which effective monitoring and prevention or treatment can be achieved. In this regard, auditory evoked potentials allow evaluation of some brainstem functions [91]. Numerous clinical, physiologic, and neuropathologic studies have appeared during the last decade; most have focused upon the brainstem, but the cerebral white matter and vagus nerve have been examined, as well.

In 1976, Naeye reported an abnormal proliferation of astroglial fibers in the brainstem of fourteen of twenty-eight SIDS victims compared with eighteen controls who were of similar race and gestational and postnatal age [87]. Interpretation of this retrospective study is difficult since microscopic tissue sections of the medulla were not standardized.

Subsequently, Takashima and colleagues observed that, compared with controls, the brainstem of SIDS cases revealed a greater density of astrocytes with astroglial fibers in the pontomedullary reticular formation, nucleus solitarius, and dorsal motor nucleus of the vagus [92]. This study is of particular interest because the central respiratory control centers were analyzed. However, the mean ages of the SIDS cases and controls, and sufficient data to determine whether there is skewing of the ages of the groups in opposite directions are not provided. The sensitivity and reliability of the analytical methods come into question when the severity of brainstem gliosis did not differ between term and prematurely born infants, or between cases with cyanotic and noncyanotic congenital heart disease. In a closely controlled study, Kinney et al. compared the severity of reactive gliosis in six anatomic brainstem regions, five of which are related to respiratory control [93]. Compared with controls, the SIDS cases revealed increased numbers of reactive astrocytes in some regions, including the inferior olivary nucleus, the nucleus of the tractus solitarius, and all six regions combined. The greatest difference, however, was seen in the inferior olivary nucleus, a region without known contribution to respiratory control. Despite relatively close matching of these two groups, there are some important differences. The SIDS cases averaged eight weeks younger than the controls; sixteen of the twenty controls apparently did not die suddenly, and a substantially lower percentage of the SIDS cases were black compared with controls (51 percent versus 75 percent). Also, two of four control infants who died suddenly and did not suffer antecedent illness had total reactive astrocyte counts greater than the median for the SIDS group. No association between gliosis and numerous specific clinical or pathologic variables such as prematurity, low birthweight, low Apgar scores, and subcortical leukomalacia could be identified. Therefore, Kinney and colleagues cautiously concluded that "the relationship of these (reactive astrocytes), if any, to SIDS remains uncertain." [93]

Not all investigators have identified brainstem gliosis in SIDS victims. Increased numbers of astrocytes were not detected by Pearson and Brandeis [94]. Furthermore, Ambler et al. identified glial reactive changes in nearly half of both the SIDS and control groups, the latter of which was composed of infants who also had died suddenly, but for known reasons [95]. They concluded that infants dying of an established cause are not suitable to serve as a control group. Using random sections of medulla and pons, Summers and Parker found no difference in the degree of brainstem gliosis in SIDS infants and controls [96].

More recently, Becker and Takashima reinvestigated the question of brainstem gliosis using immunoperoxidase techniques to identify glial fibrillary acidic protein (GFAP) [97, 98]. Compared with controls, there were increased numbers of GFAP positive glia in the reticular formation and solitary nuclei of the vagus in about 50 percent of the SIDS cases [97]. Furthermore, they demonstrated a delay in the normal loss of dendritic spines from the neurons in these same brainstem regions of SIDS infants; however, this was unaccompanied by gliosis in 20 percent to 40 percent of cases [98, 99]. In an elegant study in which cases were matched for postconceptual age, Quattrochi et al. identified significantly greater dendritic spine density in SIDS infants than in controls; furthermore, spine density declined at a faster rate in SIDS [100]. Finally, there was a significant difference in spine density between the nucleus ambiguous and nucleus solitarius, and between reticular and nonreticular formation areas in SIDS infants, but not in controls. These investigators concluded that the brainstem in SIDS victims is developmentally delayed, which may indicate pathologic injury by hypoxemia or contribute to abnormal central respiratory and arousal control [97–100].

In another paper, Takashima and colleagues compared neuronal development in the visual cortex of infants born at less than thirty-four weeks gestation with that of infants born at term [101]. This study included three SIDS cases in the study group and nine in the control group. Despite severe prematurity and birthweights below 1400 grams, the prematurely born SIDS victims had a normal number and distribution of glia and neurons and normal neuronal differentiation including the structure, number, and distribution of dendritic spines. Conversely, Quattrochi et al. demonstrated persistence of dendritic spines by neurons of the brainstem reticular system in SIDS infants compared with controls [102]. They suggested their findings indicate either an immature pattern of development or pathologic interference with maturation by hypoxemia [103].

Much of the central nervous system control of respiration is mediated via the vagus nerve. Tidal volume, respiratory rate, the mucosal irritant, and Hering-Breuer stretch receptors are dependent upon the vagus nerve [104, 105]. Sachis et al. demonstrated fewer myelinated fibers less than two microns in diameter in SIDS victims than in controls of similar postconceptual age [106]. This observation and the finding that the number of these fibers gradually increased with postconceptual age suggested that the development of the vagus nerve was delayed or abnormal. How this relates to SIDS, if at all, remains speculative; these investigators interpreted their observations as evidence that SIDS is not sudden but rather is the "terminal episode in a long pathologic process." [106]

Subcortical leukomalacia (SL) was found in 16 percent of eighty-four SIDS cases compared with 13 percent of sixty-three infants with congenital heart disease (half had a cyanotic type) and 4 percent of forty-five infants who died acutely and without antecedent respiratory, cardiovascular, or intracranial disease [107]. Rather than necrotic, SL was characterized by fewer axons and less myelin than adjacent white matter. The pathogenesis of this lesion is unknown, but the authors speculated it was a result of subcortical ischemia, especially because it occurred in the white matter of the deep sulci. The report does not indicate whether SL occurred more often in cyanotic than noncyanotic congenital heart disease, or in premature rather than term infants.

Atkinson et al. described an eight-month-old infant, an alleged victim of SIDS, who suffered a cardiopulmonary arrest and at necropsy had edema and neuronal degeneration in the dorsal nuclei of the vagus nerve, but no astroglial proliferation (compared with a single control) [108]. SIDS seems an unlikely diagnosis in this case because the clinical course included high fever, and necropsy also showed acute bronchopneumonia, acute splenitis, and bone marrow hypercellularity.

Finally, there is the intriguing paper by Gilles et al. regarding atlantooccipital instability [109]. In their investigation of postmortem head extension in infants, including victims of SIDS, they noted that vertebral artery compression can follow inversion of the posterior arch of the atlas through the foramen magnum during extension of the head. The vertebral arteries supply the brainstem and rostral cervical spinal cord. Thus, if collateral blood supply is inadequate, brainstem ischemia theoretically could cause apnea or sudden death.

Pulmonary Surfactant and Pressure Volume Characteristics

In 1982, Morley et al. reported that the surfactant from the lungs of SIDS victims contained significantly less phospholipid and dipalmitoylphosphotidylcholine than that from controls, which on average were 157 days younger than the SIDS infants [110]. Subsequently, Talbert and Southall postulated that during critical periods of lung development, defective surfactant might cause extensive pulmonary atelectasis with hypoxemia, which on occasion could be lethal [111]. This hypothesis was not supported by Fagan and Milner, who found similar pressure volume characteristics in SIDS and controls [112, 113].

Pulmonary Inflammation

Although mild peribronchiolar and focal alveolar septal lymphocytic infiltration often are seen microscopically, macroscopic consolidation of the lung is not seen in SIDS [19, 20, 38, 39]. When pneumonia is apparent to the naked eye, the death should be ascribed to pneumonia rather than to SIDS.

Laryngotracheal Lesions

Fibrinoid necrosis and inflammation have been observed with equal frequency in the vocal cords of SIDS cases and controls [114]. Laryngeal mucous gland hyperplasia has been identified in some SIDS victims, but the severity of inflammation did not differ between SIDS and control cases; no relationship was found between mucous gland hyperplasia, inflammation, and antemortem infections [115].

Cardiac Lesions

Although the bulk of current evidence favors respiratory dysfunction as the primary event in the majority of SIDS cases, cardiac disease deserves consideration. Appropriately, attention has been directed toward the conduction system and coronary arteries to account for sudden death. Cardiac arrhythmias often are presumed to be the cause of death when other lesions are not found. Schwartz and colleagues presented abundant data that a prolonged QT interval may be important in SIDS [116], but this contention has been challenged [117–121]. Haddad and colleagues suggested that infants with life-threatening apnea and considered at high risk for SIDS have increased sympathoadrenal activity manifested by tachycardia, beat-to-beat and overall heart rate variability, and a smaller QT index [122–125]. Identification of such arrhythmias is particularly cogent since many types are either treatable or preventable. The existence of arrhythmias becomes more credible if pathologic lesions can be identified in the conduction system.

Petechiae have been observed in the conduction system in SIDS, but there has been no difference in their frequency in SIDS and controls. In a comparison of thirty SIDS victims and eighteen controls by Kozakewich et al., petechiae were identified in 20 percent and 17 percent of cases, respectively [126]. In two other studies, petechiae were identified in 57 percent to 73 percent of both SIDS victims and controls [127, 128]. Although petechiae were seen only in SIDS infants in the study of Jankus, he studied only three SIDS cases and three controls [129]. The significance of these petechiae remains unknown, but they are unlikely to be the cause of death. The pathogenesis of their presence probably is similar to that of the petechiae found in the pericardium, epicardium, and thymus [39].

Intimal thickening, internal elastic lamina fragmentation, and narrowing of the lumen of the arteries supplying the conduction system have been found in some SIDS victims. These arterial lesions were identified initially by James in 10 percent of infants who died suddenly and unexpectedly; he did not specify the frequency of such lesions in SIDS cases and explained deaths [130]. Anderson and Hill identified narrowing of the atrioventricular (AV) nodal artery in five of forty SIDS victims and of the sinoatrial (SA) nodal artery in one case, but there were no controls [131]. W. R. Anderson et al. found intimal arteriopathy in 35 percent of eighteen SIDS cases compared to 10 percent of controls [128]. However, in the studies of Valdes-Dapena et al. and Lie et al., arteriopathy was not described despite examination of hundreds of microscopic sections per case [132, 133]. Interestingly, degeneration, hemosiderosis, and necrosis of the conduction system were not identified in the SIDS cases in any of these studies. The absence of lesions within the conduction system does not preclude a lethal arrhythmia in SIDS [134], but perimortem electrocardiographic evidence for such has not been documented.

Inflammatory cell infiltration of the cardiac conduction system has been identified in a few SIDS cases. These were cases in which many, if not serial, microscopic sections were obtained and in which the inflammatory infiltrates were limited to the conduction system. W. R. Anderson et al. found minor inflammatory infiltrates in the conduction system of 50 percent of both SIDS cases and controls [128]. Jankus examined several hundred microscopic sections of the conduction systems of three SIDS victims and three controls. He found extraordinarily mild lymphocytic and eosinophilic infiltration of the conduction system in SIDS but not in control cases [129]. This is in contrast to the work of Kozakewich et al., who found inflammatory infiltrates in the otherwise unaltered conduction system of two of eighteen controls but none of thirty SIDS cases [126]. The significance of these minor lesions is unknown.

James suggested that postnatal molding of the AV conduction system during infancy may cause a lethal arrhythmia [130]. Numerous investigators have made similar observations of postnatal molding, yet they have differed in their interpretations of its significance [132, 133]. For detailed descriptions and illustrations of these morphologic changes, the reader is referred particularly to the papers of James [130] and Lie et al. [133]. During the first year of life, the left side of the AV conduction system fragments into small archipelagos of fibers surrounded by dense fibrous tissue. These changes apparently occur in response to the development of high pressures in the left heart after birth. The importance of these anatomic changes remains to be clarified. James opined that one could not assume that these changes are not functionally significant because similar alterations were found in controls (also dead); this "presupposes that more was known about the exact mechanism of death in those cases than is usually the case . . . but that ubiquity could not be read as synonymous with safety or stability." [134]

Growth and Development

Most pathologists experienced in the autopsy of SIDS victims are of the opinion that these infants appear well nourished and without evidence of chronic disease [38, 39]. While it is true that infants born with low birth weights are at higher risk of SIDS [135], most victims have birth weights within normal ranges. However, closer analysis reveals that the postnatal growth of SIDS infants is slower than that of living peers [136, 137]. These findings suggest that factors contributory to SIDS have their onset prenatally and extend into postnatal life. In a more recent study, Peterson reanalyzed data from 155 SIDS victims and 270 contemporary living peers and found the retarded growth pattern of SIDS victims was similar to that of babies born to mothers who smoked during pregnancy [138]. SIDS infants did not manifest the early postnatal acceleration of growth typically seen in infants.

Other aspects of growth disturbance in SIDS have been examined. Vawter and Kozakewich found dysmorphic, dysplastic, or anomalous features in 59.6 percent of SIDS victims compared to 65.1 percent of controls who were closely matched for age [139]. Dysplastic lesions such as nevi, hemangiomas, and nodular renal blastema occurred in 14 percent of SIDS victims, but were not seen in infants dying because of trauma, and were seen in only one (5 percent) of twenty-one young infants who died of infection. These numbers are too small to permit meaningful conclusions. The mean static lung volumes in SIDS victims, expressed as either volume per body length or per unit weight of lung, were nearly identical to published normal values [140].

Compared with controls, important differences were not found in SIDS with respect to lung height, transverse or anterior-posterior thoracic diameters, rib angle with the spinal axis, or plane of the diaphragm. Domed diaphragmatic configurations, as determined by lateral chest radiographs, were seen only in SIDS victims, whereas flat diaphragms were seen in 20 percent of SIDS victims compared to 50 percent of controls. The significance of these observations remains obscure [139].

Hypoglycemia

It has been suggested that SIDS is associated with hypoglycemia [141]. Apparent pancreatic islet cell hyperplasia has been identified by a number of investigators [142–144]. Loo et al. reported no differences between SIDS and control cases with respect to pancreatic beta cell frequency and distribution and insulin content [145]. Currently available studies of hepatic glycogen content are too premature to allow meaningful conclusions [139].

Overheating

Overheating has been implicated in some cases of SIDS [146, 147]. This hypothesis is of particular interest since hypohidrotic ectodermal dysplasia, a sex-linked disorder in which heat regulation is inadequate, has been associated with sudden, unexpected death in infants [148]. More recently, Stanton found that thirty-two of thirty-four SIDS victims in England had at least one of four risk factors for overheating, including being hot or sweating when found, being found in an unusually warm environment, being excessively clothed, or having a terminal infective illness [149]. Seventeen of these cases were complicated by terminal infection with high fever and should be excluded because they apparently are explained deaths. His remaining data are inadequate to draw firm conclusions, especially when one remembers that 50 percent of sudden, unexpected deaths in England are eventually explained after complete investigation compared to only 15 percent in the United States. Last, the author admits that postneonatal febrile apnea has not been proven in humans; hence, his conclusion remains speculative, especially in cases in which the temperature was recorded at less than 40° Celsius.

Postmortem Vitamins, Hormones, and Chemistry

Body fluids and tissues have been analyzed in an attempt to identify metabolic disturbances that might account for or contribute to SIDS. Most of these studies have been hampered by the lack of ideally matched controls and postmortem deterioration of such specimens. According to Coe, the eye is relatively protected from postmortem contamination and putrefaction; therefore, the vitreous humor appears to be a more reliable fluid for analysis than either the blood or cerebral spinal fluid [150]. However, results of all of the studies must be interpreted with caution.

Hillman et al. excluded a simple vitamin D deficiency or 25-hydroxy-vitamin D deficiency as a significant factor in SIDS [151].

Read proposed that thiamine deficiency may be linked to SIDS [152]. Peterson et al. found no evidence of thiamine deficiency in SIDS victims when measured as erythrocyte transketolase activity [153]. However, elevated serum thiamine levels have been measured in some SIDS victims [154, 155]. More recently, Wyatt et al. observed no differences in thiamine levels in SIDS and controls and suggested that the elevated levels are a postmortem artifact occurring in both groups [156].

Comparing ranges in SIDS infants with the ranges established in age-matched living outpatients, Naeye et al. found SIDS infants had normal blood insulin, cortisol, growth hormone, and thyroid stimulating hormone levels [157].

Blumenfeld et al. compared vitreous humor chemistry in 127 SIDS cases, 47 children who died in the hospital, and 21 cases of acute traumatic childhood deaths [158]. Sodium (Na), potassium, chloride (Cl), calcium, magnesium (Mg), urea nitrogen (BUN), creatinine, and total protein ranges in SIDS and non-SIDS cases did not differ.

These results do not confirm previous studies, which indicated some SIDS cases have elevated Na and BUN levels [159] and Mg deficiency [160]. Naeye found no differences between SIDS infants and controls in serum Mg, phosphate, calcium, copper, and zinc levels [157]. Hillman et al. found normal serum calcium and copper levels in SIDS victims [151].

One study reported that concentrations of lead, but not calcium, were higher in the liver and ribs in SIDS infants than in non-SIDS cases [161]. However, further analysis of these data reveals that only four of sixty-six SIDS cases had lead concentrations outside of one standard deviation (SD) of the control group, and none of the SIDS cases had levels outside of two SD of the control mean. The authors were careful to conclude that "the higher lead levels found in the four- to twenty-six-week-old SIDS infants do not provide sufficient evidence to say that lead toxicity contributes to SIDS." [161] There were no differences in lung, liver, kidney, and rib levels of zinc and calcium; the SIDS cases did have significantly less lung copper and more liver magnesium than non-SIDS cases.

Future Directions

Despite the explosion of information available today, SIDS remains a poorly understood entity that can be neither reliably predicted nor prevented. This syndrome undoubtedly represents a small group of diseases; some of these remain to be defined, whereas others are well understood but present as sudden, unexpected infant death [162–167].

Intrathoracic petechiae remain the most common and undisputed finding in the majority of SIDS cases. Furthermore, they appear to correlate with sudden catastrophic death. Delineation of their pathogenesis and significance may lead to effective screening or monitoring systems, allowing earlier attempts at therapeutic intervention.

Few of Naeye's hypoxic tissue markers have been confirmed, possibly because nearly all of the studies in this area are severely limited by difficulties in acquiring ideal controls. Nevertheless, lack of general confirmation does not refute the existence of hypoxic tissue markers in individual cases. Future studies aided by more sophisticated analytical methods are indicated, especially since there is good evidence that many SIDS victims suffer prenatal and postnatal growth failure and, occasionally, subtle growth disturbances.

References

1. McNeill, J.T., and H.M. Gamer. 1938. *Medieval Handbooks of Penance,* New York: Columbia University Press. Quoted by S.G. Norvenius. The contribution of SIDS to infant mortality trends in Sweden. Presented at the seventeenth Intra-Science Symposium on Sudden Infant Death Syndrome, Santa Monica, California, February, 1984.
2. Savitt, T.L. 1979. The social and medical history of crib death. *J Fla Med Assoc* 66:853–859.
3. Trexler, R.C. 1973–74. Infanticide in Florence: New sources and first results. *History of Children's Quarterly* 1:98–116.
4. Savitt, T.L. 1975. Smothering and overlaying of Virginia slave children: A suggested explanation. *Bull Hist Med* 49:400–404.
5. Templeman, C. 1892. 258 Cases of suffocation of infants. *Edinburgh Medical Journal* 38:322–329.
6. Editorial. 1984. *Lancet* 2:1137.
7. Plater, F. 1614. Observationum in hominis affectibus plerisque-libri tress. *Basileae,* p. 172. Quoted by John Ruhrah in *Pediatrics of the Past.* 1925. New York: Paul B. Hoeber.
8. Lee, C.A. 1842. On the thymus gland: Its morbid affections, and the diseases which arise from its abnormal enlargement. *Am J Med Sci* 3:135–154.
9. Friedleben, A. 1858. Die Physiologie der Thymusdruse in Gesundheit und Krankheit vom Standpunkte Experimentellar Forschung und Klinischer Erfahrung: Ein Beitrag zur Lebensgeschichte der Kindheit. *Bietriag Zur Lebensgeschichte Der Kindheit,* Vol. 8. Frankfurt a.M.: literarische Anstalt.
10. Paltauf, A. 1889:1890. Uber Die Beziehung der Thymus zum Plotzlichen Tod. *Wiener Klinische Wochenschrift* 2:877–881; 3:172–175.
11. Quoted in Jessop, E. 1905. Sudden death and the thymus gland. *Br Med J* 2:1586.
12. Young, M., and H.M. Turnbull. 1931. An analysis of the data collected by

the status lymphaticus investigation committee. *J Pathol & Bacteriol* 34:213–258.

13. Brouardel, P. 1895. La Mort et la Mort Subite. *Balliere Paris,* p. 270 (quoted from second edition, New York: William Wood and Co., 1902).
14. Farber, S. 1934. Fulminating streptococcus infections in infancy as a cause of sudden death. *N Eng J Med* 211:154–159.
15. Goldbloom, A., and F.W. Wigglesworth. 1938. Sudden death in infancy. *Can Med Assoc J* 38:119–129.
16. Werne, J. 1942. Post mortem evidence of acute infection in unexpected death in infancy. *Am J Pathol* 18:759.
17. Werne, J., and I. Garrow. 1947. Sudden death of infants allegedly due to mechanical suffocation. *Am J Public Health* 37:675–687.
18. Werne, J., and I. Garrow. 1953. Pathologic findings in infants dying immediately after violence contrasted with those after sudden apparently unexplained death. *Am J Pathol* 29:833–851.
19. Werne, J., and I. Garrow. 1953. Sudden apparently unexplained death during infancy: 1. Pathologic findings in infants found dead. *Arch Pathol* 29: 633–675.
20. Adelson, L., and E.R. Kinney. 1956. Sudden and unexpected death in infancy and childhood. *Pediatrics* 17:663–699.
21. Ray, C.G., J.B. Beckwith, N.M. Hebestreit, and A.B. Bergman. 1970. Studies of the Sudden Infant Death Syndrome in King County Washington: I. The role of viruses. *JAMA* 211:619–623.
22. Scott, D.J., P.S. Gardner, J. McQuillin, A.N. Stanton, and M.A.P.S. Downham. 1984. Respiratory viruses and cot death. *Br Med J* 2:12–13.
23. Williams, A.L., E.C. Uren, and L. Bretherton. 1984. Respiratory viruses and sudden infant death. *Br Med J* 288:1491–1493.
24. Hall, C.B., A.E. Kopelman, R.G. Douglas, J.M. Geiman, and M.P. Meagher. 1979. Neonatal respiratory syncytial virus infection. *N Eng J Med* 300:393–396.
25. Anas, N., C. Boettrich, C.B. Hall, and J.G. Brooks. 1982. The association apnea and respiratory syncytial virus infection in infants. *J Pediatr* 101:65–68.
26. Ogra, R.L., S.S. Ogra, and P.R. Koppola. 1975. Secretory component in sudden infant death syndrome. *Lancet* 2:387–390.
27. Bruhn, F.W., S.T. Mokrohisky, and K. McIntosh. 1977. Apnea associated with respiratory syncytial virus infection in young infants. *J Pediatr* 90: 382–386.
28. Steinschneider, A. 1977. Nasopharyngitis and the sudden infant death syndrome. *Pediatrics* 60:531–533.
29. Steinschneider, A. 1975. Nasopharyngitis and prolonged sleep apnea. *Pediatrics* 56:967–971.
30. Tonkin, S. 1975. Sudden infant death syndrome: Hypothesis of causation. *Pediatrics* 55:650–661.
31. Arnon, S.S., T.F. Midura, K. Damus, R.M. Wood, and J. Chin. 1978. Intestinal infection in toxin production by Clostridium botulinum as one cause of sudden infant death syndrome. *Lancet* 1:1273–1277.
32. Arnon, S.S., K. Damus, and J. Chin. 1981. Infant botulism: Epidemiology

in relation to sudden infant death syndrome. *Epidemiol Rev* 3:45–66.

33. Arnon, S.S., K. Damus, B. Thompson, T.F. Midura, and J. Chin. 1982. Protective role of human milk against sudden death from infant botulism. *J Pediatr* 100:568–573.

34. Arnon, S.S. 1983. "Breast feeding and toxigenic intestinal infections: Missing links in SIDS?" In *Sudden Infant Death Syndrome*, ed. J.T. Tildon, L.M. Roeder, and A. Steinschneider. New York: Academic Press.

35. Arnon, S.S. 1981. "Infant botulism: Pathogenesis, clinical aspects and relation to crib death." In *Biomedical Aspects of Botulism*, ed. G.E. Lewis, Jr. New York: Academic Press.

36. Arnon, S.S., D.C. Mills, P.A. Day, R.V. Henrickson, N.M. Sullivan, and T.D. Wilkins. 1984. Rapid death of infant rhesus monkeys injected with Clostridium difficile toxins A and B: Physiologic and pathologic basis. *J Pediatr* 104:34–40.

37. Sonnabend, O.A.R., W.F.F. Sonnabend, U. Crech, G. Moltz, and T. Siegrist. 1985. Continuous microbiologic and pathological study of 70 sudden and unexpected infant deaths: Toxigenic intestinal Clostridium botulinum infection in nine cases of Sudden Infant Death Syndrome. *Lancet* 1:237–241.

38. Beckwith, J.B. 1973. Sudden Infant Death Syndrome. *Curr Probl Pediatr* 3:1–37.

39. Krous, H.F. 1984. The microscopic distribution of intrathoracic petechiae in Sudden Infant Death Syndrome. *Arch Pathol Lab Med* 108:75–76.

40. Fearn, S. 1834. Sudden and unexplained death of children. *Lancet* 2:246.

41. Berg, F.T. 1843. *Arsberattelse Ofver Spada Barnens Helso-Och Sjukvard Vid Stockholms Allmanna Barnhus Ar,* p. 144. (Kindly provided by Professor S.G. Norvenius.)

42. Handforth, C.P. 1959. Sudden unexpected death in infants. *Can Med Assoc J* 80:872–873.

43. Beckwith, J.B. 1970. "Observations of the pathological anatomy of the Sudden Infant Death Syndrome." In *Sudden Infant Death Syndrome*, ed. A.B. Bergman, J.B. Beckwith, and C.G. Ray. Proceedings of the Second International Conference on Causes of Sudden Infant Death in Infants. Seattle: University of Washington Press.

44. Farber, J.P., A.C. Catron, and H.F. Krous. 1983. Pulmonary petechiae: Ventillatory-circulatory interactions. *Pediat Res* 17:230–233.

45. Buda, A.J., J.S. Schroeder, and C. Guilleminault. 1981. Abnormalities of pulmonary wedge pressures in sleep-induced apnea. *Int J Cardiol* 1:67–74.

46. Bromberger-Barnea, B. 1981. Mechanical effects of inspiration on heart functions: A review. *Federation Proceedings* 40:2172–2177.

47. Krous, H.F., and J. Jordan. 1984. A necropsy study of distribution of petechiae in non-sudden infant death syndrome. *Arch Pathol Lab Med* 108:75–76.

48. Kuna, S.T., and J.E. Remmers. 1985. Neuronal and anatomic factors related to upper airway occlusion during sleep. *Med Clin North Am* 69:1221–1242.

49. Tonkin, S.L., J.H. Stuart, and S. Withey. 1980. Obstruction of the upper airway as a mechanism of sudden infant death: Evidence for a restricted

nasal airway contributing to pharyngeal obstruction. *Sleep* 3:375–382.
50. Beckwith, J.B. 1975. The sudden infant death syndrome: A new theory. *Pediatrics* 55:583–584.
51. Robin, P. 1934. Glossoptosis due to atresia and hypotrophy of the mandible. *Am J Dis Child* 48:541–547.
52. Couly, G., and C. LeLievre-Ayer. 1983. La crete neurale cephalique et les malformations cervico-faciales humaines. *Rev Pediatr (Paris)* 19:5–21.
53. Cozzi, F. and A. Pierro. 1985. Glossoptosis-apnea syndrome in infancy. *Pediatrics* 75:836–843.
54. Guilleminault, C., G. Heldt, N. Powell, and R. Riley. 1986. Small upper airway in near-miss sudden infant death syndrome infants and their families. *Lancet* 1:402–407.
55. Guilleminault, C., R.L. Ariagno, L.S. Forno, L. Nagel, R. Baldwin, and M. Owen. 1979. Obstructive sleep apnea and near-miss for SIDS: 1. Report of an infant with sudden death. *Pediatrics* 63:837–843.
56. Merritt, T.A., and M. Valdes-Dapena. 1984. SIDS research update. *Pediatric Annals* 13:193–207.
57. Naeye, R.L. 1973. Pulmonary arterial abnormalities in the sudden infant death syndrome. *N Engl J Med* 289:1167–1170.
58. Weibel, E.R. 1979. *Stereological Methods: 1. Practice Methods for Biological Morphometry*. London: Academic Press.
59. Wagenvoort, C.A., H.N. Neufeld, and J.E. Edwards. 1961. The structure of the pulmonary arterial tree in fetal and early post-natal life. *Lab Invest* 10:751–762.
60. Mason, J.M., L.H. Mason, M. Jackson, J.S. Bell, J.T. Francisco, and B.R. Jennings. 1975. Pulmonary vessels in SIDS. *N Engl J Med* 292:479.
61. Phat, V.N., and M. Durigan. 1976. Mort subite du nourrison: etude morphometrique des arteres pulmonaires. *Soc. D'Electroenceph. et de Neurophysiol. Clin. de Langue Franc* 6:93–96.
62. Kendeel, S.R., and J.A.J. Ferris. 1977. Apparent hypoxic changes in pulmonary arterioles and small arteries in infancy. *J Clin Pathol* 30:481–485.
63. Williams, A., G. Vawter, and L. Reid. 1979. Increased muscularity of the pulmonary circulation in victims of sudden infant death syndrome. *Pediatrics* 63:18–23.
64. Valdes-Dapena, M., M.M. Gillane, J.C. Cassady, R. Catherman, and D. Ross. 1980. Wall thickness of small pulmonary arteries: Its measurement in victims of sudden infant death syndrome. *Arch Pathol Lab Med* 104:621–624.
65. Weiler, G., and J. deHaardt. 1983. Morphometrical investigations into alterations of the wall thickness of small pulmonary arteries after birth and in cases of sudden infant death syndrome (SIDS). *Forensic Sci Int* 21:33–42.
66. Singer, D.B., and E. Tilly. 1984. Pulmonary arteries and arterioles; normal in the sudden infant death syndrome. Paper presented at the seventeenth Intra-Science Symposium, Santa Monica, California.
67. Hislop, A., and L. Reid. 1973. Pulmonary arterial development during childhood: Branching pattern and structure. *Thorax* 28:129–135.
68. Winn, K.J., and A. Steinschneider. 1982. Pulmonary artery changes in response to recurrent episodes of anoxia. *Lab Invest* 46:481–484.

69. Naeye, R.L., P. Whalen, M. Ryser, and R. Fisher. 1976. Cardiac and other abnormalities in the sudden infant death syndrome. *Am J Pathol* 82:1–8.
70. Valdes-Dapena, M.A., K. Amazon, M.M. Gillane, D. Ross, and R. Catherman. 1980. The question of right ventricular hypertrophy in sudden infant death syndrome. *Arch Pathol Lab Med* 104:184–186.
71. Naeye, R.L., R. Fisher, M. Ryser, and P. Whalen. 1976. Carotid body in the sudden infant death syndrome. *Science* 191:567–569.
72. Dinsdale, F., J.L. Emery, and D.R. Gadsdon. 1977. The carotid body: A quantitative assessment in children. *Histopathology* 1:179–187.
73. Cole, S., L.B. Lindenberg, F.M. Galioto, Jr., P.E. Howe, A.C. DeGraff, Jr., J.M. Davis, R. Lubka, and E.M. Gross. 1979. Ultrastructural abnormalities of the carotid body in sudden infant death syndrome. *Pediatrics* 63:13–17.
74. Perrin, D.G., E. Cutz, L.E. Becker, and A.C. Bryan. 1984. Ultrastructure of carotid bodies in sudden infant death syndrome. *Pediatrics* 73:646–651.
75. Perrin, D.G., E. Cutz, L.E. Becker, A.C. Bryan, A. Madapallimatum, and M.J. Sole. 1984. Sudden infant death syndrome: Increased carotid body dopamine and noradrenaline content. *Lancet* 2:535–537.
76. Nishino, T., and S. Lahiari. 1981. Effects of dopamine on chemo reflexes in breathing. *J Appl Physiol* 50:892–897.
77. Krous, H.F., A.C. Catron, and J.P. Farber. 1984. Norepinephrine-induced pulmonary petechiae in the rat: An experimental model with potential implications for sudden infant death syndrome. *Pediatr Pathol* 2:115–122.
78. Teplitz, C., and Y.C. Lim. 1974. The diagnostic significance of diffuse brown adipose tissue (B.A.T.). Transformation of adult periadrenal fat: A morphologic indicator of severe chronic hypoxemia. *Lab Invest* 30:390.
79. Naeye, R.L. 1974. Hypoxemia and the sudden infant death syndrome. *Science* 186:837–838.
80. Valdes-Dapena, M.A., M.M. Gillane, and R. Catherman. 1976. Brown fat retention in sudden infant death syndrome. *Arch Pathol Lab Med* 100:547–549.
81. Beckwith, J.B. 1983. "Chronic hypoxemia in the sudden infant death syndrome: A critical review of the data base." In *Sudden Infant Death Syndrome*, ed. J.T. Tildon, L.M. Roeder, and A. Steinschneider. New York: Academic Press.
82. Aherne, W., and D. Hull. 1966. Brown adipose tissue and heat production in the newborn infant. *J Pathol & Bacteriol* 91:223–234.
83. Emery, J.L., and F. Dinsdale. 1978. Structure of periadrenal brown fat in childhood in both expected and cot deaths. *Arch Dis Child* 53:154–158.
84. Valdes-Dapena, M.A., M.M. Gillane, D. Ross, and R. Catherman. 1979. Extramedullary hematopoiesis in the liver in sudden infant death syndrome. *Arch Pathol Lab Med* 103:513–515.
85. Kozakewich, A., A. Sytkowski, J. Fisher, G. Vawter, and F. Mandell. 1986. Serum erythropoitin in infants with emphasis on sudden infant death syndrome. *Lab Invest* 54:5p.
86. Krause, B.L., and H.R. Zielke. 1982. Activity of five enzymes and fetal hemoglobin in RBC's of infants dying from sudden infant death syndrome (SIDS). Paper presented at the International Research Conference on Sud-

den Infant Death Syndrome, June 28–30, Baltimore, Maryland.

87. Naeye, R.L. 1976. Brain-stem and adrenal abnormalities in the sudden infant death syndrome. *Am J Clin Pathol* 66:526–530.

88. Visser, J.W. 1979. Sudden Infant Death Syndrome (letter). *Arch Pathol Lab Med* 103:544–545.

89. Suzuki, T., S. Kashimura, and K. Umetsu. 1980. Sudden infant death syndrome: Histological studies on adrenal gland and kidney. *Forensic Sci Int* 15:41–46.

90. Patrick, J.R., and S.T. Patrick. 1982. Adrenal chromaffin tissue in sudden infant death syndrome. *Lab Invest* 46:12p.

91. Gupta, P.R., C. Guilleminault, and L.J. Dorfman. 1981. Brainstem auditory evoked potentials in near-miss sudden infant death syndrome. *J Pediatr* 98:791–794.

92. Takashima, S., D. Armstrong, L. Becker, and C. Bryan. 1978. Cerebral hypoprofusion in the sudden infant death syndrome? Brainstem gliosis and vasculature. *Ann Neurol* 4:257–262.

93. Kinney, H.C., P.C. Burger, F.E. Harrell, Jr., and R.P. Hudson, Jr. 1983. "Reactive gliosis" in the medulla oblongata of victims of sudden infant death syndrome. *Pediatrics* 72:181–187.

94. Pearson, J., and L. Brandeis. 1983. "Normal aspects of morphometry of brainstem astrocytes, carotid bodies and ganglia in SIDS." In *Sudden Infant Death Syndrome,* ed. J.T. Tildon, L.M. Roeder, and A.S. Steinschneider. New York: Academic Press.

95. Ambler, M.W., C. Neave, and W.Q. Sturner. 1981. Sudden and unexpected death in infancy and childhood. *Am J Forensic Med Pathol* 2:23–30.

96. Summers, C.G., and J.C. Parker, Jr. 1981. The brainstem in sudden infant death syndrome: A postmortem survey. *Am J Forensic Med Pathol* 2:121–127.

97. Becker, L.E., and S. Takashima. 1985. Chronic hypoventilation and development of brainstem gliosis. *Neuropediatrics* 16:19–23.

98. Takashima, S., and L.E. Becker. 1985. Developmental abnormalities of medullary "respiratory centers" in sudden infant death syndrome. *Exp Neurol* 90:580–587.

99. Takashima, S., T. Mito, and L.E. Becker. 1984. Neuronal development in the medullary reticular formation in sudden infant death syndrome and premature infants. *Neuropediatrics* 16:76–79.

100. Quattrochi, J.J., P.T. McBride, and A.J. Yates. 1985. Brainstem immaturity in sudden infant death syndrome: A quantitative rapid Golgi study of dendritic spines in 95 infants. *Brain Research* 325:39–48.

101. Takashima, S., L.E. Becker, and F-W. Chan. 1982. Retardation of neuronal maturation in premature infants compared with term infants of the same postconceptual age. *Pediatrics* 69:33–39.

102. Quattrochi, J., N. Baba, and L. Liss. 1980. Sudden infant death syndrome (SIDS): A preliminary study of reticular dendritic spines in infant SIDS. *Brain Research* 181:245–249.

103. Baba, N., J.J. Quattrochi, C.B. Reiner, W. Adrion, P.T. McBride, and A.J. Yates. 1983. The possible role of the brainstem in sudden infant death syndrome. *JAMA* 249:2789–2791.

104. Fleming, P.J., A.C. Bryan, and M.H. Bryan. 1978. Functional immaturity of pulmonary irritant receptors and apnea in newborn preterm infants. *Pediatrics* 61:515–518.

105. Cross, K.W., M. Klaus, W.H. Tooley, and K. Weisser. 1960. The response of the newborn baby to inflation of the lung. *J Physiol (London)* 51:551–565.

106. Sachis, P.N., D.L. Armstrong, L.E. Becker, and A.C. Bryan. 1981. The vagus nerve and sudden infant death syndrome: A morphometric study. *J Pediatr* 98:278–280.

107. Takashima, S., D. Armstrong, L.E. Becker, and J. Huber. 1978. Cerebral white matter lesions in sudden infant death syndrome. *Pediatrics* 62:155–159.

108. Atkinson, J.B., O.B. Evans, R.S. Ellison, and M.G. Netsky. 1984. Ischemia of the brainstem as a cause of sudden infant death syndrome. *Arch Pathol Lab Med* 108:341–342.

109. Gilles, F.H., M. Bina, and A. Sotrel. 1979. Infantile atlantooccipital instability: The potential danger of extreme extension. *Am J Dis Child* 133:30–37.

110. Morley, C.J., B.D. Brown, C.M. Hill, A.J. Barson, and J.A. Davis. 1982. Surfactant abnormalities in babies dying from sudden infant death syndrome. *Lancet* 1:1320–1322.

111. Talbert, D.G., and D.P. Southall. 1985. A biomodal form of alveolar behaviour induced by a defect in lung surfactant—a possible mechanism for sudden infant death syndrome. *Lancet* 1:727–728.

112. Fagan, D.G., and A.D. Milner. 1985. Pressure volume characteristics of the lungs in sudden infant death syndrome. *Arch Dis Child* 60:471–485.

113. Fagan, D.G., and A.D. Milner. 1985. Pressure volume characteristics of the lungs in sudden infant death syndrome (letter). *Arch Dis Child* 60:1104–1109.

114. Pinkham, J.R., and J.B. Beckwith. 1970. "Vocal cord lesions in the sudden infant death syndrome." In *Proceedings of the Second International Conference on Causes of Sudden Death in Infants,* ed. A.B. Bergman, J.B. Beckwith, and C.G. Ray. Seattle: University of Washington Press.

115. Fink, B.R., and J.B. Beckwith, 1980. Laryngeal mucous gland excess in victims of sudden infant death syndrome. *Am J Dis Child* 134:144–146.

116. Schwartz, P.J., M. Montemerlo, M. Facchini, P. Lalice, D. Rosti, G. Poggio, and R. Giorgetti. 1982. The QT interval throughout the first six months of life: A prospective study. *Circulation* 66:496–501.

117. Steinschneider, A. 1978. Sudden infant death syndrome and prolongation of the QT interval. *Am J Dis Child* 132:688–691.

118. Kelly, D.H., D.C. Shannon, and R.R. Liberthson. 1977. The role of the QT interval in the sudden infant death syndrome. *Circulation* 55:633–635.

119. Maron, B.J., C.E. Clark, R.E. Goldstein, and S.E. Epstein. 1976. Potential role of QT interval prolongation in sudden infant death syndrome. *Circulation* 54:423–430.

120. Guntheroth, W.G. 1982. The QT interval and sudden infant death syndrome (editorial). *Circulation* 66:502–504.

121. Montague, T.J., J.P. Finley, K. Mukelabai, S.A. Black, S.M. Rigby, C.A.

Spencer, and B.M. Horacek. 1984. Cardiac rhythm, rate and ventricular repolarization properties in infants at risk for sudden infant death syndrome: Comparison with age- and sex-matched control infants. *Am J Cardiol* 54:301–307.

122. Haddad, G.G., M.A.F. Epstein, R.A. Epstein, N.M. Mazza, R.B. Mellins, and E. Crongrad. 1979. The QT interval in aborted sudden infant death syndrome infants. *Pediatr Res* 13:136–138.

123. Haddad, G.G., E. Crongrad, R.A. Epstein, M.A.F. Epstein, H.S. Law, J.B. Katz, N.M. Mazza, and R.B. Mellins. 1979. Effect of sleep state on the QT interval in normal infants. *Pediatr Res* 13:139–141.

124. Leistner, H.L., G.G. Haddad, R.A. Epstein, T.L. Lai, M.A.F. Epstein, and R.B. Mellins. 1980. Heart rate and heart rate variability during sleep in aborted sudden infant death syndrome. *J Pediatr* 97:51–55.

125. Haddad, G.G., H.L. Leistner, T.L. Lai, and R.B. Mellins. 1981. Ventilation and ventilatory pattern during sleep in aborted sudden infant death syndrome. *Pediatr Res* 15:879–883.

126. Kozakewich, H.P.W., B.M. McManus, and G.F. Vawter. 1982. The sinus node in sudden infant death syndrome. *Circulation* 65:1242–1246.

127. Anderson, R.H., J. Bouton, C.T. Burrow, and A. Smith. 1974. Sudden death in infancy: A study of cardiac specialized tissue. *Br Med J* 2:135–139.

128. Anderson, W.R., J.F. Edland, and E.A. Schenk. 1970. Conduction system changes in the sudden infant death syndrome. *Am J Pathol* 59:35A.

129. Jankus, A. 1976. The cardiac conduction system in sudden infant death syndrome: A report on three cases. *Pathology* 8:275–280.

130. James, T.N. 1968. Sudden death in babies: New observations and the heart. *Am J Cardiol* 22:479–506.

131. Anderson, K.R., and R.W. Hill. 1982. Occlusive lesions of cardiac conducting tissue arteries in sudden infant death syndrome. *Pediatrics* 69:50–52.

132. Valdes-Dapena, M.A., M. Greene, N. Basavanand, R. Catherman, and R.C. Xtruex. 1973. The myocardial conduction system in sudden death in infancy. *N Engl J Med* 289:1179–1180.

133. Lie, J.T., H.S. Rosenberg, and E.E. Erickson. 1976. Histopathology of the conduction system in the sudden infant death syndrome. *Circulation* 53:3–8.

134. James, T.N. 1976. Sudden death of babies. *Circulation* 53:1–2.

135. Lewak, N., B.J. van den Berg, and J.B. Beckwith. 1979. Sudden infant death syndrome risk factor. *Prospective Data Review* 18:404–411.

136. Peterson, D.R., E.A. Benson, L.D. Fisher, N.M. Chinn, and J.B. Beckwith. 1974. Postnatal growth and the sudden infant death syndrome. *Am J Epidemiol* 99:389–394.

137. Jorgensen, T., F. Biering-Sorensen, and J. Hilden. 1982. Sudden death in Copenhagen 1956–1971: IV. Infant development. *Acta Paediatr Scand* 71:183–189.

138. Peterson, D.R. 1981. Sudden infant death syndrome: Reassessment of growth retardation in relation to maternal smoking and the hypoxia hypothesis. *Am J Epidemiol* 113:583–589.

139. Vawter, G.F., and H.P.W. Kozakewich. 1983. "Aspects of morphologic vari-

ation amongst SIDS victims." In *Sudden Infant Death Syndrome*, ed. J.T. Tildon, L.M. Roeder, and A. Steinschneider. New York: Academic Press.

140. Fagan, D.G. 1969. "Functional development of the human lung." In *The Anatomy of the Developing Lung*, ed. J. Emery. London: William Heineman Medical Books.

141. Sturner, W.Q., and J.B. Susa. 1980. SIDS and liver phosphoenolpyruvate carboxykinase. *Forensic Sci Int* 16:19–28.

142. Pollak, J.M., and J.S. Wigglesworth. 1976. Islet-cell hyperplasia and sudden infant death. *Lancet* 2:570–571.

143. Pollak, J.M., A. Aynsley-Green, S.R. Bloom, and J.S. Wigglesworth. 1978. Nesidioblastosis as a cause of sudden neonatal death. *Scand J Gastroenterol* (supplement) 49:143.

144. Cox, J.M., G. Guelpa, and M. Terrapon. 1976. Islet-cell hyperplasia and sudden infant death. *Lancet* 2:739–740.

145. Loo, S., H.P.W. Kozakewich, R.A. Wald, and G.F. Vawter. 1982. SIDS and nesidioblastosis. *Lab Invest* 46:10p.

146. Stanton, A.N., D.J. Scott, and M.A.P.S. Downham. 1980. Is overheating a factor in some unexpected infant deaths? *Lancet* 1:1054–1057.

147. Sunderland, R., and J.L. Emery. 1981. Febrile convulsions and cot death. *Lancet* 2:176–178.

148. Bernstein, R., I. Hatchuel, and T. Jenkins. 1980. Hypohidrotic ectodermal dysplasia in sudden infant death syndrome. *Lancet* 2:1024.

149. Stanton, A.N. 1984. Overheating and cot death. *Lancet* 2:1199–1201.

150. Coe, J.I. 1969. Postmortem chemistries on human vitreous humor. *Am J of Clin Pathol* 51:741–750.

151. Hillman, L.S., M. Erickson, and J.G. Haddad, Jr. 1980. Serum 25-hydroxyvitamin D concentrations in sudden infant death syndrome. *Pediatrics* 65:1137–1139.

152. Read, D.J.C. 1978. The aetiology of the sudden infant death syndrome: Current ideas on breathing and sleep and possible links to deranged thiamine neurochemistry. *Aust N Z J Med* 8:322–336.

153. Peterson, D.R., R.F. Labbe, G. van Belle, and N.M. Chinn. 1981. Erythrocyte transketolase activity and sudden infant death. *Am J Clin Nutr* 34:65–67.

154. Davis, R.E., G.C. Icke, and J.M. Hilton. 1982. High serum thiamine and the sudden infant death syndrome. *Clin Chim Acta (Amsterdam)* 123:321–328.

155. Davis, R., G. Icke, and J. Hilton. 1980. High thiamine levels in sudden infant death syndrome (letter). *N Engl J Med* 303:462.

156. Wyatt, D.T., M.M. Erickson, R.E. Hillman, and L.S. Hillman. 1984. Elevated thiamine levels in SIDS, non-SIDS, and adults: Postmortem artifact. *J Pediatr* 104:585–588.

157. Naeye, R.L., R. Fisher, H.R. Ruben, and L.M. Demers. 1980. Selected hormone levels in victims of sudden infant death syndrome. *Pediatrics* 65:1134–1136.

158. Blumenfeld, T.A., C.H. Mantell, R.L. Catherman, and W.A. Blanc. 1979. Postmortem vitreous humor chemistry in sudden infant death syndrome and in other causes of death in childhood. *Am J Clin Pathol* 71:219–223.

159. Emery, J.L., P.G.F. Swift, and E. Worthy. 1974. Hypernatremia and Uraemia in unexpected death in infancy. *Arch Dis Child* 49:686–692.
160. Cadell, J.L. 1972. Magnesium deprivation in sudden unexpected infant death. *Lancet* 2:258–262.
161. Erickson, N.M., A. Pocklis, G.E. Gantner, A.W. Dickinson, and L.S. Hillman. 1983. Tissue mineral levels in victims of sudden infant death syndrome: I. Toxic metals—lead and cadmium. *Pediatr Res* 17:779–784.
162. Pauli, R.M., C.I. Scott, E.R. Wassman, Jr., E.F. Gilbert, L.A. Leavitt, J. Ver Hoeve, J.G. Hall, M.W. Partington, K.L. Jones, A. Sommer, W. Feldman, L.O. Langer, D.L. Rimoin, J.T. Hecht, and R. Lebovitz. 1984. Apnea and sudden unexpected death in infants with achrondroplasia. *J Pediatr* 104:342–348.
163. Potter, J.M., and J.M.N. Hilton. 1983. Type I hyperlipoproteinemia presenting as sudden death in infancy. *Aust N Z J Med* 13:381–383.
164. Cagle, P., and C. Langston. 1984. Pulmonary veno-occlusive disease as a cause of sudden infant death. *Arch Pathol Lab Med* 108:338–340.
165. Sun, C-C.J., and T. Smith. 1984. Sudden infant death with congenital cytomegalic inclusion disease. *Am J Forensic Med Pathol* 5:65–67.
166. Dunne, J.W., C.G. Harper, and J.M.N. Hilton. 1984. Sudden infant death syndrome caused by poliomyelitis. *Arch Neurol* 41:775–777.
167. Carlson, R.A., S. Arya, and E.F. Gilbert. 1985. Budd-Chiari Syndrome presenting as sudden infant death. *Arch Pathol Lab Med* 109:379–380.

3

The Mechanism of Death in Sudden Infant Death Syndrome

J. BRUCE BECKWITH, M.D.

Anatomical studies of SIDS victims traditionally have been disappointing as a means for explaining these tragic deaths. Indeed, the failure of a complete postmortem examination to account for the death is an integral part of the most popular working definition of SIDS [1]. That a young and seemingly vigorous life could end so suddenly, without obvious lesions to account for the death, has challenged and frustrated investigators of this problem. Many workers have become disillusioned with autopsy as a means of solving the dilemma of SIDS and view the procedure merely as a means of ruling out definable causes of death and as a source of materials for laboratory investigations.

Although disappointing in terms of demonstrating "the cause" of SIDS, the postmortem examination does have potential value as a means of better understanding the mechanism of death. Most pathologic research of SIDS has concentrated upon the search for etiologic factors such as infectious agents, toxins, or genetic abnormalities, or the quest for evidence of preexistent disease states. These are important subjects for investigation, but no less important is the determination of the way, or ways, in which these babies die. Establishment of the "how" of these deaths could make the search for the "why" much more efficient. This chapter focuses specifically upon pathologic investigations of the mechanism, or mechanisms, of SIDS.

Ultimate Mechanisms of Sudden Death

The dying human approaches the final moments by an almost infinite variety of pathways, and at dramatically different rates. These pathways ultimately converge at a single point—death of the organism. Just prior to that convergence point, these paths have resolved into a small number of routes—the exact number of "final" mechanisms depends upon the specific point in the process one wishes to examine. For example, if one accepts a definition of death (i.e., the death of autonomous individuals not connected to external life support devices) as the permanent cessation of circulation or of electrical activity of the heart, it follows that the agonal event in all deaths is cardiac arrest. The question thus resolves not into one of the ultimate event in the dying process but the penultimate one. Many lethal events are in fact initiated by cardiac dysfunction or arrest. In other cases, however, cardiac arrest is the secondary effect of some other antecedent form of catastrophe; the most common, at least in sudden death, is hypoxia. A leading authority of forensic pathology concluded that all sudden deaths ultimately resolve into one of three "final" mechanisms, namely circulatory cessation, respiratory cessation, or exsanguination [2]. Some would add neurologic mechanisms to this list, but it can be argued that these ultimately lead to death by a respiratory or cardiac mechanism.

With respect to SIDS, in which the possibility of exsanguination can be discarded, the question as to the final mechanism of death becomes: Does effective respiration stop prior to effective circulation, or does circulatory dysfunction inaugurate the final episode?

Clues to the Agonal Physiology of SIDS—Intrathoracic Petechiae

Whereas postmortem studies of SIDS victims have been disappointing in terms of demonstrating the "cause" of death, they have revealed a surprisingly repetitive spectrum of relatively minor changes. The consistency of these changes was one of the principle justifications for viewing SIDS as a distinctive entity [2–13]. These relatively consistent findings include minor inflammatory changes in the respiratory tract, congestive pulmonary edema, unclotted blood, and intrathoracic petechial hemorrhages. These latter hemorrhages form the crux of our thesis and are reviewed in some detail.

Intrathoracic petechiae have been mentioned repeatedly as being exceptionally prominent in a majority of SIDS victims. One of the first to emphasize them was Fearn, who in 1834 described two infants, aged five and six months, found dead in bed without signs of antecedent illness. The only abnormality noted at postmortem examination was the presence of numerous "spots of extravasated blood" on the surfaces of the thymus, lungs, and heart [14]. One of these babies shared a bed with an adult, but in the second case there was no possibility, from the history or the circumstances under which the body was found, of external suffocation. Fearn ended his report of these two deaths with the plea that someone enlighten him as to the cause of the blood spots as an explanation for how these babies might have died so suddenly and inexplicably. (SIDS researcher Dr. Abraham Bergman proposed that the petechiae so characteristic of SIDS victims should be called "Fearn's spots.")

Most authors have been content merely to mention that intrathoracic petechiae usually are prominent and characteristic in SIDS victims, but

TABLE 3.1 Frequency of Intrathoracic Petechiae in SIDS and Controls

Author	Number of SIDS Victims	Percent with Petechiae	Comment
Werne and Garrow, 1953[8]	31	80	Petechiae absent or sparse in infants dying of suffocation, CO asphyxia, burns, or drowning.
Jacobsen and Voigt, 1956[15]	97	95	Rarely seen in infanticide or accidents.
Geertinger, 1968[16]	80	79	Seen in only 6 of 43 controls.
Marshall, 1970[17]	162	68	Present in 29% of 42 controls.
Beckwith, 1970[18]	109	87	Noted relative sparing of cervical thymus.
Krous, 1984[19]	100	85	

several have documented their frequency. Table 3.1 presents the incidence of these findings in several large series. Petechiae are not merely present in a majority of SIDS victims; they have been emphasized repeatedly as a characteristic and distinctive finding. For example, Geertinger, a forensic pathologist with wide experience in the investigation of sudden infant death, stated, "This (the presence of intrathoracic petechiae) may be considered the most obvious feature typical of SUD (SIDS). When the thorax is opened at autopsy and the conspicuous petechiae on thymus, pericardium, and pleurae meet the eye, the examiner can feel reasonably convinced that this probably will be the only significant finding in the whole postmortem examination" [16].

Despite the prominence of intrathoracic petechiae in a majority of SIDS victims and their paucity in controls dying of identifiable causes, few authors have been willing to consider them of any pathogenic significance. A brief consideration of the history of this topic should partially explain this reluctance.

Intrathoracic petechiae have been the subject of lively controversy since they were first emphasized as being diagnostic of suffocation by Ambroise Tardieu in a series of monographs beginning in 1859, and summarized in his classic monograph on infanticide [20]. Tardieu clearly distinguished cases of generalized petechiae, often attributable to such systemic causes as toxemias or poisonings, from those in which cutaneous petechiae were limited to the head and neck and, internally, to the pleura and pericardium. He proposed that these localized petechiae were diagnostic of suffocation, and they have since been known as "Tardieu spots."

Brouardel's monumental 1987 monograph of death by various forms of mechanical asphyxia critically reviewed the evidence from the literature and from his extensive personal experience and laboratory experimentation [21]. He was especially interested in testing the proposition of Donders that these lesions were the result of violent inspiratory efforts. On page 20 of Brouardel's monograph, freely translated from the French, we find the following important but generally overlooked observations:

I have, with M. Descoust, undertaken the study of this question (Donder's proposal), using a variety of experimental manipulations. Our most typical experiment was as follows: In a vigorous dog, we placed a window in the parietal wall of the thorax to permit visualization of the visceral pleura. Then, we forcefully applied a mask of soft wax to the face of the dog. In resisting this, the animal made vigorous inspiratory efforts, yet the pleura remained pale; then it suddenly and instantaneously became covered with spots at the precise moment of onset of the second stage of asphyxia, namely respiratory contractions (gasping). We repeated the experiment with numerous variations, such as strangling or hanging the subject, and the result was always the same; subpleural ecchymoses appeared immediately preceding death [21].

Brouardel's lengthy and critical analysis of the problem is rich with observations that, if more generally known, would have prevented some of the experimental design flaws of studies eight decades later. Among his many observations and conclusions, the following, freely translated from the French, deserve special note:

1. Intrathoracic petechiae occur in several types of violent deaths, such as some cases of suffocation and hanging. However, in many cases of hanging and of unequivocal infant suffocation, admitted by the mother, these hemorrhages are absent.

2. They occur more readily in some species than in others. For example, they can be produced with ease by suffocating rabbits, but are more difficult to produce in dogs by this means.

3. In the suffocated human, they seem to occur much more readily in the newborn, with a decreasing trend through childhood, adulthood, and senescence.

4. They are seen in certain clinical conditions, as well, notably epileptic seizures, diptheria, respiratory infections, and certain poisonings.

Brouardel's research led him to the generalization that "the presence of subpleural and subpericardial ecchymoses is an excellent sign (of suffocation), but not a pathognomonic one. You should not follow the formulation of Tardieu and conclude, on the basis of these alone, that a crime has been committed." [21] Tragically, many forensic scientists of succeeding decades failed to note these wise dictates, with the result that a vast number of erroneous convictions for homicide were based upon expert testimony that "Tardieu spots" proved death by suffocation. This unfortunate situation was brought to a halt by an influential paper of Gordon and Mansfield in 1955 [22], supported by an almost equally influential editorial [23], in which intrathoracic petechiae were debunked as signs of asphyxia by suf-focation. These authors demonstrated that petechiae may arise or become more prominent after death and concluded that these lesions have virtually no significance. This opinion has been widely quoted in modern texts of forensic pathology and can be considered as the orthodox dogma of pres-ent medicolegal circles. Certainly, this view is preferable to the over-zealous interpretation of petechiae as a sign of suffocation (or of their ab-sence as evidence to the contrary). But have we gone too far in so zealously rejecting a thesis only because it was propounded with un-justified zeal at an earlier time? Are there specific circumstances under which these petechiae might be viewed reasonably as pathogenetically significant?

At the Second International Conference on Causes of Sudden Death in Infants in 1969, as a young and enthusiastic investigator of the pathologic anatomy of these tragic deaths, I presented what was perhaps my only original observation on the subject—the striking sparing of the dorsum of the cervical lobes of the thymus [18]. This, and other studies to be pre-sented later, had led me to conclude that marked increase in intrathoracic negative pressure was the only logical means by which this peculiar dis-tribution of petechiae could be explained. I anticipated that this paper would spur a flurry of efforts to confirm or refute our observations and interpretations. We were prepared for either support or disproof, but not for apathy. Our conclusions were cited often enough, but our data and spe-cific observations apparently were poorly understood. Before discussing the work that followed, I would like to resurrect some of the major points of that paper in the hope that they can be clarified to a larger audience.

The central point of our observations was that it was not the mere pres-ence of petechiae that was important, but their distribution. Those who would argue for nonspecific or generalized pathogenic mechanisms (such as anoxia, agonal venous hypertension, or endotoxemia) for the formation of petechiae must be prepared to account for this very specific and predict-able pattern of distribution.

Of the three organs whose surfaces are noted repeatedly to be involved by petechiae—heart, lungs, and thymus—only the latter is partially out-side the chest and in a position to be somewhat shielded from the effects of excess negative pressure in the thorax. The topographic anatomy of the thymus offers several features of great relevance to the negative pressure concept. In most glands, the left innominate vein—a sizable structure in the infant—passes transversely across its posterior aspect at the thoracic inlet, usually being firmly adherent to or even partially embedded in the thymus. On its anterior surface, the thoracic portion of the thymus has a "bare area" of variable width, depending upon the points of the anterior pleural reflections onto the chest wall. These may be several centimeters apart, or they may meet in the midline.

We postulated that elevated negative pressure in the pleural cavities would be transmitted across the anterior pleural reflection into the areolar tissue in front of the thymic "bare area." From there, the measure would be transmitted upward (and downward), decreasing as the distance from the pleural cavities increased. On the ventral surface of the thymus, there is no anatomical barrier to upward transmission of this pressure gradient into the cervical portion; however, on the dorsal side, the innominate vein should dampen the effects of pressure transmission into the neck. Since the entire gland is normally drained by a single vein, with no separate circulation to its cervical and thoracic portions, this organ seemed to afford an excellent opportunity to examine the negative pressure thesis.

In 1970, we showed that the portions of cervical lobe immediately rostral to the innominate vein are impressively less involved by petechiae than is the remainder of the gland [24]. Of ninety-five glands with petechiae of the thoracic lobes, fifty-seven showed complete sparing of the dorsum of the cervical lobes; in eighty-six the density was greater in thoracic than cervical lobes, and in the remaining nine they were of equal density, none having a greater degree of involvement in the cervical portion. Figure 3.1 shows the dorsum of the excised thymuses of five SIDS victims, illustrating the typical appearances of this sparing. Figure 3.2 illustrates a frequent appearance—numerous petechiae laterally on surfaces in contact with the pleura, but diminishing numbers centrally in the anterior "bare area."

In 18 percent of the cases, we encountered petechiae of the parietal pleura on the diaphragm, but in none were they found on its peritoneal surface, or elsewhere in the abdomen. Thus, the principle emerged that the petechiae usually seen in SIDS victims involved all surfaces with the thorax and none outside the chest. No known characteristic of circulatory anatomy could explain how thymus, heart, and lung could be regularly involved, yet all other organs and tumors be spared. We have searched in vain for an alternate explanation to the negative pressure concept, and to our knowledge no other investigator has provided another explanation for this unique distribution.

Two important findings of our study were presented in the 1969 proceedings. First, rather large pleural petechiae occasionally are distributed in a pattern corresponding to dependent livor (Figure 3.3). We suggested that these pleural hemorrhages occur post mortem, perhaps through vascular ruptures that occur agonally. We wondered if the lower blood pressures of the pulmonary circulation retarded the tendency to hemorrhagic extravasation until after death. On the other hand, fine, "splinter" hemorrhages of the pleura, often seen in SIDS victims, do not seem to have a dependent distribution. Thymic and epicardial petechiae show no predilection for dependent distribution and might arise by mechanisms different from those that cause petechiae in the lungs.

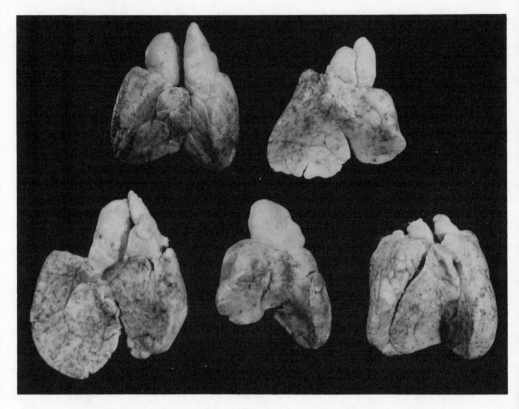

FIGURE 3.1. Dorsal view of thymus glands from five victims of SIDS, illustrating the relative sparing of the cervical lobes by petechiae.

Another observation of relevance to this discussion was made when we sacrificed three anesthetized adult baboons by tracheal occlusion [24]. In the first two, despite seemingly vigorous respiratory efforts, no hemorrhages occurred. In the third, we took care to occlude the airway at end-expiration, and in this animal myriads of minute splinter hemorrhages studded the surfaces of the lungs and heart. In this circumstance, the animal presumably is able to generate maximal negative pressures, suggesting a possible explanation for the lack of petechiae in true suffocation victims [24, 25].

Our observations seemed to implicate upper airway obstruction— perhaps end-expiratory obstruction—as an immediate mechanism of death in SIDS. This seemed a point worthy of intensive investigation, yet only a few related papers subsequently appeared. The first, and most widely quoted, was published by Guntheroth et al. in 1973 [26]. These authors attempted to test our hypothesis by sacrificing elderly adult rats by six defined mechanisms, including tracheal occlusion, immersion in 100

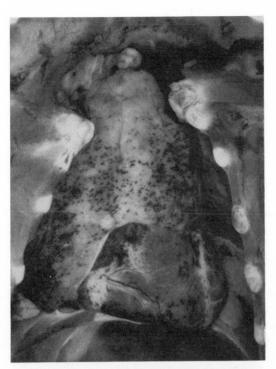

FIGURE 3.2. Opened thorax of SIDS victim, showing numerous petechiae on surfaces of heart and thymus. The thymic petechiae are more densely concentrated laterally over the thoracic lobes than centrally, over the "bare area" (see text), which in this instance was over 2.0 cm in width.

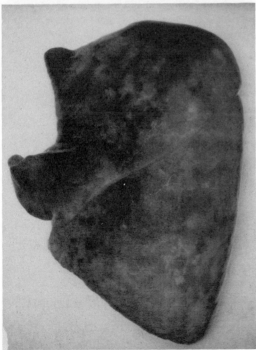

FIGURE 3.3. Same case as in Figure 3.2. Lung petechiae are concentrated ventrally in this baby who died face down and had ventral livor mortis. Pulmonary petechiae sometimes show this distribution, suggesting that they might occur after death. However, other intrathoracic petechiae in SIDS do not show a dependent distribution and presumably occur by another pathway.

percent nitrogen, cardiac arrest, and succinylcholine-induced respiratory paralysis. Petechiae were studied only on the lungs, and other body surfaces were not investigated. No attempt was made to occlude the airways at end-expiration, and there was no documentation of the degree of negative pressures generated. Some animals in all study groups developed petechiae, their incidence being lowest in the airway occlusion group and highest in the nitrogen-induced hypoxia group. These authors thus concluded that hypoxia was the most important factor leading to petechiae, and that vigorous respiratory efforts potentiated this effect.

In 1980, the same group of investigators reported on their subsequent unsuccessful attempt to replicate the earlier study [27]. In this study, they found that 100 percent nitrogen failed to produce petechiae; the only difference in study design was that rats in the second study were younger. Postulating that infections might have been present in the older subjects of the earlier study, the investigators inoculated the airways of rats with Sendaivirus. Six days after inoculation, they repeated the study and observed petechiae, especially in the nitrogen-immersed group. An additional defect of this investigation was the failure to document microscopically the severity of respiratory infection in the study animals; this variable alone could have materially affected their results.

Species differences in susceptibility are of concern in such studies. Brouardel observed important differences in results from different animal species [21]. Rabbits, as he pointed out, seem to be quite susceptible to petechial formation with airway occlusion. Farber and colleagues were able to document this in an important and elegant series of observations in which they used repeated end-expiratory tracheal obstruction in rabbits with simultaneous recording of pulmonary wedge pressure, systemic blood pressure, and intratracheal negative pressure [28]. They found numerous petechiae in the lungs, but few or none in the heart, thymus, or abdomen, suggesting that the dynamics of formation of pulmonary petechiae might differ from those of the systemic circuit. Of extreme interest, however, was their documentation of a direct relationship between number of petechiae and the pressure differential between pulmonary vessels and intratracheal pressure. In another study, they found rats to be resistant to petechial formation by airway occlusion [29].

Campbell and Read documented again in rabbits that repeated tracheal obstruction produced numerous pulmonary petechiae, and that they did not occur with apneic asphyxia induced by barbituate [30]. Intracardiac electrocution and a rapid injection of noradrenaline also produced petechiae, and they concluded that circulatory pressures play a role in the genesis of pulmonary petechiae.

Other animal studies could be cited, but the extent to which these can be generalized to human SIDS victims remains dubious. Therefore, it is most germane to review in this context two recent postmortem studies of

SIDS by Krous and collaborators. In one of these, the topography of petechiae was analyzed microscopically [19]. In the heart and thymus, petechiae showed a striking predilection for surfaces oriented toward intrapleural negative pressure. Pulmonary petechiae, conversely, were more numerous within lobules than peripherally, a distribution suggesting that pulmonary venous pressure elevation was directly involved in their genesis. Krous postulated that acute left ventricular failure was responsible for lung hemorrhages, but not for thymic or epicardial ones. He quoted studies from his laboratory and those of others in which increased intrathoracic negative pressure, by afterloading the left ventricle, reducing its compliance, and increasing preload of that chamber, could explain this result. His conclusion that lung hemorrhages and hemorrhages of the systemic circulation may be formed by somewhat different mechanisms is in accord with our observations, cited earlier, relating differences in distribution with respect to postmortem dependency. This conclusion also could be related to his observations of ready production of lung hemorrhages by tracheal occlusion, without thymic or epicardial lesions in the rabbit model.

In a companion paper, Krous and Jordan documented that, in pediatric autopsies of non-SIDS victims, localization of petechiae to the intrathoracic surfaces was correlated with conditions of airway obstruction [31]. When these hemorrhages were more widespread, there was no such correlation.

It is apparent that more work needs to be done in the area of agonal physiology before the inferences derived from observations of petechial distribution may be considered firm. However, a substantial body of evidence clearly exists to support the thesis that upper airway obstruction is an important part of the final event and perhaps is the ultimate cause of SIDS.

Proposed Mechanisms of Airway Obstruction in SIDS

Marked increases in intrathoracic pressures imply that airway obstruction occurs in the presence of vigorous respiratory efforts. We would further localize the probable site of obstruction to the upper airway, for several reasons:

1. Obstruction at the bronchiolar level should give an asthmalike picture, in which marked increases in negative pressure are not seen.
2. Obstruction at the tracheal or bronchial level should be due to obstructing foreign material in these rigid cartilaginous tubes, yet this is not seen in SIDS (except for postmortem passage of gastric contents into the airway), especially when positive pressure resuscitation has been used.

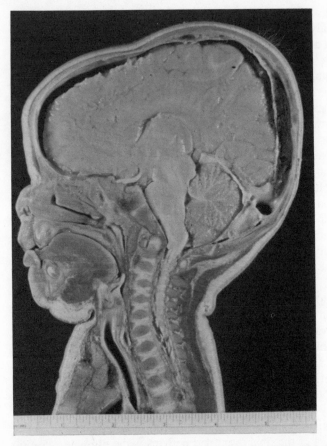

FIGURE 3.4. Sagittal hemisection of SIDS victim. The subject was frozen in the face down position prior to preparation of the section. Note the small caliber of the pharyngeal airway in this position.

3. Obstruction at the laryngeal or pharyngeal level can occur due to local mechanical factors, yet not be apparent during postmortem dissection.

The anatomy of the sleeping infant affords some insight into possible sites of such an obstruction. Figure 3.4 is a sagittal frozen section of a SIDS victim, three months of age. The body was placed in the face down, prone position in which he was found. The extremely small dimensions of the pharyngeal airway in this situation are evident. This vulnerability to positional factors suggests one possible mechanism of airway obstruction, but reflex muscular activity also could occlude the same region easily. Tonkin's important research showed how readily this region of the airway collapses when a baby is inspiring against a nasal obstruction [32], and

Shaw pointed out the possibility of nasal obstruction as well [33]. Finally, the demonstration that obstructive forms of sleep apnea occur in infants affords us another clue that such a mechanism could explain a rapidly lethal episode during sleep in an apparently healthy infant [34]. Obstructive apnea is especially intriguing to us in view of the fact that such spells usually have their onset at the end of expiration, affording maximum opportunity for generating intrathoracic negative pressure.

In conclusion, a substantial body of evidence suggests that the mechanism of SIDS might be upper airway obstruction. Those who would implicate a cardiac or other mechanism for the onset of the lethal episode must be prepared to account for the frequency and the distribution of petechiae in SIDS.

It would seem that Fearn, in 1834, was correct in drawing attention to these hemorrhagic spots in the chests of suddenly dead infants and asking of his colleagues how such hemorrhages might form [14]. Perhaps, 150 years later, we are finally beginning to attempt an answer to his question— an answer that potentially can bring us close to an understanding of how these babies die.

References

1. Beckwith, J.B., A.B. Bergman, C.E. Gardner, R. Steele, J.R. Patrick, T.K. Marshall, J.T. Miller, and R.J. Wedgwood. 1970. "Discussion of terminology and definition of Sudden Infant Death Syndrome." In *Sudden Infant Death Syndrome: Proceedings of the Second International Conference on Causes of Sudden Death in Infants,* ed. A.B. Bergman, J.B. Beckwith, and C.G. Ray. Seattle: University of Washington Press.

2. Davis, J.H. 1980. "Asphyxial deaths." In *Modern Legal Medicine, Psychiatry and Forensic Science,* ed. W.J. Curran, A.L. McGarry, and C.S. Petty. Philadelphia: F.A. Davis Co.

3. James, T.N. 1968. Sudden death in babies: New observations on the heart. *Am J Cardiol* 22:479–506.

4. James, T.N. 1976. Sudden death in babies. *Circulation* 99:277–282.

5. James, T.N. 1985. Crib death. *J Amer Coll Cardiol* 5:1185–1187.

6. Marino, T.A., and B.M. Kane. 1985. Cardiac atrioventricular junctional tissues in hearts from infants who died suddenly. *J Amer Coll Cardiol* 5:1178–1184.

7. Bharati, S., E. Krongrad, and M. Lev. 1985. Study of the conduction system in a population of patients with Suddent Infant Death Syndrome. *Pediatr Cardiol* 6:29–40.

8. Werne, J., and I. Garrow. 1953. Sudden apparently unexplained death during infancy. I. Pathologic findings in infants found dead. *Am J Pathol* 29:633–652.

9. Adelson, L., and E.R. Kinney. 1956. Sudden and unexpected death in infancy and childhood. *Pediatrics* 17:663–697.

10. Adelson, L. 1965. "Specific studies of infant victims of sudden death." In *Sudden Death in Infants*, ed. R.J. Wedgwood and E.P. Benditt. U.S. Public Health Service Publication No. 1412.

11. Valdes-Dapena, M. 1982. The pathologist and the Sudden Infant Death Syndrome. *Am J Pathol* 106:118–131.

12. Beckwith, J.B. 1973. The Sudden Infant Death Syndrome. *Curr Prob Pediatr* 3(8):1–36. Reprinted by U.S. Department of Health, Education and Welfare as Publication No. (HSA)-76-5137, 1976.

13. Sturner, W.Q. 1977. "Sudden unexpected infant death." In *Forensic Medicine: Trauma and Environmental Hazards*, ed. C.G. Tedeschi. Philadelphia: W.B. Saunders.

14. Fearn, S.W. 1834–35. Sudden and unexplained death of children. *Lancet* 1:246.

15. Jacobsen, T., and J. Voigt. 1956. Cited by Geertinger.

16. Geertinger, P. 1968. *Sudden Death in Infancy.* Springfield, Ill.: Charles C Thomas.

17. Marshall, T.K. 1970. "The Northern Ireland Study: Pathology Findings." In *Sudden Infant Death Syndrome: Proceedings of the Second International Conference on Causes of Sudden Death in Infants*, ed. A.B. Bergman, J.B. Beckwith, and C.G. Ray. Seattle: University of Washington Press.

18. Beckwith, J.B. 1970. "Observations on the pathological anatomy of the Sudden Infant Death Syndrome." In *Sudden Infant Death Syndrome: Proceedings of the Second International Conference on Causes of Sudden Death in Infants*, ed. A.B. Bergman, J.B. Beckwith, and C.G. Ray. Seattle: University of Washington Press.

19. Krous, H.F. 1984. The microscopic distribution of intrathoracic petechiae in Sudden Infant Death Syndrome. *Arch Pathol Lab Med* 108:77–79.

20. Tardieu, A. 1868. *Etude Medico-Legale sur l'Infanticide.* Paris: J.-B. Bailliere et Fils.

21. Brouardel, P. 1897. *La Pendaison, la Strangulation, la Suffocation, la Submersion.* Paris: J.-B. Bailliere et Fils.

22. Gordon, I., and R.A. Mansfield. 1955. Subpleural, subpericardial and subendocardial hemorrhages. A study of their incidence at necropsy and of the spontaneous development, after death, of subpericardial petechiae. *J Forensic Med* 2:31–50.

23. Editorial. 1955. Tardieu spots in asphyxia. *J Forensic Med* 2:1–4.

24. Beckwith, J.B. 1970. "Pathology discussion: Mechanism of death in SIDS." In *Sudden Infant Death Syndrome: Proceedings of the Second International Conference on Causes of Sudden Death in Infants*, ed. A.B. Bergman, J.B. Beckwith, and C.G. Ray. Seattle: University of Washington Press.

25. Garrow, I., and J. Werne. 1953. Sudden apparently unexplained death during infancy. III. Pathologic findings in infants dying immediately after violence, contrasted with those after sudden apparently unexplained death. *Am J Pathol* 29:833–845.

26. Guntheroth, W.G., D. Breazeale, and G.A. McGough. 1973. The significance of pulmonary petechiae in crib death. *Pediatrics* 52:601–603.

27. Guntheroth, W.G., I. Kawabori, D. G. Breazeale, L.E. Garlinghouse, and

G.L. Van Hoosier. 1980. The role of respiratory infection in intrathoracic petechiae. *Am J Dis Child* 134:364–366.

28. Farber, J.P., A.C. Catron, and H.F. Krous. 1982. Pulmonary petechiae: Ventilatory-circulatory interactions. *Pediatr Res* 17:230–233.

29. Krous, H.F., A.C. Catron, and J.P. Farber. 1984. Norepinephrine-induced pulmonary petechiae in the rat: An experimental model with potential implications for Sudden Infant Death Syndrome. *Pediatr Pathol* 2:115–122.

30. Campbell, C.J., and D.J.C. Read. 1980. Circulatory and respiratory factors in the experimental production of lung petechiae and their possible significance in the Sudden Infant Death Syndrome. *Pathology* 12:181–188.

31. Krous, H.F., and J. Jordan. 1984. A necropsy study of distribution of petechiae in non-Sudden Infant Death Syndrome. *Arch Pathol Lab Med* 108:75–76.

32. Tonkin, S.L., J. Partridge, D. Beach, and S. Whiteney. 1979. The pharyngeal effect of partial nasal obstruction. *Pediatrics* 63:261–271.

33. Shaw, E.B. 1970. Sudden unexpected death in infancy syndrome. *Am J Dis Child* 119:416–418.

34. Guilleminault, C., R. Ariagno, R. Korobkin, L. Nagel, R. Baldwin, S. Coons, and M. Owen. 1979. Mixed and obstructive sleep apnea and near-miss SIDS: II. Near-miss and normal control infants, comparison over age. *Pediatrics* 64:882–891.

4

The Potential Role of Airway Obstruction in Sudden Infant Death Syndrome

BRADLEY T. THACH, M.D.

During the past thirty years, the search for the cause, or causes, of SIDS has followed two main paths. Some investigators have employed classic epidemiologic and pathologic methods that could uncover clues; others have developed numerous "SIDS theories." Such theories have led to many studies of developmental physiology directed toward understanding mechanisms potentially related to SIDS. The "SIDS theory" approach also has led to intense interest in experimental or clinical "SIDS models," defined as naturally occurring or experimentally induced disorders potentially leading to sudden death under circumstances similar to those of SIDS. This chapter addresses possibly the oldest of the numerous SIDS theories—the airway obstruction theory. Several subdivisions of this theory have emerged and can be categorized as "external" and "internal" obstruction theories. Additionally, in recent years, "muscular contraction" and "muscular relaxation" theories have been proposed. The relevance of these various theories and "SIDS models" to SIDS itself is critically evaluated.

Historical Background

Suffocation caused by obstruction of the nose and mouth has long been associated with rapid death. Accidental smothering of the newborn is a significant cause of infant mortality in some domesticated species [1]. Early explanations of sudden and unexpected deaths in infants viewed suffocation from external sources as the probable cause. Reference to the accidental smothering of an infant trapped beneath his sleeping parent appears in the Bible [2]. Such "laying over" was considered the major cause of sudden death in infants until recent times [3]. In fact, cases in which accidental laying over is presumed to have occurred still appear in the medical literature [4]. On the other hand, Guntheroth pointed out that accidental laying over as a cause of death virtually always has been a presumed diagnosis [3]. Procurement of convincing evidence for suffocation

62

in this manner is exceedingly rare. In the majority of SIDS cases, it can be shown that the infant was sleeping alone, and hence laying over has not been considered a major cause of SIDS in recent times. Additionally, the idea that an infant could be suffocated by bedclothing was at one time prevalent. This theory was rejected by Wooley who showed that the high premeability to oxygen of most fabrics would make suffocation from bedclothing unlikely and concluded that suffocation was not the major cause of SIDS [5]. Nevertheless, one cannot exclude accidental suffocation and laying over as causes of some SIDS deaths. Current diagnostic and investigative techniques are inadequate to indicate how much of what is currently diagnosed as SIDS might be caused by these mechanisms [4, 6].

The concept that suffocation might be due to internal obstruction of the airway is relatively new. In 1954, Beinfield drew a connection between sudden death in infants with choanal atresia and SIDS [7, 8], suggesting that death in choanal atresia might be a model for SIDS. Shortly thereafter, Crosse and Young, and also Illingworth, proposed that many unexplained cyanotic attacks in young infants might be due to "obstruction of the respiratory tract by mucus or other material" [9, 10]. Such thinking provided the background for Shaw's proposal that nasal obstruction due to infection could be "the trigger mechanisms" for asphyxial deaths in SIDS [11].

The past fifteen years have seen the rapid development of several neuromuscular theories for airway obstruction as a cause of SIDS. The first of such theories probably is attributable to Stowens who published an article in 1957 suggesting that laryngospasm might be a cause of SIDS [12]. The laryngospasm theory subsequently was modified and developed by Shaw, Handforth, and Berman [11, 13, 14]. The concept that asphyxiation could result from the relaxation of airway-maintaining muscles came later. A postural mechanism for airway obstruction was suggested by Cross and Lewis, who noted that slight pressure on the mandible, forcing it backward, could completely obstruct the airway of sleeping infants [15]. This theme received substantial further development by Tonkin [16] and later by Stark and Thach, who showed that either external pressure [17] or spontaneous postural changes of the head and neck [18] could lead to prolonged episodes of apnea and bradycardia in young infants.

The origins of the idea that SIDS might be attributed to abnormal control of respiration can be traced to an article appearing in Lancet in 1923 [19]. In that year, Still published observations on "apparently healthy infant(s) found dead in (their) cots." He made detailed observations of "attacks of arrested respiration" in young infants, many of whom subsequently died during repeat episodes. Because postmortem examination failed to reveal a cause of death, Still proposed that "some affection of the respiratory center" was the cause of these attacks and could explain infant deaths that might otherwise be attributed to overlaying. Almost fifty years later, Weitzman and Graziani proposed that obstructive apnea due to abnormal regulation of pharyngeal airway muscles might be a cause of prolonged apneic spells and of SIDS [20]. Shortly thereafter, Guilleminault et al. [21] and Steinschneider and Rabuzzi [22] made polygraphic recordings documenting obstructive apnea episodes during sleep in infants with a past history of "near miss SIDS" episodes, thereby providing objective evidence in support of Weitzman's theory.

The notion that inspiratory suction pressure in the pharynx could be a critical factor leading to obstructive apnea was first introduced by Remmers et al. in studies of adult patients with obstructive sleep apnea syndrome [23]. Soon after publication of these observations, a number of clinical and experimental studies strongly supported the airway suction concept. These studies established yet another theoretical mechanism for airway obstruction in SIDS [24–29].

The Nasal Obstruction Theory

In 1968, Shaw suggested that obstruction of the nasal passages due to mucous secondary to an otherwise mild upper respiratory infection might cause sufficient asphyxia to "trigger" a fatal spasm of the larynx [11]. In informal experiments, he found that only 50 percent of newborn infants responded to nasal occlusion by breathing through the mouth. The remainder attempted in vain to breathe through their noses until the nasal obstruction was relieved. Shaw termed such infants "obligate nose breathers" and viewed them as being at increased risk for suffocation from nasal obstruction. Swift and Emery repeated Shaw's experiments but maintained the nasal occlusion for twenty-five seconds [30]. They found that 13 percent of newborn infants failed to respond to nasal occlusion with oral breathing. In more recent studies, Rodenstein and co-workers obstructed the nasal airway of nineteen infants of various ages [31]. All infants eventually established oral breathing provided sufficient time was allowed for them to do so. In this study, sleep and immaturity seemed to be factors that delayed arousal and establishment of oral breathing. Thus, the infant can no longer be deemed an "obligate nose breather" but still clearly is a "preferential nose breather" [32]. In support of Shaw's concept, however, it has been established that in certain situations life-threatening apnea can occur as a result of upper airway obstruction by secretions. Thus, severe cyanotic episodes in young infants have been reported to result from secretions in the nose and pharynx [10, 33]. Also, obstruction of an infant's nose by medical devices or as a consequence of malformation of the nares reportedly causes apnea and cyanosis [34, 35]. Internal nasal obstruction due to hematoma, enlarged adenoids, and other abnormalities is a frequently reported cause of obstructive sleep apnea in pediatric patients (Table 4.1) [36]. In fact, as previously mentioned, sudden death in

TABLE 4.1 Sites of Airway Narrowing and Primary Diagnoses in the Narrow Upper Airway Obstructive Sleep Apnea Syndrome

Presumed Location of Airway Narrowing	Condition
Nostrils	Fetal Warfarin Syndrome
Nose	Nasal Septal Hematoma
	Choanal Atresia or Stenosis
	Crouzon Disease
	Nasal Septal Deviation
Nasopharynx	Adenoid Hypertrophy
	Obesity
	Post Palatoplasty
Pharynx	Mandibular Hypoplasia
	(Pierre Robin Syndrome, Treacher Collins Syndrome,
	Cornelia Delang Syndrome, and others)
	Down's Syndrome
	Achondroplasia
	Tonsillar Hypertrophy

circumstances somewhat similar to SIDS has been reported in infants with nasal obstruction secondary to choanal atresia or surgery involving the soft palate and producing partial nasopharyngeal obstruction [7, 8, 37].

Regarding the sudden infant death syndrome per se, Shaw's theory has been tested by French et al., who performed radiographic studies of the upper airway in 100 consecutive SIDS cases [38]. In 97 percent of these cases, the nasal passages were patent and were similar in diameter to those of controls. Although highly relevant, this study should be considered within the context of two limitations. First, as noted by Cross and others, the diameter of the nasal passages is largely a function of the volume of the submucosal vascular bed [39, 40]. Postmortem reduction in volume of the nasal vascular bed would be expected to occur secondary to the postmortem fall in blood pressure. This would lead to shrinkage of the nasal mucosa, and hence a state of total nasal obstruction existing prior to death might not be present in the postmortem examination. Second, French et al.'s study was done with the neck in an unnatural hyperextended posture, which greatly increases the diameter of the pharyngeal airway and thus could have dislodged mucous or other material obstructing the nasopharynx [41]. Additionally, it should be mentioned that according to current thinking concerning the mechanism for obstructive sleep apnea, any increase in nasal resistance can produce pharyngeal closure. Hence, obstruction in the nose need not be total in order to trigger complete airway obstruction in the pharynx, a concept in keeping with Shaw's original theory. Therefore, Shaw's general theory remains worthy of consideration and further study.

The Airway Muscle Spasm Theory

Upper Airway-Constricting Muscles: Relevant Physiology

The upper airway serves many functions relating to respiration, feeding, speech, and regulation of chest and abdominal pressure [42, 43]. The neuromuscular mechanisms underlying these functions are extremely complex. The internal configuration of the pharyngeal airway alone is controlled by no less than twenty-four sets of paired muscles. Still other muscles control the narial, posterior oral, and laryngeal regions of the upper airway. Based on their anatomical position, most of these muscles can be classified as either airway-constricting or airway-dilating muscles.

A series of muscular sphincters in the nasopharynx, oropharynx and larynx is capable of completely closing the upper airway at these several sites [42, 44]. These sphincters are regulated by precise timing mechanisms. For example, during swallowing, both the velopharyngeal and the laryngeal-constricting muscles close the airway in a precisely timed sequence spanning less than one second [45, 46]. In contrast, during vomiting, the oropharynx is widely patent, whereas the nasopharynx and larynx are tightly closed [47]. Additionally, a variety of functions including singing, coughing, crying, "grunting" respiration, lifting, and abdominal expulsive maneuvers require narrowing, or complete closure, of the laryngeal airway in order to maintain an elevated abdominal and thoracic pressure—the familiar Valsalva maneuver [44, 48]. This role of the Valsalva maneuver is clearly appreciated during coughing. However, only relatively recently has the Valsalva maneuver been appreciated as a mechanism for thoracic fixation to facilitate forceful limb movements [49]. The normal motor acts of swallowing, regurgitation, and Valsalva maneuver figure prominently in several pathologic syndromes of airway obstruction leading to asphyxia in young infants.

Upper airway protective mechanisms involving the pharynx and larynx include coughing, sneezing, and swallowing [50]. Laryngeal closure and apnea also are protective mechanisms. In the newborn in particular, Johnson and co-workers showed that certain types of chemical stimulation of the larynx provoke not only swallowing but also laryngeal constriction and prolonged apnea [51, 52]. Recent studies in human infants showed that this chemoreflex can cause swallowing and central apnea [53] and may be a common triggering mechanism for prolonged mixed and obstructive apnea in preterm infants [54, 55]. According to Sasaki and co-workers, there are fundamentally two forms of airway protective laryngeal closure reflexes [56, 57]. The first is termed "the glottic closure reflex" [57, 58]. In anesthetized animals, a variety of mechanical and chemical stimuli applied locally in the larynx or at more distal sites in the body will produce glottic closure at the level of the vocal cords and the area of the epiglottic folds [59, 60]. Laryngeal closure ends abruptly with removal of the stimulus. According to Suzuki and Sasaki, a second form of glottic closure, which is more sustained and is termed "laryngospasm," is characterized by laryngeal closure that persists even after removal of the stimulus [56]. From an electrophysiologic standpoint, laryngospasm is distinguished from glottic closure reflex by a sustained after-discharge of the laryngeal constricting muscles. In animals, laryngospasm, unlike the glottic closure reflex, is seen only with direct stimulation of laryngeal mucosa or electrical stimulation of the superior laryngeal nerve. Hyperthermia, maturation, increased oxygen or decreased carbon dioxide, and decreased lung volume facilitate laryngospasm produced by laryngeal nerve stimulation [61–63]. However, from the standpoint of relevance for SIDS, such laryngospasm usually produces only transient laryngeal closure. In the animal model, a falling arterial oxygen saturation and a rising arterial carbon dioxide tension usually lead to reversal of the laryngospasm and reopening of the airway before severe asphyxia develops. Thus, Taylor et al. were unsuccessful in their attempts to produce lethal laryngospasm in young monkeys by using continuous laryngeal nerve stimulation [64]. Fatal airway closure was possible only with sustained stimulation of the motor nerves to the laryngeal-constricting muscles.

Airway Muscle Contraction and Spasm: Models for SIDS

Laryngospasm during General Anesthesia. During administration of a general anesthetic, a respiratory condition clinically termed "laryngospasm" frequently is encountered. Although laryngospasm occurs in 1 percent of surgical procedures employing a general anesthetic, detailed clinical descriptions are few [65]. The underlying pathophysiology of this condition is unclear. As mentioned, some authorities feel that laryngospasm and the glottic closure reflex are distinctly different entities from a standpoint of pathophysiology. In clinical practice, these two conditions probably are viewed frequently as one and the same. Olsson has given surgical laryngospasm a purely operational definition, "Laryngospasm is considered to be present when inflation of the lungs is hindered or made impossible by an unwanted muscular action of the larynx and when other cases such as bronchospasm or an occluding tongue are excluded [65]. In this form of laryngospasm, blood and secretions in the larynx often are implicated as the triggering stimuli. Of possible relevance to SIDS, children one to three months old have been found to be at increased risk for this complication as are asthmatics and patients with local airway inflammatory conditions or infections [65]. Although some authors consider laryngospasm to be life-threatening, others have not viewed it as a particularly serious condition [65]. Hence, in most cases, laryngospasm is said to be a transient phenomenon that disappears as asphyxia due to respiratory obstruction increases [66]. Cardiac arrest during anesthesia-related laryngospasm has been reported, although it is said to be relatively rare.

Also of possible relevance for SIDS are recent reports of acute hemorrhagic pulmonary edema appearing within minutes or hours after anesthetic-induced laryngospasm and upper airway obstruction from other causes [67, 68].

Pharyngeal Spasm with Local Anesthesia. Clinical observations in humans and animal studies suggest that the sensations from respiratory airflow in the upper airway are an important stimulus for regulation of tone of upper airway muscles [69, 70]. In the rabbit, upper airway mucosal mechanoreceptors responsive to airway pressure changes appear to be essential for maintaining airway patency [70]. If the rabbit's nose, pharynx, and larynx are treated with topical anesthetic, thereby eliminating responses to airway pressure, the animal is unable to open its pharyngeal airway and rapidly dies from asphyxiation caused by airway obstruction. Physiologic measurements and a direct observation suggest that airway closure is caused by contraction of pharyngeal-constricting muscles. At autopsy, these rabbits revealed intrathoracic petechiae similar to those found in SIDS victims.

Infectious, Toxic, and Metabolic Conditions Associated with Pharyngeal and Laryngeal Spasm. In the past, severe and often fatal spasm of the pharynx and larynx was encountered frequently in several diverse and now rare disorders, including rabies [71, 72], tetanus [73, 74], hypocalcemic tetany [75], and strychnine poisoning [76]. Although generalized spasms of other muscles in the body are characteristic of all of these disorders, sudden death often has been attributed to episodes of pharyngeal and/or laryngeal spasms causing upper airway obstruction. In the case of strychnine poisoning, the basis for the muscular spasm is related to loss of function of inhibitory postsynaptic pathways in the central nervous system [76]. The muscular spasms in tetanus are similar to those in strychnine poisoning. Like strychnine, the tetanus neurotoxin, tetanospasmin, also blocks synaptic transmission in the central nervous system [77]. In all of these disorders, the relaxation of muscles following a physiologic contraction appears to be inhibited. Thus, in rabies and in hypocalcemic tetany, pharyngeal and laryngeal spasm similar to those in tetanus or strychnine poisoning often are initiated by swallowing [72, 78]. Prolonged spasm occurs with failure of the pharyngeal and laryngeal constrictors to relax after completion of the swallow.

Laryngeal Spasm Associated with Upper Respiratory Tract Infections. Certain infections producing upper airway inflammation have been associated with spasm of airway-constricting muscles producing severe airway obstruction. These infections include infectious laryngitis (croup syndrome) and pertussis [78, 79]. Respiratory obstruction is characterized by inspiratory stridor. In these conditions, some degree of airway obstruction no doubt is due to mucosal edema. However, because stridor and impairment to inspiratory flow frequently are sudden in onset and may be episodic, a significant component of the airway obstruction in these disorders has been attributed to laryngeal spasm [78, 79]. Cornwell and associates [80], also Bosma [81], and more recently Pickens and associates [82], made detailed observations of "near miss SIDS" episodes in several young infants in whom coughing secondary to upper respiratory tract infection coincided with obstructive or mixed apneic episodes. Episodes of prolonged and complete airway obstruction leading to marked asphyxia were documented. Guilleminault and Ariagno reported a young infant with pertussis infection whose first manifestation of the disease was prolonged sleep apnea [83]. In the past, death during paroxysms of coughing associated with pertussis was not uncommon in infants under six months of age [78]. Death attributed to acute laryngeal obstruction still occurs occasionally in infants with croup [79].

Laryngospasm Associated with Gastroesophageal Reflux and Regurgitation Episodes. Herbst et al. and Spitzer et al. found a temporal relation between occult reflux of gastric contents into the esophagus and episodes of obstructive or mixed apnea in young infants [84, 85]. These authors suggested that the origin of the obstruction was laryngospasm. Menon et al. studied infants during overt regurgitation episodes and found an increased incidence of prolonged mixed and obstructive apnea immediately following these episodes [86]. More recent studies of infants in whom upper airway chemoreflexes were stimulated with a small volume of fluid introduced into the airway strongly support the role of a reflex mechanism in the apnea following regurgitation [54, 55] (Figure 4.1). Although the clinical diagnosis of gastroesophageal reflux and its management in relation to apneic spells is controversial and doubtless will continue to be so, collectively these several observations suggest that symptomatic upper airway obstruction secondary to reflux or regurgitation of gastric contents into the pharynx does occur in certain infants.

Velopharyngeal Sphincter Closure Associated with Swallowing During Prolonged Mixed and Obstructive Apnea. Recently, a number of investigators have noted that the typical apneic spell in preterm infants and in some full-term infants with idiopathic apnea is associated with obstructed inspiratory efforts [18, 87–89] and with swallowing [57, 90–92]. The obstructed breaths during such spells appear to have at least two different mechanisms. One type of obstructed breath immediately precedes swallowing and appears to be an intrinsic component of the normal swallowing mechanism [91]. During such "swallow breaths," the nasopharyngeal airway is occluded by contraction of the velopharyngeal sphincter.

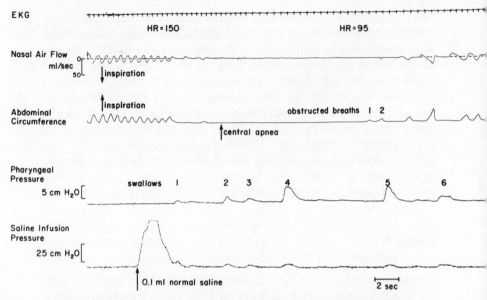

EKG

HR = 150   HR = 95

Nasal Air Flow
ml/sec
inspiration

inspiration

Abdominal
Circumference
obstructed breaths 1 2

central apnea

Pharyngeal
Pressure
5 cm H₂O
swallows   1   2   3   4   5   6

Saline Infusion
Pressure
25 cm H₂O

0.1 ml normal saline   2 sec

FIGURE 4.1. Polygraphic tracings of heart rate and respiratory activity in a sleeping preterm infant. The tracings show an episode of apnea, upper airway obstruction, and swallowing following infusion of a .1 ml bolus of saline into the pharynx via an indwelling nasopharyngeal catheter. Note the swallow three seconds after the bolus and the central apnea. Several more swallows occur with two obstructed breaths occurring late in the spell. The obstructed breaths are evidenced by abdominal respiratory excursions without nasal airflow. Note the decrease in heart rate from 150 bpm to 95 bpm and the spontaneous recovery from the spell. There was absent oral ventilation during the episode as indicated by an oral carbon dioxide monitor (tracing not shown). The infusion pressure indicates duration of stimulus delivery and does not reflect pharyngeal pressures. In similar studies, responses of this kind are more frequently seen with water than with saline, indicating that chemoreceptors in the airway are important in mediating these reflex responses [55]. (From Pickens, et al, [54]. With permission).

Upper Airway Closure during Breathholding Spells. Breathholding spells are a well known and very common cause of acute asphyxia in young infants. The pathophysiology of such spells is complex [36, 93, 94]. Typically, spells begin with a sudden, painful stimulus or emotional disturbance. The infant frequently cries out and then holds its breath, performing a Valsalva maneuver [95]. According to several accounts, the Valsalva maneuver is followed by obstructed inspiratory efforts [78, 96]. Cyanosis usually is present and frequently is intense. In severe breathholding spells, the infant rapidly loses consciousness, becomes limp and areflexic. A brief seizure secondary to hypoxic cerebral depression often occurs. Although typically first observed in infants nine months to two years of age, the breathholding spell is known to occur in younger infants and is believed to account for some near miss SIDS episodes in this younger age group [36, 97, 98]. During "pale breathholding spells," a variant of the "blue breathholding spell," the Valsalva maneuver also occurs, but sudden sinus bradycardia may be the primary cause for loss of consciousness [97]. "Blue" and "pale" spells may occur in the same infant.

A seemingly closely related type of apneic spell recently was described in preterm infants during "squirming" motor activity [99]. Such spells constitute a significant portion of apneic episodes otherwise known as "apnea of prematurity" [99, 100]. These spells often result in cyanosis and bradycardia and may require medical intervention to terminate the episode. In addition to the marked slowing of respiration associated with the Valsalva maneuver, obstructed inspiratory efforts have been documented during such spells. Unlike breathholding spells in the older infant, crying seldom occurs at the start of the spell, and these episodes associated with squirming often occur in infants who are sleeping. Peabody and coworkers [100, 101] have characterized episodes of "disorganized breathing" in preterm and older infants, which are associated with cyanosis and have features similar both to breathholding spells and to "squirming spells." Disorganized breathing episodes also occur during sleep. It is likely that these three varieties of obstructive apnea (i.e., squirming spells, disorganized breathing, and breathholding spells) are closely related. Kahn and co-workers found an increased incidence of subsequent development of breathholding spells in near miss SIDS infants suggesting a relationship between the two disorders. [102].

Seizure-Related Laryngospasm. Occasionally, acute asphyxial episodes associated with inspiratory stridor have been attributed to an epileptic seizure [103–105]. In these cases, a spasm of upper airway muscles is presumed to be the sole manifestation of the seizure. Such obstructive episodes usually have been termed "laryngospasm," although the pathophysiological mechanisms involved and site of obstruction often have been ill defined. Kelly and Shannon reported five young infants with recurrent near miss SIDS episodes [106, 107]. The mechanism of the asphyxial episodes was believed to be laryngospasm based on difficulties that parents encountered in attempting to ventilate the infants. In one case, a narrow glottic aperture was observed during direct laryngoscopy [106]. One of these infants died and SIDS was diagnosed.

The Airway Muscle Relaxation Theory

Upper Airway-Dilating Muscles: Relevant Physiology

Unlike the nasal or tracheal airways, which are supported by a rigid framework of bone or cartilage, the pharyngeal airway lacks intrinsic rigidity. Its walls are composed of soft tissue and muscle. It is easily collapsed by neck flexion, posterior movement of the mandible, or external pressure over the hyoid bone [17]. It also is readily collapsed by suction within the airway [29, 41, 108–110]. If the airway-maintaining muscles are paralyzed, very slight reductions in pressure within the airway lumen (−1 cm H_2O or less), similar to those occurring during normal inspiratory efforts, are sufficient to cause airway collapse. The more easily collapsed region is the oropharynx. The entrance to the larynx at the level of the aryepiglottic folds also is readily collapsed by pressure. Mechanical support of these compliant areas of the upper airway derives from the numerous muscles surrounding the pharynx. Muscle tone prevents airway collapse during neck flexion or during inspiration [23, 111]. For example, mimicking tongue muscle contraction by applying mechanical tension to the genioglossus and geniohyoid muscle tendon dilates the pharyngeal airway, making it more rigid and more resistant to collapse by negative pressure [28, 41]. Furthermore, electrical stimulation of individual airway muscles results in similar improvement in upper airway stability [112]. The genioglossus, geniohyoid, sternohyoid, sternothyroid, and thyrohyoid muscles have been identified as muscles with airway-stabilizing function [41, 112, 113]. These muscles are phasically active in inspiration. Thus, they increase airway rigidity during the inspiratory phase of the respiratory cycle, when pharyngeal pressure is negative and airway rigidity is required [114–116].

These observations support a model for pharyngeal airway maintenance illustrated in Figure 4.2. On one side of an imaginary fulcrum is diaphragmatic contractile force and nasal resistance. These two forces determine the degree of fall in pharyngeal pressure (airway suction force) during inspiration. Opposing the airway suction force is the contractile force of airway-dilating muscles. This model demonstrates that any increase in nasal resistance or in diaphragmatic activity that is not matched by an appropriate increase in airway muscle activity will tip the balance toward airway closure. Changes in neck posture are analogous to shifting the position of the fulcrum. An increase in flexion of the neck requires an increase in tone of the pharyngeal dilators to keep the airway patent. Furthermore, the model indicates that constriction of the airway resulting in limitation of inspiratory airflow "upstream" from the pharynx would increase inspiratory suction in the pharynx and tip the balance of forces toward pharyngeal closure. The alae nasi muscles regulate the caliber of the nasal airway during inspiration [117, 118]. The tensor muscles of the soft palate presumably act in a similar fashion [119]. Thus, any decrease in inspiratory activity of these muscles would promote pharyngeal airway closure. As mentioned, increased nasal resistance due to edema, increased volume of the nasal vascular bed, or nasal obstruction from secretions would favor pharyngeal closure. Once pharyngeal closure occurs, mucosal adhesion of the collapsed walls of the airway is an additional

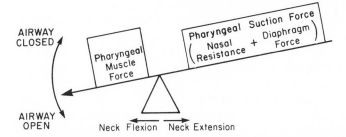

FIGURE 4.2. A schematic model of pharyngeal airway maintenance illustrating the balance of opposing forces that affect airway diameter. Airway constricting (suction force) and airway dilating forces (pharyngeal muscles) are shown on either side of a fulcrum. Like a playground seesaw, the interaction is dynamic; for example, a sudden increase in nasal resistance or diaphragm force during the course of an inspiration can result in airway closure in a fraction of a second. Change in neck posture shifts position of the fulcrum and thus can bias the balance toward airway closure or airway patency.

force acting to maintain obstruction [29, 41]. Surface tension forces thus constitute an added load on airway-maintaining muscles, and increased tension in the muscles appears to be required to overcome this "sticking" effect between airway walls.

Figure 4.2 shows that the inspiratory activity of the diaphragm and upper airway dilating muscles must be matched carefully in order to insure the balance of forces required for airway patency. From studies in infants and adults with obstructive sleep apnea, we know that airway closure can occur rapidly during the middle of an inspiratory effort [108, 110]. Thus, the balance between airway dilating and airway constricting forces is often fragile and can be upset rapidly. A number of reflex mechanisms maintain this balance. For example, chemoreceptor stimuli (either increased arterial carbon dioxide or decreased oxygen) stimulate the airway-dilating muscles [114, 120, 121]. This effect might tend to correct an imbalance of forces acting on the airway and would favor airway patency. Stimuli resulting from suction pressures in the nose, pharynx, or larynx rapidly stimulate activity in the upper airway-dilating muscles [122, 124]. Also, pharyngeal suction pressure causes a rapid reduction of diaphragm activity that would promote airway patency by decreasing the suction pressures during inspiration [123, 125–128]. The upper airway receptors for this reflex appear to be superficially located in the airway mucosa [127, 129].

Central nervous system arousal and reflex postural changes in response to asphyxia are additional airway-maintaining responses. Arousal has a potent effect on stimulating airway dilating muscles. During arousal produced by nonspecific stimuli or asphyxia, the phasic activity of these airway-dilating muscles increases disproportionately compared to diaphragm activity [23, 120]. Reflex control of neck posture is yet another factor in airway patency. In animal studies, hyperextension of the neck occurs when asphyxia becomes marked [130] and appears to be reflexive. Studies in infants and adults suggest that neck extension increases the tone of the pharyngeal walls and favors airway patency.

Even during severe asphyxia, when hypoxic coma supervenes and many reflexes are suppressed, regulation of upper airway-dilating muscles appears to be maintained in a manner favoring airway patency. In the rabbit model, the upper airway muscles appear to be maximally recruited during asphyxial gasps [131]. Such activity would favor reopening of the airway even if the other mechanisms had failed. Gasping thus can be viewed as a "fail-safe" mechanism for recovery from obstructive apnea.

Relaxation of Airway-Dilating Muscles: Models for SIDS

Upper Airway Obstruction Associated with General Anesthesia. As discussed, airway obstruction during general anesthesia may be increased by enhanced tone in the laryngeal-constricting muscles. Paradoxically, upper airway obstruction in the anesthetized patient also quite commonly results from decreased tone in the pharyngeal-dilating muscles. Thus, Safar et al. concluded that airway obstruction during anesthesia was due to "flaccid pharyngeal walls" and a "relaxed tongue." [132] They also observed that obese patients were much more prone to obstruction than non-obese patients. This observation links sleep obstructive apnea, which commonly occurs in obese patients, to obstruction induced by anesthesia. In both cases, the underlying basis for the obstruction appears to be depression of activity of upper airway-dilating muscles. The model depicted in Figure 4.2 illustrates how such events would lead to airway obstruction.

Obstructive Sleep Apnea Associated with a Narrow Upper Airway. In 1934, Robin described a syndrome of impaired ventilation in infants born with an underdeveloped mandible [133]. He attributed the problem to airway obstruction from backward movement of the tongue, causing intermittent pharyngeal occlusion ("glossoptosis"). A variety of other pediatric syndromes of obstructive apnea closely resemble Robin's glossoptosis syndrome from the standpoint of pathophysiology and symptomatology. These syndromes have in common anatomical narrowing of the nasal or pharyngeal airway [36] (Table 4.1).

The pathophysiology of the obstructive episodes is similar to that proposed by Remmers and co-workers for adults with obstructive sleep apnea syndrome [23]. When the lumen of the nasopharyngeal airway is reduced in diameter by enlarged adenoids, for example, resistance to air flow is increased and inspiratory suction increases downstream for the constriction. Periodically, this suction overcomes the force exerted by the airway-

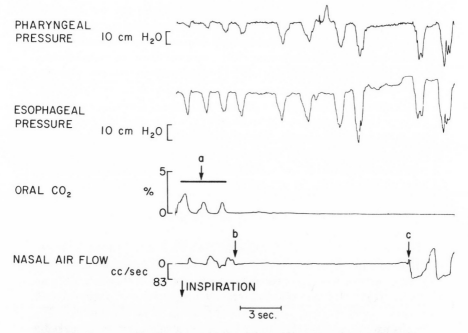

FIGURE 4.3. Tracings illustrating timing and site of pharyngeal airway closure during an episode of spontaneous obstructive apnea in a young infant with Pierre Robin syndrome. Airflow is occurring through both nose and mouth prior to the obstructive episode (arrow a). Then the infant suddenly closes his mouth (arrow b). With the next inspiratory effort, nasal airflow begins but soon returns to zero, signifying airway closure. The next four breaths are obstructed (note inspiratory efforts but no respiratory airflow). Spontaneous recovery occurs at arrow c. The site of airway closure is in the pharynx above the tip of the pharyngeal pressure catheter (from Roberts et al., [110]).

maintaining muscles and the walls of the oropharynx collapse inward (Figure 4.3). Such obstructive episodes characteristically occur during sleep [134–136], probably because the airway-maintaining muscles have reduced activity during sleep [137]. Hence, glossoptosis in infants with obstructive sleep apnea apparently results from the inability of the tongue muscles to overcome pharyngeal suction forces [26, 110]. In some infants, no obvious source of airway narrowing can be found. Therefore, motor control of tongue muscles or airway maintaining reflexes may be abnormal in these infants [128, 138].

Patients usually are symptomatic at birth when the cause of the upper airway narrowing is a congenital defect, such as mandibular hypoplasia or choanal stenosis. Apneic episodes in these infants are similar to those in adults with sleep apnea syndrome from the standpoint of their cyclic recurrence and spontaneous termination. As a rule, many spells occur in a single night. A typical episode of obstruction in these patients lasts three to twenty seconds. Sinus bradycardia may occur during the episode and appears to be the result of an interaction between hypoxic chemoreceptor stimuli and lung inflation reflexes [139]. Arterial desaturation always accompanies such episodes [135, 140]. Spontaneous recovery from the episode is often associated with signs of arousal such as a startle. Episodes of decreased ventilation presumed to be caused by partial airway obstruction "hypopneas" also occur in these infants [134–136, 140]. Some of these hypopneas result from marked narrowing or a complete closure of the airway in mid-inspiration, so that only the early part of the inspiratory effort contributes to effective ventilation [110]. Hypopnea and snoring probably have a similar pathophysiologic mechanism [110]. After three to four months of age, a history of loud snoring is almost universal in the infants with this form of sleep apnea. Why snoring is less frequent prior to three months of age is unclear.

A number of factors can increase the severity of obstructive episodes in children with the narrow upper airway syndrome. For example, micrognathic infants usually have more symptoms when they are sleeping supine. This may reflect efforts of gravity on the tongue or increased neck flexion. Upper respiratory infection appears to worsen symptoms. The mechanism is unclear [141]. In adults, seasonal allergic rhinitis markedly increases the number and duration of obstructive episodes [142]. Thus, upper respiratory infection and rhinitis may increase symptoms on the basis of increased nasal resistance produced by congestion and inflammation.

Recent findings indicate that growth retardation and developmental delay are caused by the obstructive apnea syndrome in infants [135, 136]. Also, *cor pulmonale,* which can rapidly progress to pulmonary edema, has long been recognized as part of the syndrome [140]. With maturation, the varied symptoms and also the sleep apnea tend to become less severe. Recently, Roberts and co-workers developed a test of pharyngeal airway maintaining ability and have documented that progressive improvement in airway maintenance tends to occur with maturation in infants with Pierre Robin syndrome [110].

Unlike older patients with obstructive sleep apnea syndrome, young infants with Pierre Robin syndrome have had a very high mortality (20–30 percent) even in recent times [143]. Deaths in such infants often occur suddenly and unexpectedly when the infants appear to be improving and have been discharged from the hospital [144–146]. In these cases, evidence of aspiration of gastric contents is sometimes seen at postmortem examination. Other cases have only minimal findings associated with intrathoracic petechiae and pulmonary edema similar to those seen in SIDS cases [146]. Acute airway obstruction is the presumed, although un-proven, cause of these deaths.

Apnea of Prematurity. Idiopathic apneic spells in seemingly healthy in-fants were first described by G. S. Still in 1923 [19]. Still observed that if the infant did not rapidly resume breathing, it soon became deeply cyano-tic. Still, and subsequently others, noted that if resuscitation is delayed, such infants have a marked risk of dying during prolonged apneic spells [78, 147, 148]. In infants with recurrent apneic spells, Stevens noted pro-gressively longer delays in spontaneous recovery from apnea [148]. Ac-cording to Stevens, fatal apneic spells were like non-fatal spells in every respect except that spontaneous recovery failed to occur.

Subsequent investigators clearly established the extraordinary suscep-tibility of preterm infants to such apneic spells [149]. The incidence of apneic spells in preterm infants is associated with maturity [36]; more than 80 percent of infants with a birth weight less than 1,000 grams will have one or more apneic spells during the postnatal period. The frequency of spells is highly variable, but spells usually have ceased by the time the infant reaches a postconceptional age of forty weeks.

A rapid fall in heart rate usually occurs five to ten seconds after the onset of apnea, and cyanosis usually is present by twenty seconds. In most cases, recovery from spells is spontaneous. When spontaneous recovery fails to occur, stimulating the infant by gently patting or rubbing the limbs usually is followed by resumption of ventilation. In the rare spell that does not respond to stimulation, cardiopulmonary resuscitation rapidly im-proves oxygenation and nearly always is followed by spontaneous ventila-tion within one to two minutes [147, 149].

A number of factors may suddenly "trigger" an apneic spell in the sus-ceptible preterm infant. Neck flexion, either caused by handling the infant or as a result of the infant's spontaneous movements, increases the risk of an apneic spell [17, 18]. Most spells occur while the infant is asleep. About a third of all spells occur during sudden episodes of increased mo-tor activity or squirming [99]. Additionally, hiccups have been observed to initiate apneic spells in preterm infants [150]. In other infants, spells may be associated with feedings or episodes of regurgitation [86, 92, 151, 152]. The presence of swallowing in the majority of spells suggests that the air-way chemoreflex is an important triggering mechanism [54, 55, 91].

In addition to these several factors that seem to trigger spells acutely, a host of predisposing factors appear to increase susceptibility to spells. Ap-neic episodes are increased during the recovery period following general anesthesia [153] and when room or incubator temperature is rapidly in-creasing [154]. Upper respiratory tract infections (e.g., respiratory syncy-tial virus, pertussis) may precipitate or exacerbate apneic spells [155,

156]. In other infants, anemia or bacterial septicemia may be associated with apneic spells. In fact, a host of conditions causing compromise of cardiopulmonary function are clinically recognized as causes of increased severity or frequency of apneic spells in the susceptible preterm infant.

Apnea of prematurity previously was thought to result from total cessation of diaphragmatic activity. Recently, it has been found that one or more inspiratory efforts without air flow usually occur during an apneic spell in these infants [18, 87–89]. Half of all spells begin with such obstructed breaths. Usually this obstruction is followed by cessation of all respiratory effort; then, in most spells, obstructive breaths occur again toward the end of the spell. Since these spells consist both of obstructed breaths (i.e., "obstructive apnea") as well as respiratory pauses (i.e., "central apnea"), they are called "mixed apnea." In preterm infants, mixed apnea is more common than central or obstructive apnea [91]. Any given infant usually has a combination of these types of apnea. The site of obstruction frequently is in the pharynx [158]. The mechanism responsible for this obstruction is complex and still is not completely resolved. As mentioned, it seems likely that when obstruction occurs in association with squirming episodes, with swallowing, or with regurgitation episodes, at least some of the obstructed breaths are due to airway closure produced by contraction of airway-constricting muscles. However, the experience with neck flexion as both a triggering and a predisposing factor for apneic spells in preterm infants [18] and experience with the therapeutic effects of positive end-expiratory pressure [89] suggest that relaxation of airway-dilating muscles also may contribute to airway obstruction in apnea of prematurity. That is, apneic spells in preterm infants appear to involve a combination of active closure mechanisms and also the passive closure mechanisms induced by suction.

Recent studies suggest that the incidence of apnea in the preterm infant is more closely related to neurologic maturation than to chronologic age. Thus, Henderson-Smart showed that apnea in the preterm infant is more closely related to maturation of auditory brain stem pathways than it is to gestational or postnatal age [159]. Likewise, Gerhardt and Bancalari found that degree of maturity of pulmonary stretch reflexes and ventilatory responses to carbon dioxide is a better predictor of risk for apneic spells in the preterm infant than is the infant's postconceptional age [160, 161]. Thus, apnea of prematurity appears to be linked to immaturity of the nervous system. From all that has been said, it seems likely that the different forms of obstructive apnea (muscular airway constriction and passive airway collapse) result from failure of the complex regulatory mechanisms controlling the function of airway constricting and airway dilating muscles. From this perspective, it is not surprising to find causal mechanisms for apnea involving both airway constrictors and airway dilators in the preterm infant with an immature nervous system.

Evaluation of the Airway Obstruction Theories for SIDS

Strengths of the Airway Obstruction Hypothesis for SIDS

The plethora of theories for SIDS occasionally has created more confusion than enlightenment. Nevertheless, formulation of theories is essential to progress, and since the cause, or causes, of SIDS remain unknown, the testing, formulation, and revision of theories must continue. Additional support for any given theory may be provided by more recent research findings. The strength of any SIDS theory is measured by its compatibility with generally accepted facts regarding the syndrome. Thus, the primary strengths of the airway obstruction hypothesis for SIDS result from the fact that it potentially explains a number of generally accepted facts relating to SIDS; further, the theory is supported by recent findings.

Death in SIDS is sudden. In most cases, the infant is dead when first discovered. The maximal duration from onset of recognizable fatal symptoms until death in SIDS is unknown but is not likely to be much longer than one to two hours. In many cases when the parent has checked the infant just prior to death, one can deduce that death likely has occurred within ten to fifteen minutes. The time course of death from airway obstruction in the human infant, based on animal studies and clinical observations, is compatible with that in SIDS. In the rabbit model, asphyxial coma occurs within eighty seconds of airway obstruction and death occurs within three to four minutes [70, 162].

Death in SIDS is silent and signs of struggle, although sometimes present, frequently are absent. Although inspiratory stridor classically is associated with laryngospasm, with severe spasm, stridor is absent [66]. In the preterm infant, prolonged apnea spells, including obstructive and mixed spells, usually are silent. In many infants, acute airway obstruction often is associated with arousal and struggling prior to severe asphyxia. However, other infants have been observed to develop marked hypoxia and bradycardia secondary to airway obstruction without struggling [17, 92].

As defined, the cause of death in SIDS is still unknown after a complete postmortem examination has been performed. The pulmonary edema and intrathoracic petechiae that characterize SIDS are compatible with death caused by acute upper airway obstruction [13, 70, 163–165]. The specificity of intrathoracic petechiae as an indication of airway obstruction, as opposed to other mechanisms of death, has been much debated [3]. A number of detailed studies performed by Krous and colleagues utilizing new approaches to this problem strongly supported Beckwith's suggestion that the petechiae specifically indicate upper airway obstruction as the cause of death in SIDS [163, 164, 166]. This highly pertinent topic is discussed in more detail in Chapter 2.

Most studies indicate that the majority of SIDS deaths occur when the infant is presumed to have been asleep [3]. Several of the "SIDS models" are characterized by obstructive or mixed apnea, which occur primarily during sleep. From this standpoint, the airway obstruction theory is compatible with SIDS epidemiology. Furthermore, a high percentage of SIDS infants not only have a history of mild respiratory tract infection prior to death but also have morphologic evidence of mild upper respiratory tract infection at the time of postmortem examination [167, 168]. As indicated in the earlier discussion, upper respiratory tract infections have been clearly established as a predisposing factor for asphyxial episodes associated with both active and passive airway closure mechanisms (e.g., croup syndrome, narrow upper airway syndrome). Additionally, SIDS infants have slowed postnatal growth, which is potentially compatible with obstructive sleep apnea as a cause [169].

Clinical observations suggest that the sequence of physiologic events leading to death in SIDS is readily reversible if intervention occurs in time. As Bergman and others have noted, relatively few SIDS deaths are actually witnessed [167, 170]. In striking contrast, the sudden and unexpected "near death" of infants in the SIDS age range is witnessed relatively often [169]. Often such infants respond to simple stimulation. Many others respond to resuscitation administered by parents inexperienced in cardiopulmonary resuscitation. Most of these "near miss" infants are not found to have a diagnosable disease that could account for the "near death" episode. It is assumed that, had they died during the episode, postmortem examination would have revealed no cause for death and the pathologist's diagnosis would have been SIDS. That these infants would have died had they not been resuscitated is suggested by the asphyxial brain injury that is sometimes sustained during the episodes and also by the relatively high risk for subsequent SIDS death [171–174]. Accordingly, the near miss SIDS syndrome has been accepted widely as an important model for SIDS. Indeed, some have suggested that the near miss SIDS syndrome is a "nonlethal form" of SIDS [3]. From the standpoint that the asphyxial episodes associated with obstructive sleep apnea or apnea of prematurity are readily reversible by stimulation alone, they would appear to be better models for SIDS and for near miss SIDS than fatal metabolic or cardiac disorders, such as arrhythmias, which usually do not respond to stimulation or simple resuscitation measures.

Additional recent findings suggest an association between near miss SIDS and obstructive sleep apnea. Obstructive sleep apnea potentially would explain the high risk for subsequent SIDS deaths in such infants since such apnea tends to be recurrent. Guilleminault and associates [175] found more brief episodes of obstructive sleep apnea in near miss SIDS infants than in controls, an observation that has been confirmed by Rosen et al. and Kahn et al [174, 176]. Also, Guilleminault noted that 5 percent of near miss SIDS infants subsequently develop typical sleep obstructive apnea syndrome at nine months to two years of age, suggesting a relationship between the two disorders [177]. Likewise, Kahn observed that near miss SIDS infants have an increased incidence of snoring at one to two years of age compared with control infants, which suggests upper airway narrowing or neuromuscular abnormalities in near miss infants [178].

With respect to SIDS itself, several recent findings suggest abnormalities of neuromuscular regulation of the pharynx and larynx in SIDS victims. Guilleminault performed extensive respiratory studies of an infant with increased brief obstructive and mixed apneic episodes who subsequently died of SIDS [179]. Others reported prolonged obstructive or mixed apnea in infants who later died of SIDS [92, 107]. Additionally, a number of SIDS victims have a past history of respiratory disorders possibly linked to airway obstruction. In retrospective studies of SIDS infants, Mandell found a history of apnea or unexplained cyanotic episodes prior to death in 22 percent [180]. Likewise, Beal found that 5 percent of SIDS infants had a history of breathholding spells prior to death and an additional 11 percent had a past history of choking or apneic spells [181].

Other observations suggest altered pharyngeal or laryngeal function in SIDS. Stark and Nathansen, and also Golub and co-workers, reported abnormal crying patterns in infants who subsequently died of SIDS [182, 183]. Stark's patient and Golub's two patients had acoustical features in the cry that suggested constriction of the vocal tract. Supporting these findings, Naeye reported that substantially more infants with SIDS than controls had a past history of weak or otherwise abnormal cry [184]. Additionally, Steinschneider found more brief apnea (obstructive and/or central) during feeding in infants who ultimately died of SIDS than in control infants [185].

Finally, it should be mentioned that Naeye and co-workers [186], and also Becker and co-workers [187], accumulated substantial morphologic evidence of chronic hypoxia in SIDS victims, which they view as consistent with recurrent apneic or obstructive episodes prior to death. This important topic is treated in depth in Chapter 2.

Weaknesses of the Airway Obstruction SIDS Theory

Death in SIDS occurs in young infants over a discrete age range with a pronounced peak incidence near three months of age. Aside from the fact that respiratory tract infections occur more commonly at this age as maternally acquired immunity begins to disappear, the airway obstruction hypothesis offers no clear explanation for this well-established age distribution. As mentioned, sudden death in the Pierre Robin syndrome often occurs at two to three months, when respiratory symptoms and overall regulation of pharyngeal patency seem to be improving. This clinical observation suggests that some factor other than neural maturation, such as respiratory infection, is important in sudden death resulting from obstructive apnea during sleep.

A second, perhaps more important, deficiency of the airway obstruction theory for SIDS is the failure to explain the unexpected nature of SIDS. The majority of the clinical SIDS models we have described have alarming symptoms or obvious abnormalities that precede fatal airway obstruction episodes. Thus, sudden death in the Pierre Robin syndrome frequently has been described as quite unexpected. Yet there is a clear history of abnormality in these infants prior to death. Occasionally, respiratory infections, such as pertussis, may present first with severe apnea and airway obstruction [83]. The respiratory infection models for SIDS may be the strongest of the SIDS models with respect to absence of alarming signs or symptoms prior to death. As Carpenter and Emery pointed out, whether or not sudden death in an infant is expected or could have been anticipated totally depends on the observational skills and experience of the infant's caretaker [188]. Thus, in SIDS we are unable to distinguish between absence of symptoms and failure to detect symptoms. Symptoms of serious illness in the young infant often are more subtle than those in the adult; signs suggesting impending respiratory failure from upper airway obstruction, such as respiratory retractions, mild cyanosis, stridor, or stertor might be detected and their significance appreciated by some parents but not by others.

In the final analysis, the chief difficulty with the airway obstruction theory for SIDS, and all other SIDS theories, is that the supporting evidence is indirect. A major criterion for any proof of cause and effect is documentation of a temporal sequence between the purported cause and its effect. Whereas certain steps in the proposed sequence of events in which upper airway obstruction leads ultimately to death in SIDS have been directly observed in infants, other key steps in this sequence have not. Obstructive sleep apnea leading to acute asphyxia has been observed and documented repeatedly in young infants. However, detailed observations of the complete chain of events in which upper airway obstruction leads to a death that is then diagnosed as SIDS by the pathologist are extremely rare [107]. Although one can explain the failure of parents and health workers to have observed such SIDS deaths on the basis of the ease with which such infants are resuscitated, nevertheless, a cause and effect relationship between SIDS and airway obstruction does not meet traditional criteria for proof due to lack of sufficient documentation.

Koch's criteria for establishing causation for an infectious disease require that the organism first be isolated in pure culture, then characterized, and finally that it be cultured from every case [189]. By analogy, to fulfill similar criteria for airway obstruction and SIDS, we would have to characterize and classify more accurately the various forms of airway obstruction, and then document the fatal obstructive event in every SIDS case, either by recordings or by specific postmortem evidence. Because the classification of airway obstruction is incomplete, the first of Koch's criteria is only partially fulfilled. Lacking a consensus regarding what constitutes a specific postmortem marker for fatal airway obstruction, and lacking observations made during SIDS deaths, we have yet to fulfill the second criterion.

A second approach to proving that airway obstruction causes SIDS could use criteria more recent than Koch's for proving causation in disease. This approach demands proof that removal of the purported cause be followed by reduction in frequency of the disease [189]. Preventing SIDS is the primary goal of home monitoring programs for infants believed to be at risk for apnea and airway obstruction. It has yet to be proven that such monitoring reduces the risk of SIDS [190]. Therefore, this criterion for proof of cause in SIDS has yet to be fulfilled.

References

1. Glastonbury, J.R.W. 1977. Preweaning mortality in the pig. *Australian Veterinary Journal* 53:310–314.
2. Bible. I. Kings 3:16.
3. Guntheroth, W.G. 1982. *Crib Death: The Sudden Infant Death Syndrome.* Mount Kisko, N.Y.: Futura Publishing Co.
4. Bass, M., R.E. Kravath, and L. Glass. 1986. Death-scene investigations in sudden infant death. *N Engl J Med* 315:100–105.
5. Wooley, P.V. 1945. Mechanical suffocation during infancy: A comment on its relation to the total problem of sudden death. *J of Pediatr* 26:572–575.
6. Thach, B.T. 1986. Sudden infant death syndrome: Old causes rediscovered (editorial). *N Engl J Med* 315:126–128.
7. Beinfield, H.H. 1954. A forgotten cause of infant suffocation: The possible relation between atresia of the posterior nares to asphyxia neonatorum and sudden infant death. *J Inter Coll Surg* 22:447–455.
8. Beinfield, H.H. 1965. Ways and means to reduce infant mortality due to suffocation: Importance of choanal atresia. *JAMA* 209:1493–1497.
9. Crosse, V.M., and W.F. Young 1954. In *Disease of Infancy and Childhood,* 2nd ed., ed. L. Parsons and S. Barling. New York: Oxford University Press.
10. Illingworth, R.S. 1957. Cyanotic attacks in newborn infants. *Arch Dis Child* 32:328–332.
11. Shaw, E.B. 1968. Sudden unexpected death in infancy syndrome. *Am J Dis Child* 116:115–119.
12. Stowens, D. 1957. Sudden unexpected death in infancy. *Am J Dis Child* 94:674–681.
13. Handforth, C.P. 1959. Sudden unexpected death in infants. *Can Med Assoc J* 80:872–873.
14. Bergman, A.B. 1970. "Summary statement." In *Sudden Infant Death Syndrome,* ed. A.B. Bergman, J.B. Beckwith, and C.G. Ray. Seattle: University of Washington Press.
15. Cross, K.W., and S.R. Lewis. 1971. Upper respiratory obstruction and cot death. *Arch Dis Child* 46:211–213.

16. Tonkin, S. 1975. Sudden infant death syndrome: Hypothesis of causation. *Pediatrics* 55:650–661.
17. Stark, A.R., and B.T. Thach. 1976. Mechanisms of airway obstruction leading to apnea in newborn infants. *J Pediatr* 89:982–985.
18. Thach, B.T., and A.R. Stark. 1979. Spontaneous neck flexion and airway obstruction during apneic spells in preterm infants. *J Pediatr* 94:275–281.
19. Still, G.F. 1923. Attacks of arrested respiration in the newborn. *Lancet* 1:431–432.
20. Weitzman, E.D., and L. Graziani. 1974. "Sleep and the sudden infant death syndrome: A new hypothesis." In *Advances in Sleep Research*, ed. E.D. Weitzman. New York: Spectrum Publications.
21. Guilleminault, C., R. Peraita, M. Souquet, and W.C. Dement. 1975. Apneas during sleep in infants: Possible relationship with sudden infant death syndrome. *Science* 190:677–679.
22. Steinschneider, A., and D.D. Rabuzzi. 1976. Apnea and airway obstruction during feeding and sleep. *Laryngoscope* 86:1359–1366.
23. Remmers, J.E., W.J. deGroot, E.K. Sauerland, and A.M. Anch. 1978. Pathogenesis of upper airway occlusion during sleep. *J Appl Physio: Resp Environ Exercise Physiol* 44:931–938.
24. Strohl, K.P., N.A. Saunders, N.T. Feldman, and M. Hallett. 1978. Obstructive sleep apnea in family members. *N Engl J Med* 299:969–973.
25. Harper, R.M., and E.K. Sauerland. 1978. "The role of the tongue in sleep apnea." In *Sleep Apnea Syndromes*, ed. C. Guilleminault and W.C. Dement. New York: Alan R. Liss.
26. Tonkin, S.L., J. Partridge, D. Beach, and S. Whiteney. 1979. The pharyngeal effect of partial nasal obstruction. *Pediatrics* 63:261–271.
27. Cozzi. F., R. Albani, and E. Cardi. 1979. A common pathophysiology for sudden cot death and sleep apnea, "The vacuum-glossoptosis syndrome." *Medical Hypotheses* 5:329–338.
28. Brouillette, R.T., and B.T. Thach. 1979. A neuromuscular mechanism maintaining extrathoracic airway patency. *J Appl Physiol* 46:772–779.
29. Wilson, S.L., B.T. Thach, R.T. Brouillette, and Y.K. Abu-Osba. 1980. Upper airway patency in the human infant: Influence of airway pressure and posture. *J Appl Physiol Resp: Environ Exercise Physiol* 48:500–504.
30. Swift, P.G.F., and J.L. Emery. 1973. Clinical observations on response to nasal occlusion in infancy. *Arch Dis Child* 48:947–951.
31. Rodenstein, D.O., N. Perlmutter, and D.C. Stanescu. 1985. Infants are not obligatory nasal breathers. *Am Rev Resp Dis* 131:343–348.
32. Miller, M.J., R.J. Martin, W.A. Carlo, J.M. Fouke, and K.P. Strohl. 1984. Oral ventilation occurs in term neonates during spontaneous breathing or nasal obstruction (abstract). *Am Rev Resp Dis* 129:A207.
33. Deuel, R.K. 1973. Polygraphic monitoring of apneic spells. *Arch Neurol* 28:71–76.
34. Kang, H., and E. Mazzi. 1976. Apnea resulting from obstruction of the nares by an eye shield. *J Pediatr* 89:652.
35. Hall, J.G., R.M. Pauli, and K.M. Wilson. 1970. Maternal and fetal sequelae of anticoagulation during pregnancy. *Am J Med* 68:122–140.

36. Thach, B.T. 1985. Sleep apnea in infancy and childhood. *Med Clin North Am* 69:1289–1315.
37. Kravath, R., C. Pollak, B. Borowiecki, and E. Weitzman. 1980. Obstructive sleep apnea and death associated with surgical correction of velo-pharyngeal incompetence. *J Pediatr* 96:645–648.
38. French, J.W., J.B. Beckwith, C.B. Graham, and W.G. Guntheroth. 1972. Lack of postmortem radiographic evidence of nasopharyngeal obstruction in the sudden infant death syndrome. *J Pediatr* 81:1145–1148.
39. Cross, K.W. 1974. "Response to upper airway obstructions." In *SIDS 1974: Proceedings of the Francis E. Camps International Symposium on Sudden and Unexpected Death in Infancy,* ed. by R.R. Robinson. Toronto: The Canadian Foundation for the Study of Infant Deaths.
40. Haight, J.J., and P. Cole. 1984. Reciprocating nasal airflow resistances. *Acta Oto-Laryngologica* (Stockh) 84:416–421.
41. Reed, R., J.L. Roberts, and B.T. Thach. 1985. Factors influencing regional patency and configuration of the upper airway in human infants. *J Appl Physiol* 58:635–644.
42. Bosma, J.F. 1975. "Introduction to the symposium." In *Symposium on Development of Upper Respiratory Anatomy and Function: Implications for Sudden Infant Death Syndrome,* ed. J.F. Bosma and J. Showacre. Washington, D.C.: U.S. Government Printing Office.
43. Harding, R. 1984. Function of the larynx in the fetus and newborn. *Ann Rev Physiol* 46:645–659.
44. Pressman, J.J. 1941. Sphincter action of the larynx. *Arch Otolaryngol* 33:351–377.
45. Gryboski, J.D. 1969. Suck and swallow in the premature infant. *Pediatrics* 43:96–102.
46. Wilson, S.L., B.T. Thach, R.T. Brouillette, and Y.K. Abu-Osba. 1981. Coordination of breathing and swallowing in human infants. *J Appl Physiol: Resp Environ Exercise Physiol* 50:851–858.
47. Menon, A., G. Schefft, and B.T. Thach. 1985. Airway protective and abdominal expulsive mechanisms during infantile regurgitation. *J Appl Physiol* 59:716–721.
48. Fink, R. 1973. The curse of Adam: Effort closure of the larynx. *Anesthesiology* 39:325–326.
49. Grillner, S., J. Nilsson, and A. Thorstensson. 1978. Intra-abdominal pressure changes during natural movement in man. *Acta Physiolog Scand* 103:275–283.
50. Thach, B.T., and A. Menon. 1985. Pulmonary protective mechanisms in human infants. *Am Rev Resp Dis* 131:(Suppl.) S55–S58.
51. Storey, A.T., and P. Johnson. 1975. Laryngeal water receptors initiating apnea in the lamb. *Exp Neurol* 47:42–55.
52. Harding, R., P. Johnson, and M.E. McClelland. 1980. Respiratory function of the larynx in developing sheep and the influence of sleep state. *Resp Physiol* 40:165–179.
53. Perkett, E.A., and R.L. Vaughn. 1982. Evidence for a laryngeal chemoreflex in some human preterm infants. *Acta Paediatr Scand* 71: 969–972.
54. Pickens, D.L., G. Schefft, and B.T. Thach. 1988. Prolonged apnea associ-

ated with upper airway protective reflexes in apnea of prematurity. *Am Rev Resp Dis* 137:113–117.

55. Davies, A.M., J.S. Koenig, and B.T. Thach. Upper airway chemoreflex responses to saline and water in preterm infants. *J Appl Physiol* (in press).
56. Suzuki, M., and C.T. Sasaki. 1977. Laryngeal spasm: A neurophysiologic redefinition. *Ann Otol* 86:150–157.
57. Ikari, T., and C.T. Sasaki. 1980. Glottic closure reflex: Control mechanisms. *Ann Otol* 89:220–224.
58. Rex, M.A.E. 1970. A review of the structural and functional basis of laryngospasm and a discussion of the nerve pathways involved in the reflex and its clinical significance in man and animals. *Br J Anaesth* 42:891–899.
59. Rex, M.A.E. 1970. The production of laryngospasm in the cat by volatile anesthetic agents. *Br J Anaesth* 42:941–947.
60. Rex, M.A.E. 1971. Laryngospasm and respiratory changes in the cat produced by mechanical stimulation of the pharynx and respiratory tract: Problems of intubation in the cat. *Br J Anaesth* 43:54–57.
61. Haraguchi, S., R. Fung, and C.T. Sasaki. 1983. Effect of hyperthermia on the laryngeal closure reflex: Implications for the sudden infant death syndrome. *Ann Otol Rhinol Laryngol* 92:24–28.
62. Nishino, T., T. Yonezawa, and Y. Honda. 1981. Modification of laryngospasm in response to changes in $PaCO_2$ and PaO_2 in the cat. *Anesthesiology* 55:286–291.
63. Sasaki, C.T. 1979. Development of laryngeal function: Etiologic significance in the sudden infant death syndrome. *The Laryngoscope* 89:1964–1982.
64. Taylor, M., D. Sutton, C.R. Larson, O.A. Smith, and R.C. Lindeman. 1976. Sudden death in infant primates from induced laryngeal occlusion. *Arch Otolaryngol* 102:291–296.
65. Olsson, G.L., and B. Hallen. 1984. Laryngospasm during anesthesia. A computer aided incidence study in 136,929 patients. *Acta Anaesth Scand* 28:567–575.
66. Stephen, C.R., E.W. Ahlgren, and E.J. Bennett. 1970. *Elements of Pediatric Anesthesia.* 2nd ed. Springfield, Ill.: Charles C Thomas.
67. Jackson, F.N., V. Rowland, and G. Corssen. 1980. Laryngospasm-induced pulmonary edema. *Chest* 78:819–821.
68. Lee, K.W., and J.J. Downes. 1983. Pulmonary edema secondary to laryngospasm in children. *Anesthesiology* 59:347–349.
69. Tagaki, Y., J.V. Irwin, and J.F. Bosma. 1966. Effect of electrical stimulation of the pharyngeal wall on respiratory action. *J Appl Physiol* 21:454–462.
70. Abu-Osba, Y.K., O.P. Mathew, and B.T. Thach. 1981. An animal model for airway sensory deprivation producing obstructive apnea with postmortem findings of Sudden Infant Death Syndrome. *Pediatrics* 68:796–800.
71. Nelson, W.E., ed. 1964. *Textbook of Pediatrics,* 18th ed. Philadelphia: W.B. Saunders.
72. Koprowski, H. 1967. "Viral diseases that may involve the central nervous system." In *Cecil-Loeb Textbook of Medicine,* ed. P.B. Beeson and W.M. McDermott. Philadelphia: W.B. Saunders.

73. Rothstein, R.J., and F.J. Baker. 1978. Tetanus: Prevention and treatment. *JAMA* 240:675–676.
74. Laforce, F.M., L.S. Young, and J.V. Bennett. 1969. Tetanus in the United States (1965–1966): Epidemiologic and clinical features. *N Engl J Med* 280:569–574.
75. Harrison, H.E. 1968. In *Pediatrics*, ed. H.L. Barnett and A.H. Einhorn. New York: Appleton-Century-Crofts.
76. Esplin, D.W., and B. Zablocka. 1969. "Central nervous system stimulants." In *The Pharmacological Basis of Therapeutics*, 5th ed. ed. L.S. Goodman and A. Gilman. New York: Macmillan Publishing Company.
77. Stoll, B.J. 1979. Tetanus. *Pediatr Clin North Am* 26:415–431.
78. Peiper, A. 1963. Cerebral Function in Infancy and Childhood. New York: Consultants Bureau.
79. McCracken, G.H., and H.F. Eichenwald. 1975. "Acute infections of the larynx and trachea." In *Nelson Textbook of Pediatrics*, 10th ed. ed V.C. Vaughan and R.J. McKay. Philadelphia: W.B. Saunders.
80. Cornwell, A.C., and E.D. Weitzman. 1979. Respiratory and cardiac events recorded during a "near miss" episode observed in-hospital: A case report (abstract). *Sleep Research* 8:178.
81. Bosma, J.F. 1960. Glossopharyngeal respiration as a part of focal seizures of the pharyngeal area in an infant. *Acta Paediatr Scand* 123 (Suppl): 56–61.
82. Pickens, D.L., G.L. Schefft, and B.T. Thach. 1987. Prolonged apnea in infants with respiratory syncytial virus (RSV) infection is similar to apnea of prematurity and laryngeal chemoreflex (LC) apnea. *Pediatr Res* 21:504A.
83. Guilleminault, C. and R.L. Ariagno. 1978. Why should we study the infant in "near miss for sudden infant death"? *Early Hum Dev* 2: 207–218.
84. Herbst, J.J., L.S. Book, and S.D. Minton. 1979. Gastroesophageal reflex causing respiratory distress and apnea in newborn infants. *J Pediatr* 95: 763–768.
85. Spitzer, A.R., J.T. Boyle, N.M. Tuchman, and W.W. Fox. 1984. Awake apnea associated with gastroesophageal reflux: A specific clinical syndrome. *J Pediatr* 104:200–205.
86. Menon, A., G. Schefft, and B.T. Thach. 1985. Apnea associated with regurgitation in infants. *J Pediatr* 106:625–629.
87. Milner, A.D., A.W. Boon, R.A. Saunders, and I.E. Hopkin. 1980. Upper airway obstruction and apnea in preterm babies. *Arc Dis Child* 55: 22–26.
88. Dransfield, D.A., A.R. Spitzer, and W.W. Fox. 1983. Episodic airway obstruction in premature infants. *Am J Dis Child* 137:441–443.
89. Miller, M.J., W.A. Carlo, and R.J. Martin. 1985. Continuous positive airway pressure selectively reduces obstructive apnea in preterm infants. *J Pediatr* 106:91–94.
90. Bellgaumkar, T.K., and K.E. Scott. 1976. Apnea in premature infants: Recording by arterial catheter. *European J Pediatr* 123:301–305.
91. Menon, A., G. Schefft, and B.T. Thach. 1984. Frequency and significance of swallowing during prolonged apnea in infants. *Am Rev of Resp Dis* 130:969–973.

92. Roberts, J.L., O.P. Mathew, and B.T. Thach. 1985. Observations made on severe apneic spells in two infants at risk for sudden death. *Early Hum Dev* 10:261–271.
93. Gauk, E.W., L. Kidd, and J.S. Prichard. 1963. Mechanisms of seizures associated with breathholding spells. *N Engl J Med* 268:1436–1441.
94. Lombroso, C.T., and P. Lerman. 1967. Breathholding spells (cyanotic and pallid infantile syncope). *Pediatrics* 39:563–581.
95. Maulsby, R., and P. Kellaway. 1964. "Transient hypoxic crises in children." In *Neurological and Electroencephalographic Correlative Studies in Infancy,* ed. P. Kellaway and I. Petersen. New York: Grune and Stratton.
96. Bridge, E.M., S. Livingston, and C. Tietze. 1943. Breath-holding spells. *J Pediatr* 23:539–561.
97. Stephenson, J.B.P. 1978. Reflex anoxic seizures ('while breath-holding') non-epileptic vagal attacks. *Arch Dis Child* 53:193–200.
98. Brooks, J.G. 1982. Apnea of infancy and sudden infant death syndrome. *Am J Dis Child* 136:1012–1023.
99. Abu-Osba, Y.K., R.T. Brouillette, S.L. Wilson, and B.T. Thach. 1982. Breathing patterns and transcutaneous oxygen tension during motor activity in preterm infants. *Am Rev Resp Dis* 125:382–387.
100. Peabody, J.L., G.A. Gregory, M.M. Willis, A.G.S. Philip, and J.F. Lucey. 1979. Failure of conventional monitoring to detect apnea resulting in hypoxemia. *Birth Defects* 15:275–284.
101. Peabody, J., R. Huch, and A. Huch. 1979. Sleep apnea syndromes. *Lancet* 1:219.
102. Kahn, A., J. Riazi, and D. Blum. 1983. Oculocardiac reflex in near miss sudden infant death syndrome. *Pediatrics* 71:49–52.
103. Amir, J., S. Ashkenazi, T. Schonfeld, R. Weitz, and M. Nitzan. 1983. Laryngospasm as a single manifestation of epilepsy. *Arch Dis Child* 58:151–153.
104. Ravindran, M. 1981. Temporal lobe seizure presenting as "laryngospasm." *Clinical Electroencephalography* 12:139–140.
105. Hooshmand, H. 1972. Apneic seizures treated with atropine. *Neurology* 22:1217–1221.
106. Kelly, D.H., K.S. Krishamoorthy, and D.C. Shannon. 1980. Astrocytoma in an infant with prolonged apnea. *Pediatrics* 66:429–431.
107. Kelly, D.H., and D.C. Shannon. 1981. Episodic complete airway obstruction in infants. *Pediatrics* 67:823–827.
108. Issa, F.Q., and C.E. Sullivan. 1984. Upper airway closing pressures in obstructive sleep apnea. *J Appl Physiol* 57:520–527.
109. Issa, F.Q., and C.E. Sullivan. 1984. Upper airway closing pressures in snorers. *J Appl Physiol* 57:528–535.
110. Roberts, J.L., W.R. Reed, O.P. Mathew, A. Menon, and B.T. Thach. 1985. Assessment of pharyngeal airway stability in normal and micrognathic infants. *J Appl Physiol* 58:290–300.
111. Hyland, R.H., M.A. Hutcheon, A. Perl, G. Bowes, N.R. Anthonisen, N. Zamel, and E.A. Phillipson. 1981. Upper airway occlusion induced by diaphragm pacing for primary alveolar hypoventilation: Implications for the pathogenesis of obstructive sleep apnea. *Am Rev Resp Dis* 124:180–185.

112. Roberts, J.L., W.R. Reed, and B.T. Thach. 1984. Pharyngeal airway stabilizing function of the sternohyoid and sternothyroid muscles of the rabbit. *J Appl Physiol: Resp Environ Exercise Physiol* 57:1790–1795.
113. Van de Graaff, W.B., J. Mitra, K.P. Strohl, J. Salamone, and N.S. Cherniack. 1982. Respiratory activity and reflexes of hyoid muscles in the dog. *Federation Proceedings* 41:1507.
114. Onal, E., M. Lopata, and T.D. O'Connor. 1981. Diaphragmatic and genioglossal electromyogram responses to isocapnic hypoxia in humans. *Am Rev Resp Dis* 124:215–217.
115. Patrick, G.B., K.P. Strohl, S.B. Rubin, and M.D. Altose. 1982. Upper airway and diaphragm muscle responses to chemical stimulation and loading. *J Appl Physiol* 53:1133–1137.
116. Roberts, J.L., W.R. Reed, O.P. Mathew, and B.T. Thach. 1982. Control of respiratory activity of upper airway dilating muscle (genioglossus) in infants (abstract). *Pediatr Res* 16:305A.
117. Strohl, K.P., C.F. O'Cain, and A.S. Clutsky. 1982. Alae nasi activation and nasal resistance in healthy subjects. *J Appl Physiol* 52:1432–1437.
118. Carlo, W.A., R.J. Martin, E.N. Bruce, K.P. Strohl, and A.A. Fanaroff. 1983. Alae nasi activation (nasal flaring) decreases nasal resistance in preterm infants. *Pediatrics* 72:338–342.
119. Anch, A.M., J.E. Remmers, E.K. Sauerland, and W.J. deGroot. 1981. Oropharyngeal patency during waking and sleep in the Pickwickian syndrome: Electromyographic activity of the tensor veli palatine. *Electromyography and Clinical Neurophysiology* 21:317–330.
120. Brouillette, R.T., and B.T. Thach. 1980. Control of genioglossus muscle inspiratory activity. *J Appl Physiol* 49:801–808.
121. Onal, E., M. Lopata, and T.D. O'Connor. 1981. Diaphragmatic and genioglossal electromyogram responses to CO_2 rebreathing in humans. *J Appl Physiol* 49:638–642.
122. Mathew, O.P., Y.K. Abu-Osba, and B.T. Thach. 1982. Influence of upper airway pressure changes on genioglossus muscle respiratory activity. *J Appl Physiol* 52:438–444.
123. Van Lunteren, E., W.B. Van de Graaff, D.M. Parker, J. Mitra, M.A. Haxhiu, K.P. Strohl, and N.S. Cherniack. 1984. Nasal and laryngeal reflex responses to negative upper airway pressure. *J Appl Physiol* 56:746–752.
124. Hwang, J.C., W.M. St. John, and D. Bartlett. 1984. Afferent pathways for hypoglossal and phrenic responses to changes in upper airway pressure. *Resp Physiol* 55:341–354.
125. Mathew, O.P., Y.K. Abu-Osba, and B.T. Thach. 1982. Influence of upper airway pressure changes on respiratory frequency. *Resp Physiol* 49:223–233.
126. Mathew, O.P., and J.P. Farber. 1983. Effect of upper airway negative pressure on respiratory timing. *Resp Physiol* 54:259–268.
127. Mathew, O.P., Y.K. Abu-Osba, and B.T. Thach. 1982. Genioglossus muscle responses to upper airway pressure changes: Afferent pathways. *J Appl Physiol* 52:445–450.
128. Thach, B.T., P.A. Menon, and G. Schefft. 1985. Negative upper airway pressure decreases inspiratory airflow and tidal volume in tracheostomized

sleeping human infants (abstract). *Am Rev Resp Dis* 131:A295.
129. Fisher, J.T., and G.S. Sant' Ambrogio. 1985. Airway and lung receptors and their reflex affects in the newborn. *Pediatric Pulmonology* 1:112–126.
130. Lawson, E.E., and B.T. Thach. 1977. Respiratory patterns during progressive asphyxia in newborn rabbits. *J Appl Physiol* 43:468–474.
131. Mathew, O.P., B.T. Thach, Y.K. Abu-Osba, R.T. Brouillette, and J.L. Roberts. 1984. Regulation of upper airway maintaining muscles during progressive asphyxia. *Pediatr Res* 18:819–822.
132. Safar, P., L.S. Escarraga, and F. Chang. 1959. Upper airway obstruction in the unconscious patient. *J Appl Physiol* 14:760–764.
133. Robin, P. 1934. Glossoptosis due to atresia and hypotrophy of the mandible. *Am J Dis Child* 48:541–547.
134. Guilleminault, C., F.L. Eldridge, F.B. Simmons, and W.C. Dement. 1976. Sleep apnea in eight children. *Pediatrics* 58:23–30.
135. Brouillette, R.T., S.K. Fernbach, and C.E. Hunt. 1982. Obstructive sleep apnea in infants and children. *J Pediatr* 100:31–40.
136. Yitzchak, F., R.E. Kravath, C.P. Pollak, and E.D. Weitzman. 1983. Obstructive sleep apnea and its therapy: Clinical and polysomnographic manifestations. *Pediatrics* 71:737–742.
137. Sauerland, E.K., and R.M. Harper. 1976. The human tongue during sleep: Electromyographic activity of the genioglossus muscle. *Exp Neurol* 51:160–170.
138. Mallory, S.B., and J.L. Paradise. 1979. Glossoptosis revisited: On the development and resolution of airway obstruction in the Pierre Robin syndrome. *Pediatrics* 46:946–948.
139. Zwillich, C.W., T. Devlin, D.M. White, N.J. Douglas, J.V. Weil, and R.J. Martin. 1982. Bradycardia during sleep apnea: Its characteristics and mechanism. *Am Rev Resp Dis* 125:234.
140. Mauer, K.W., R.A. Staats, and K.D. Olsen. 1983. Upper airway obstruction and disordered nocturnal breathing in children. *Mayo Clinic Proceedings* 58:349–353.
141. Monroe, C.W., and K. Ogo. 1972. Treatment of micrognathia in the neonatal period. *Plastic Reconstruction Surgery* 50:317–325.
142. McNicholas, W.T., S. Tarlo, P. Cole, N. Zemel, R. Rutherford, D. Griffen, and E.A. Phillipson. 1982. Obstructive apneas during sleep in patients with seasonal allergic rhinitis. *Am Rev Resp Dis* 126:625–629.
143. Heaf, D.P., P.J. Helms, R. Dinwiddie, and D.J. Matthew. 1982. Nasopharyngeal airways in Pierre Robin Syndrome. *J Pediatr* 100:698–703.
144. Williams, A.J., M.A. Williams, C.A. Walker, and P.G. Bush. 1981. The Robin anomalad (Pierre Robin Syndrome)—a follow-up study. *Arch Dis Child* 56:663–668.
145. Dennison, W.M. 1965. The Pierre Robin Syndrome. *Pediatrics* 36:336–341.
146. Forest, H., and A.G. Graham. 1963. The Pierre-Robin syndrome. *Scottish Medical Journal* 8:16–24.
147. Girling, D.J. 1972. Changes in heart rate, blood pressure and pulse pressure during apneic attacks in newborn babies. *Arch Dis Child* 47:405–410.

148. Stevens, M.H. 1965. Sudden unexplained death in infancy. *Am J Dis Child* 110:243–247.

149. Daily, W.J.R., M. Klaus, and H.B. Meyer. 1969. Apnea in premature infants: Monitoring-incidence, heart rate changes, and an effect of environmental temperature. *Pediatrics* 43:510–518.

150. Brouillette, R.T., B.T. Thach, Y.K. Abu-Osba, and S.L. Wilson. 1980. Hiccups in infants: Characteristics and effects on ventilation. *J Pediatr* 96:219–225.

151. Rosen, C.L., D.G. Glaze, and J.D. Frost. 1984. Hypoxemia associated with feeding in the preterm infant and full term neonate. *Am J Dis Child* 138:623–628.

152. Guilleminault, C., and S. Coons. 1984. Apnea and bradycardia during feeding in infants weighing >2000 gm. *J Pediatr* 104:932–935.

153. Steward, D.J. 1982. Preterm infants are more prone to complications following minor surgery than are term infants. *Anesthesiology* 56:304–306.

154. Perlstein, H., K. Edward, and J. Sutherland. 1970. Apnea in premature infants and incubator air temperature changes. *N Engl J Med* 282:461–466.

155. Brechor, F.W., S.T. Mokrohisky, and K. McIntosh. 1977. Apnea associated with respiratory syncytial virus infection in young infants. *J Pediatr* 90:382–386.

156. Church, N.R., N.G. Anas, C.B. Hall, and J.G. Brooks. 1980. Respiratory syncytial virus related to apnea in infants. *Am J Dis Child* 138:247–250.

157. Roberts, J.L., O.P. Mathew, and B.T. Thach. 1982. The efficacy of theophylline in premature infants with mixed and obstructive apnea and apnea associated with pulmonary and neurologic disease. *J Pediatr* 100:968–970.

158. Mathew, O.P., J.L. Roberts, and B.T. Thach. 1982. Pharyngeal airway obstruction in preterm infants during mixed and obstructive apnea. *J Pediatr* 100:964–968.

159. Henderson-Smart, D.J. 1983. Clinical apnea and brain stem neural function in preterm infants. *N Engl J Med* 308:353–357.

160. Gerhardt, T., and E. Bancalari. 1984. Apnea of prematurity: I. Lung function and regulation of breathing. *Pediatrics* 74:58–62.

161. Gerhardt, T., and E. Bancalari. 1984. Apnea of prematurity: II. Respiratory reflexes. *Pediatrics* 74:63–66.

162. Thach, B.T., and E.E. Lawson. 1979. Death from upper airway obstruction: Decreased survival in 33-day-old rabbits (abstract). *Pediatr Res* 13:542.

163. Farber, J.P., A.C. Catron, and H.F. Krous. 1983. Pulmonary petechiae ventilatory-circulatory interactions. *Pediatr Res* 17:181–182.

164. Krous, H.F., and J. Jordan. 1984. A necropsy study of distribution of petechiae in non-sudden infant death syndrome. *Arch Pathol Lab Med* 108:75–76.

165. Campbell, C.J., and D.J.C. Read. 1980. Circulatory and respiratory factors in the experimental production of lung petechiae and their possible significance in the sudden infant death syndrome. *Pathology* 12:181–188.

166. Krous, H.F. 1984. The microscopic distribution of intrathoracic petechiae in sudden infant death syndrome. *Arch Pathol Lab Med* 108:77–79.

167. Froggatt, P., M.A. Lynas, and G. MacKenzie. 1971 Epidemiology of sud-

den unexpected death in infants ("Cot death") in Northern Ireland. *British Journal of Preventive and Social Medicine* 25:119–134.

168. Valdes-Dapena, M.A. 1967. Sudden and unexpected death in infancy: A review of the world literature. *Pediatrics* 39:123–138.

169. Valdes-Dapena, M., and A. Steinschneider. 1983. Sudden infant death syndrome (SIDS), apnea and near miss for SIDS. *Emergency Medicine Clinics of North America* 1:27–43.

170. Bergman, A.B. 1970. "Sudden infant death syndrome in King County, Washington: Epidemiologic aspects." In *Sudden Infant Death Syndrome: Proceedings of the Second Conference on Causes of Sudden Death in Infants,* ed. A.B. Bergman, J.B. Beckwith, and C.G. Ray. Seattle: University of Washington Press.

171. Kelly, D.H., D.C. Shannon, and K. O'Connell. 1978. Care of infants with near miss sudden infant death syndrome. *Pediatrics* 61:511–514.

172. Ariagno, R.L., C. Guilleminault, R. Korobkin, M. Owen-Boeddiker, and R. Baldwin. 1983. Near-miss for sudden infant death syndrome infants: A clinical problem. *Pediatrics* 71:726–730.

173. Jeffrey, H.E., P. Rahilly, and D.J.C. Read. 1983. Multiple causes of asphyxia in infants at high risk for sudden infant death. *Arch Dis Child* 58:92–100.

174. Rosen, C.L., J.D. Frost, and G.M. Harrison. 1983. Infant apnea: Polygraphic studies and follow-up monitoring. *Pediatrics* 71:731–736.

175. Guilleminault, C., R.L. Ariagno, R. Korobkin, L. Nagel, R. Baldwin, S. Coons, and M. Owen. 1979. Mixed and obstructive sleep apnea and near miss for Sudden Infant Death Syndrome: 2. Comparison of near miss and normal control infants by age. *Pediatrics* 64:882–891.

176. Kahn, A., D. Blum, P. Waterschoot, E. Engleman, and P. Smets. 1982. Effects of obstructive sleep apneas on transcutaneous oxygen pressure in control infants, siblings of sudden infant death syndrome victims and near miss infants: Comparison with effects of central sleep apneas. *Pediatrics* 70:852–857.

177. Guilleminault, C., M. Souquet, R.L. Ariagno, R. Korobkin, and F.B. Simmons. 1984. Five cases of near-miss Sudden Infant Death Syndrome and development of obstructive sleep apnea syndrome. *Pediatrics* 73:71–78.

178. Kahn, A., E.P. Verstraeten, and D. Blum. 1984. Preliminary report on neurodevelopmental screening in children previously at risk for sudden infant death syndrome. *J Pediatr* 105:666–668.

179. Guilleminault, C., R.L. Ariagno, L.S. Forno, L. Nagel, R. Baldwin, and M. Owen. 1979. Obstructive sleep apnea and near miss for SIDS: 1. Report of an infant with sudden death. *Pediatrics* 63:837–843.

180. Mandell, F. 1981. Cot deaths among children of nurses: Observations of breathing patterns. *Arch Dis Child* 56:312–314.

181. Beal, S.M. 1983. "Some epidemiological factors about Sudden Infant Death Syndrome (SIDS) in South Australia." In *Sudden Infant Death Syndrome,* ed. J.T. Tildon, L.M. Roeder, and A. Steinschneider. New York: Academic Press.

182. Stark, R.E., and S.N. Nathansen. 1975. "Unusual features of cry in an infant dying suddenly and unexpectedly." In *Development of Upper Respira-*

tory Anatomy and Function, W3F049 No. 29, ed J.F. Bosma and J. Showacre. Bethesda, MD: National Institutes of Health.
183. Golub, H.C., and M.J. Corwin. 1982. Infant cry: A clue to diagnosis. *Pediatrics* 69:197–201.
184. Naeye, R.L., J. Messmer, T. Specht, and T.A. Merritt. 1976. Sudden infant death syndrome temperament before death. *J Pediatr* 88:511–515.
185. Steinschneider, A., S.L. Weinstein, and E. Diamond. 1982. The sudden infant death syndrome and apnea/obstruction during sleep and feeding. *Pediatrics* 70:858–863.
186. Naeye, R.L. 1983. "Pathologists' role in SIDS research: The unfinished task." In *Sudden Infant Death Syndrome,* ed. J.T. Tildon, L.M. Roeder, and A. Steinschneider. New York: Academic Press.
187. Becker, L.E. 1983. "Neuropathological basis for respiratory dysfunction in Sudden Infant Death Syndrome." In *Sudden Infant Death Syndrome,* ed J.T. Tildon, L.M. Roeder, and A. Steinschneider. New York: Academic Press.
188. Carpenter, R.G., and J.L. Emery. 1974. "The identification and follow-up of high risk infants." In *SIDS 1974,* ed. R.R. Robinson. Toronto: Canadian Foundation for the Study of Infant Deaths.
189. Schlesselman, J.J. 1982. *Case Control Studies.* New York: Oxford University Press.
190. Southall, D.P. 1983. Home monitoring and its role in the sudden infant death syndrome. *Pediatrics* 72:133–138.

5

Sleep-Related Respiratory Function and Dysfunction in Postneonatal Infantile Apnea

CHRISTIAN GUILLEMINAULT, M.D.

Interest in postneonatal infantile apnea during sleep, thought to be responsible for some cases of sudden infant death syndrome (SIDS), initially began in two independent research groups. In 1972, Steinschneider reported on five infants whose autopsies supported the diagnosis of SIDS [1]. Within this group were two siblings of SIDS victims who had long episodes of postneonatal sleep apnea. At the Sleep Research Society national meeting in the same year, we described one child with obstructive sleep apnea [2]. In a subsequent article published in 1973 [3], we linked this sleep-related respiratory pathology to an infant who, during polygraphic monitoring, had long sleep apneic events; this infant later died and was labeled a SIDS victim. We hypothesized that sleep apnea occurred in some SIDS victims and that it may have existed, unsuspected by the medical team, long before the infants died. This hypothesis was based on the reports of the autopsy results.

The autopsy results, some of which were summarized at the 1969 international SIDS conference [4], were (1) the presence of intrathoracic petechiae that dot the surfaces of the lung, pericardium, and thymus; (2) mild pulmonary congestion and edema, neither of which accounted for death; (3) minor microscopic inflammatory infiltrates in the lung and upper airway; (4) evidence of chronic hypoxemia [5, 6] (this has been largely unconfirmed [7]); and (5) hypo- or hyperplasia of the carotid body [8, 9].

At the same 1969 conference, Guntheroth reported that parents had found some infants limp and not breathing—in a state close to death—although subsequent investigations in the hospital revealed no pathologic clues; these infants later died and were called SIDS victims [10]. They were at first called "near miss death" infants and then, by extension, "near miss SIDS" infants. Because we do not know the underlying pathology of SIDS itself, the term "near miss SIDS" is at least as vague, and the group of infants under this label is very poorly defined. This term, however, does indicate that an infant had an episode that the parents considered life threatening; they found their infants blue or pale, limp, and not breathing, and had to stimulate them rigorously, often with mouth-to-mouth resuscitation. However, the term does not encompass a clearly delineated disease; the description of the event itself should alert the physician to potential risks for the infant, but the infant's prognosis will be unclear.

It was reported initially that up to 10 percent of near miss SIDS infants die of SIDS [11]. On the basis of autopsy results, other reports, including ours, have indicated that occasionally a near miss SIDS infant dies of SIDS [12]. Before the advent of home monitoring, only five of 178 near miss SIDS infants in our own infant population died and were labeled as SIDS victims after autopsy. Two were between five and six-and-a-half months of age, and three were between ten and twenty-one months of age. (Only the five month old had an autopsy with multiple serial histologic analyses, including serial brain stem slides [12].) Since 1978, only one of 255 near miss SIDS infants has died as a SIDS victim; this infant died in 1984 at five months of age, despite monitor alarms and both the mother's and paramedics' attempts at resuscitation. (The mother had been trained in cardiopulmonary resuscitation and had resuscitated the infant previously.)

The idea that the chronic hypoxia found in near miss SIDS infants may be present in some SIDS victims, supported by anecdotal reports of long sleep-related apneic episodes in both near miss and SIDS infants, has led to the various systematic investigations of normal infants and near miss SIDS infants. In particular, investigations of respiration and ventilatory functions during sleep have been conducted. Protocols have varied, depending upon the research group performing the study. Unfortunately, some reports have combined older premature infants with full-term infants, rendering comparisons of data across research groups difficult.

Breathing Patterns during Sleep in Normal Infants

To understand the pathologic condition, one must recognize the normal patterns, but few studies have examined the development over time of respiratory patterns during sleep. Presently, there is no study that delineates the normal range for states of alertness, circadian organization, age, sex, and weight of infants. Data have been collected that consider age, state of alertness, and time during one twenty-four hour cycle, but only two studies have considered these variables and the infants' sex [13, 14]. Depending on the investigator and the year of the study, techniques used to monitor breathing in infants have varied greatly. The most sophisticated studies have monitored states of alertness, breathing patterns, and oxygen tension or saturation. There has been great variation in the methodology for monitoring breathing patterns. In some studies, chest and/or abdominal movements were the only controlled variables; in others, airflow at the nostrils and mouth also was monitored simultaneously. The duration of the monitoring period has varied to the extent that some results are of only limited interest because the recording period was so short. Some data have been obtained with home monitors but without a method for recording upper airway problems or the state of alertness.

In 1982, Hoppenbrouwers found ten references on normative data for breathing pauses in full-term infants [15]. One team monitored thirty infants for twenty-four-hour periods at regular intervals between three weeks and six months of age [16]. Two teams monitored a total of eighty-five fullterm infants for twelve nocturnal hours [17, 18, 19]; fifty-three of these were followed on a monthly basis for the first six months of life [17, 18]. The other team used only impedance pneumograms, and the studies were limited in time and scope, investigating infants only during daytime naps [19]. The techniques used by Coup et al. [20] were at greatest variance with those reviewed by Hoppenbrouwers. They monitored only activity patterns and thoracoabdominal movements automatically on seventy-nine infants at monthly intervals during the first five months of life. The overall results show a certain heterogeneity, in part because the definition of an apneic episode was so vague. There was no general agreement as to how long an interruption of respiration should last for an episode to be considered an apnea; there was no standard method for measuring an apnea; and there was no standard strategy for analyzing the apnea. As Hoppenbrouwers points out, the effects of posture and temperature during the recording are addressed rarely, and when they are, they generally are considered only during the newborn period. This is unfortunate for, as Beal recently reported, more than 90 percent of SIDS victims in Western Australia are found prone [21]. We do not know the significance of this finding because we do not know the number of infants placed in the prone position during the first weeks of life. In a recent study, apnea rate and duration were not affected by sleeping position [22]. Another issue is determining the impact of apnea on blood gases. No study, of course, has been performed with arterial lines, but most of the longitudinal studies were performed without transcutaneous oxygen and carbon dioxide tension electrodes ($tcPO_2$ and $tcPCO_2$), which were unavailable at the time [23–25]. We have used a Waters Instrument ear oximeter intermittently but have not accumulated a large normative data base on the variation of $tcPO_2$ and $tcPCO_2$ with simultaneous polygraphic monitorings obtained longitudinally between one and six months of age [12]. Despite these drawbacks, one can find areas of agreement.

Apnea during sleep is a common phenomenon in normal infants. Overall, apneas occur most frequently during the newborn period and appear to decrease most noticeably between forty and fifty-two weeks gestational age (GA) [26].

Three types of sleep apnea occur in infancy: "central" (or diaphragmatic), "obstructive" (or upper airway), and "mixed" (an event with a central and an obstructive component) (Figures 5.1, 5.2, and 5.3). Most mixed

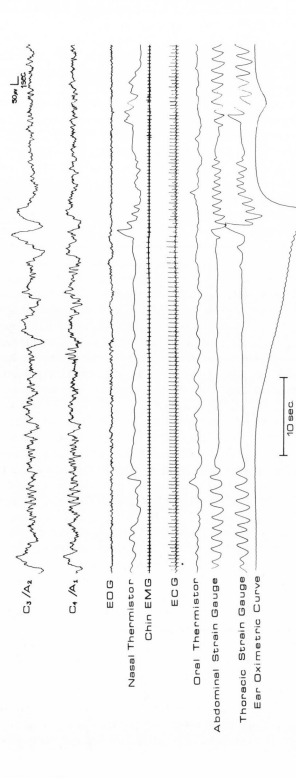

FIGURE 5.1. A thirty-two-second central apnea during NREM sleep in a male four-week-old, full-term, near miss SIDS infant. Note the slow drop in oxygen saturation measured by ear oximetry (Waters Instrument Co.) [30].

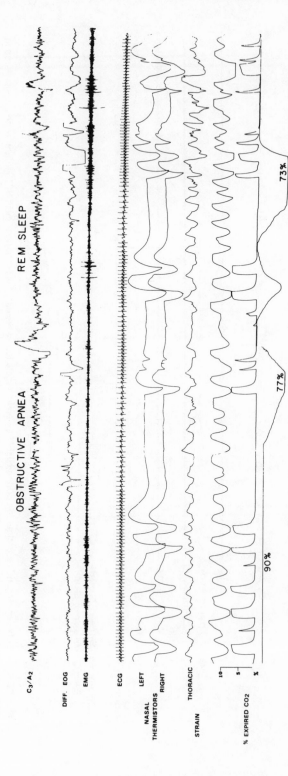

FIGURE 5.2. Obstructive sleep apneas during REM sleep in a male fourteen-week-old, full-term, near miss SIDS infant. Oxygen desaturation, measured by ear oximetry (Waters Instrument Co.), and bradycardia occur with each apneic event.

98

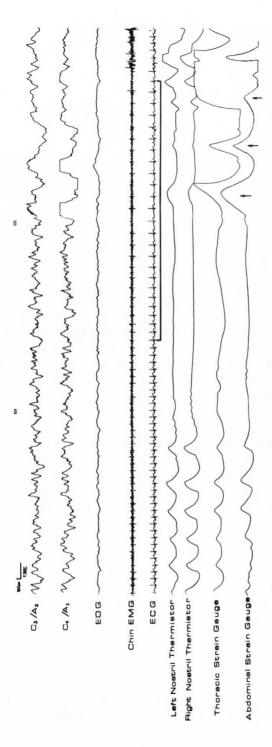

FIGURE 5.3. Mixed apnea recorded in a female full-term, ten-week-old, near miss SIDS infant. No abdominal or thoracic movements occur during the first part of the apnea, and there is no airflow through nasal and oral thermistors (Channels 4 and 7 from top). The infant's thoracic movements then increase. (The observer reported an obvious struggle for breath at this point.) Head movements occur during the obstructive component of the mixed apnea, and bradycardia develops [30].

99

events begin as central apneas, but when diaphragmatic movements resume, there is no air exchange at the nose and mouth because of an occluded upper airway. Electromyographic (EMG) studies during mixed apneas indicate that there are no EMG discharges in the genioglossus muscle during the central component [27, 28]. This finding suggests that not only the diaphragm but also other muscles involved in respiration, including those that help maintain a patent upper airway, may be inactive during a central apnea. Because of this lack of muscle tone, the orohypopharynx collapses. When diaphragmatic movements resume, the negative transpharyngeal pressure related to diaphragmatic inspiratory effort hinders an immediate return to normal upper airway patency.

Can a mixed apneic episode begin with an obstructive event and end with a central one? Although this is hypothetically possible, no good examples have been published, perhaps because of the limitations of polygraphic monitoring when invasive techniques are not used. Infants with Pierre Robin syndrome or Crouzon's syndrome who have obvious mandibular malformations initially may have central apnea with upper airway apnea developing during sleep when they are older [29].

Can an abrupt obstruction induce a reflex central apnea? Could this one obstructed breath go unnoticed unless monitored with an esophageal balloon or transducer? More work is needed to resolve this issue. We observed one case of unusual mixed apnea; in the middle of a typical upper airway obstruction, which occurred during a burst of rapid eye movement (REM) in REM sleep, diaphragmatic effort suddenly was inhibited [30]. This is the only time we have observed a mixed event that began with an upper airway obstruction (Figure 5.4).

In addition to apneas, there are events that we call "hypopneas." These occur when the upper airway does not collapse completely or when diaphragmatic movement decreases but does not cease. These incomplete events have an impact on oxygen tension, inducing hypoventilation. (Other researchers have labeled them differently, but the phenomenon is the same.)

Paradoxical breathing, the decoupling of chest wall and abdominal respiratory movements following loss of intercostal muscle activity during active (REM) sleep, is a common phenomenon in newborn infants. Normally, it does not lead to any change in oxygen and carbon dioxide tensions, since diaphragmatic effort increases and maintains adequate ventilation. Paradoxical breathing, however, may become pathologic if diaphragmatic fatigue occurs, a phenomenon not yet well documented. It also may be observed with an obstructed airway.

These respiratory events during sleep vary greatly in duration. Events as short as two or three seconds have been identified as apneas in very young infants. Coup et al. [20] preferred to use the term "missed breaths" and considered two "missed-breath apnea" or four "missed-breath apnea"

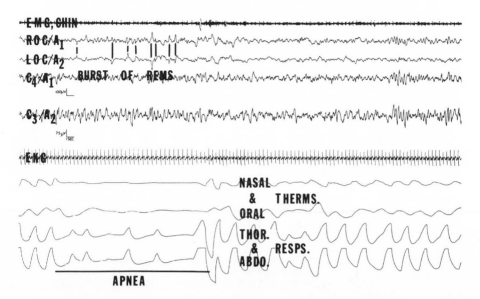

FIGURE 5.4. A mixed apnea during REM sleep in a male seven-week-old, full-term, near miss SIDS infant. The infant has an initial obstructive apnea with persistent diaphragmatic movement but no airflow. During a burst of rapid eye movement in REM sleep, a sleep-related mechanism interferes, inhibiting diaphragmatic effort for one breath in the middle and one breath at the end of the apnea [30].

during sleep. This approach, based on a computer-analyzed recording, has one advantage — respiratory rate changes with age, and the duration of an inspiration–expiration cycle will change over time. Depending on the basic respiratory cycle, therefore, the computer can calculate the number of missed breaths for a given age. Unfortunately, Coup et al. studied only central sleep apnea.

Despite problems with the duration of sleep apnea, most authors agree that no sleep apnea longer than fifteen seconds has been polygraphically monitored (with constant observation) in normal infants up to six months of age, and sleep apnea between ten and fifteen seconds is rare to exceptional. Obstructive sleep apnea is rarely noted in normal infants under six months of age. Obstructive sleep apneas of ten seconds or longer have not been reported in normal infants, and episodes between six and ten seconds are observed only rarely. They may be observed more frequently in association with a "cold," "runny nose," or clear pharyngitis. The degree of flexion of the neck during sleep also may be a factor [31].

We investigated the frequency and type of sleep apnea in a group of normal, full-term infants at ages ranging between forty weeks and six months using twenty-four-hour polygraphic monitoring [16] (Table 5.1). We divided our results by type and duration of apneic event and presented

TABLE 5.1 Respiratory Pauses: 24-Hour Indices

		3–6 Sec			6–10 Sec		
		Central	Mixed and Obstructive	Periodic Breathing	Central	Mixed and Obstructive	Periodic Breathing
3 Weeks							
Control n = 10	R	10.01±3.25	0.38±0.24	10.54±8.61	3.07±0.89	0.29±0.24	4.13±5.60
	NR	3.10±1.79	0.22±0.20	4.68±5.82	2.50±0.44	0.18±0.30	3.46±5.35
	TST	6.97±2.44	0.31±0.18	7.43±7.05	2.87±0.45	0.24±0.26	3.69±5.08
6 Weeks							
Control n = 10	R	9.85±2.59	0.98±1.43	7.89±8.03	2.70±1.58	0.49±1.05	1.84±2.79
	NR	4.29±1.97	0.37±0.21	4.12±6.23	1.97±0.97	0.29±0.39	4.42±10.28
	TST	7.10±1.57	0.66±0.66	6.11±7.15	2.46±1.15	0.38±0.61	3.26±6.45
3 Months							
Control n = 9	R	11.20±4.64	0.48±0.74	7.56±2.82	2.66±2.22	0.24±0.29	1.54±1.52
	NR	3.00±1.00	0.11±0.18	1.08±0.73	1.78±1.05	0.06±0.37	0.53±0.37
	TST	6.08±2.28	0.28±0.46	3.43±1.08	2.18±1.49	0.13±0.13	0.93±0.58
4½ Months							
Control n = 10	R	9.64±3.52	0.26±0.30	17.17±4.75	1.54±1.17	0.15±0.23	1.26±0.85
	NR	2.52±1.22	0.10±0.16	0.70±0.81	1.15±0.97	0.02±0.06	0.25±0.33
	TST	4.80±1.53	0.15±0.21	2.67±1.76	1.31±0.93	0.07±0.11	0.57±0.45
6 Months							
Control n = 9	R	10.96±3.79	0.38±0.69	12.63±9.97	2.81±2.11	0.09±0.19	2.54±2.09
	NR	2.31±0.96	0.07±0.09	0.95±1.01	2.16±1.02	0.00±0.00	0.44±0.45
	TST	4.77±1.35	0.17±0.24	4.16±2.96	2.34±0.93	0.03±0.93	0.03±0.05

This table presents the mean (and standard deviations from the mean) number of respiratory pauses during sleep during the 24-hour period for each age group. The apnea index used is equal to the number of respiratory events, divided by sleep time, multiplied by 60 (60 minutes). Abbreviations used are R, rapid eye movement sleep; NR, nonrapid eye movement sleep TST, total sleep time; X, mean.

the data by minutes of sleep. Although a larger population sampling may have yielded slightly different results, this table is in overall agreement within the findings of other groups.

Determining the importance of periodic breathing (PB) in relation to near miss SIDS and SIDS is a complex issue, and the areas of agreement are limited. Although all researchers do not agree on an exact definition of PB, all do agree that a certain amount of PB during sleep is normal (Figure 5.5). Our team used Parmelee's definition of PB as a minimum of two central events lasting less than ten seconds within twenty seconds of each other [32]. Kelly and Shannon's definition, although similar, differs in that they used three or more apneic pauses of three or more seconds with respiratory interruptions of twenty seconds or less [19]. In normal infants, PB most commonly occurs during REM sleep but also is seen during nonrapid eye movement (NREM) sleep. Within our infant population, there was a large variation across infants for the appearance of PB. Kelly and Shannon believe that, despite its presence in normals, PB may be important when considering pathology. This is an area of controversy mainly because PB can be the result of more than one set of mechanisms. During

>10 Sec		>15 Sec		Total Periodic Breathing	Total Pauses (Central, Mixed and Obstructive)			Total Pauses Mixed and Obstructive
		Central	Mixed and Obstructive		>3 Sec	>6 Sec	>10 Sec	
0.50±0.56	0.05±0.08	0.00 0.00	0.00 0.00	14.66±14.04	28.97±16.79	8.04±6.02	0.56±0.61	0.73±0.42
0.91±1.09	0.06±0.08	0.00 0.00	0.00 0.00	8.13±11.07	15.99±13.09	7.10±6.51	0.97±1.15	0.45±0.44
0.73±0.72	0.07±0.09	0.00 0.00	0.00 0.00	11.12±12.04	22.31±14.59	7.60±5.84	0.80±0.79	0.62±0.40
0.07±0.21	0.11±0.31	0.00 0.00	0.03±0.10	9.72±10.78	23.95±15.25	5.23±5.38	0.21±0.61	1.61±2.87
0.60±1.19	0.08±0.14	0.00 0.00	0.00 0.00	8.53±16.47	16.12±17.59	7.35±11.45	0.68±1.20	0.74±0.57
0.36±0.66	0.10±0.21	0.00 0.00	0.01±0.04	9.37±13.50	20.45±15.54	6.58±7.98	0.48±0.78	1.16±1.49
0.10±0.21	0.06±0.12	0.00 0.00	0.00 0.00	9.10±3.73	23.84±8.66	4.60±3.38	0.16±0.31	0.78±0.81
0.18±0.18	0.00 0.00	0.00 0.00	0.00 0.00	1.61±0.92	6.75±1.85	2.55±1.38	0.18±0.18	0.17±0.20
0.16±0.19	0.02±0.05	0.00 0.00	0.00 0.00	4.36±1.48	13.41±4.35	3.42±2.17	0.18±0.23	0.43±0.49
0.05±0.10	0.00 0.00	0.00 0.00	0.00 0.00	8.44±5.42	20.07±8.81	2.99±1.87	0.05±0.10	0.40±0.50
0.34±0.48	0.00 0.00	0.00 0.00	0.00 0.00	0.95±1.09	5.09±3.32	1.76±1.58	0.35±0.49	0.13±0.23
0.24±0.32	0.00 0.00	0.00 0.00	0.00 0.00	3.24±2.12	9.81±4.40	2.19±1.64	0.24±0.34	0.23±0.32
0.14±0.30	0.00 0.00	0.00 0.00	0.00 0.00	15.17±11.73	29.55±16.47	5.58±4.13	0.14±0.30	0.47±0.81
0.28±0.32	0.00 0.00	0.00 0.00	0.00 0.00	1.41±1.42	6.24±2.49	2.91±1.24	0.29±0.32	0.07±0.09
1.01±0.65	0.24±0.30	0.00 0.00	0.00 0.00	5.17±3.52	12.73±5.09	3.63±1.49	0.25±0.30	0.20±0.27

REM sleep, PB usually is related to REM sleep mechanisms and is associated with the phasic events of this sleep state. But PB also can be related to the oscillating ventilation seen particularly in newborns and in early infancy. Waggener et al. [33] analyzed the oscillating breathing patterns that can lead to PB; the duration of central apnea depends upon the cycle time, amplitude, and coexistence of any oscillators. Oscillations of expired minute ventilation (VE) are characteristic of the respiratory control system [33]. The stability of this system controls the amplitude of oscillations. This means that the less stable the control system, the greater the amplitude of the oscillations. PB can be considered an index of risk; in specific cases it is not a normal finding because alterations in the respiratory blood gas feedback control system can render this system more unstable and induce an oscillating breathing pattern. This occurs when there is an increase in the gain of the control loop (mediated by the carotid body chemoreceptor) and in circulatory delay time. Because hypoxia increases the gain of the peripheral chemoreceptors, it is not surprising that an increase in PB has been observed in pathologic conditions [19]. As Waggener et al. emphasized, however, ventilatory oscillations exist in healthy infants and

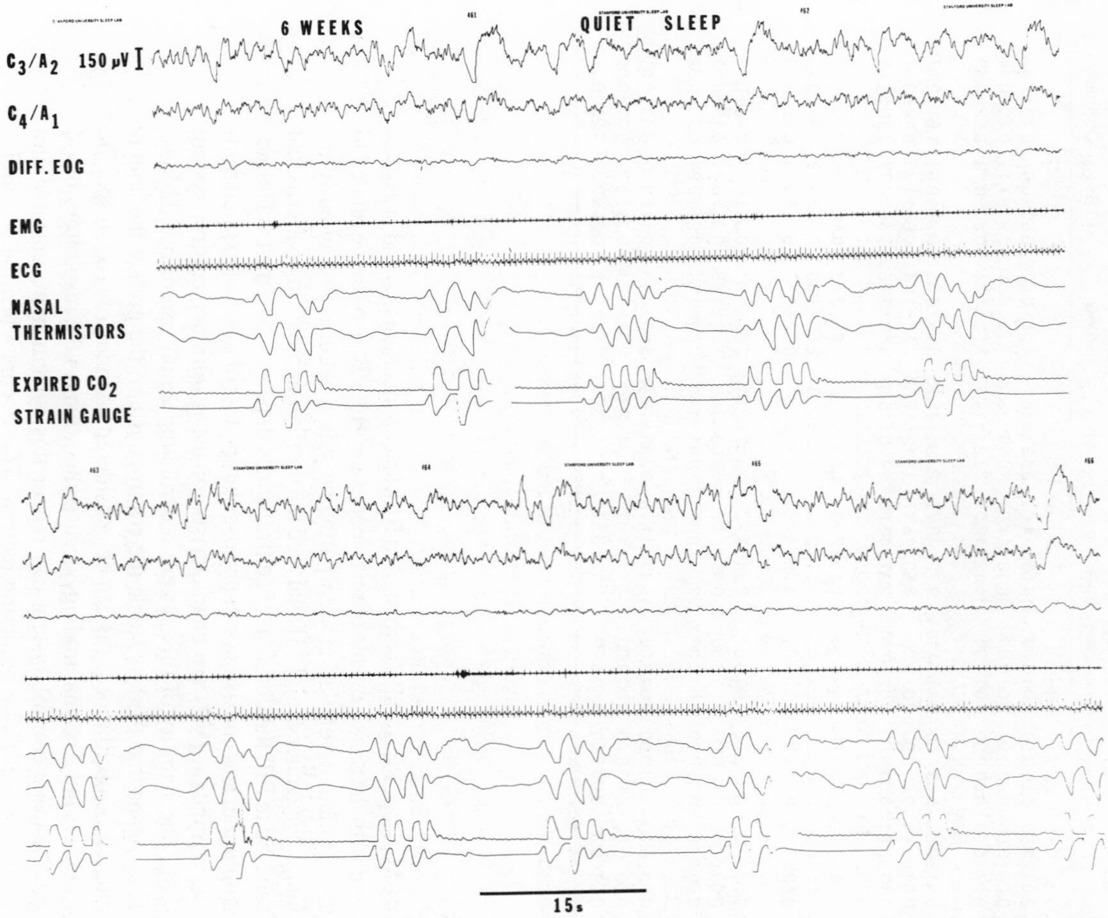

FIGURE 5.5. Periodic breathing during quiet (NREM) sleep in a male six-week-old, full-term, normal infant. This child, who is now seven years old, has developed normally and has never had any cardiorespiratory problems during sleep.

do not indicate any abnormality or pathologic condition. If the stability of a respiratory control system is fragile (the result of prematurity, delayed maturation in a full-term infant) or rendered unstable (the result of hypoxia) so that PB may be easily induced, PB also may occur without these events. A physiologic system other than blood gas feedback control, such as blood pressure control, may lead to PB. Finally, oscillatory patterns mean that there will be not only cessations of breathing but also initiations of breathing at the end of the pause programmed into the oscillation. Pathology may appear if this second component is impaired.

Researchers generally agree that PB occurs in normal infants during sleep; whether it indicates risk, especially as a frequent occurrence, is subject to controversy. Polygraphic observations of PB are not in themselves a reason for concern; what is of concern is the cause of PB and its impact on oxygen tension.

Until recently, little research had been conducted on feeding apnea in infants who are awake or drowsy. Since Steinschneider's group [34, 35] studied this issue in preterm and near miss SIDS infants, some of whom later died of SIDS, it has received more attention (Figure 5.6). Johnson and Salisbury [36] demonstrated that normal newborns have cyanosis and apnea while sucking a cow-milk formula. Mathew et al. [37] also found that full-term newborns and young infants with normal development had apnea and bradycardia during wakeful feeding periods.

In summary, normal infants have apnea during sleep and while awake and feeding. These apneas are most common in the newborn period and early infancy, and their frequency decreases with age. Long apneas, particularly those longer than fifteen seconds, usually are not observed; obstructive apneas, even lasting six to ten seconds, are rare.

Breathing Patterns during Sleep in Near Miss SIDS Infants and Siblings of SIDS Victims

Near miss SIDS infants and siblings of SIDS victims may be at greater risk for a SIDS event than the general infant population. The determination of "greater risk" is based on a series of case studies, and the increase in the percentage of risk is a controversial issue. It is obvious, however, that most near miss SIDS infants and siblings of SIDS victims survive past twelve months of age. Nevertheless, investigating these populations can give some insight into underlying discrete breathing differences that, if combined with other factors, may increase the risk of respiratory arrest. Some pertinent observations also may support the hypothesis that abnormal breathing patterns exist, particularly during sleep, that can have an impact on the cardiovascular system and lead to sudden death.

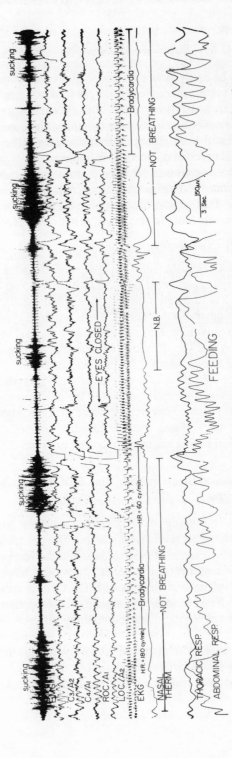

FIGURE 5.6. Example of repetitive apnea during feeding while awake in a male three-week-old, full-term, near miss SIDS infant. Note the bradycardia from 180 to 60 beats/minute in association with feeding apnea.

Near Miss SIDS Infants

Systematic polygraphic monitoring of near miss SIDS infants has shown that some infants have long (>15 seconds) central, mixed, and obstructive apnea [16, 19, 38] (Figures 5.1, 5.2, and 5.3).

Central Apnea. From an analysis of more than 500 twenty-four-hour recordings of full-term, near miss SIDS infants, we found that long central apneas do occur but in less than 1 percent of the population. Other authors also have noted these long central events. When these infants are evaluated while awake, they have normal lungs, normal thoracoabdominal musculature, and a normal command of breathing. When they are investigated during sleep, however, abnormalities can be identified.

These infants can be divided into several subgroups.

1. Shannon et al. [39] initially observed, and others [40, 41] have confirmed, that a very small group have a central congenital alveolar hypoventilation syndrome (CCHS). Because of the complete respiratory arrests, severe cyanosis, and rapidly developing cardiac failure, CCHS should be easy to identify. If it is associated with Hirschsprung's disease or another autonomic nervous system dysfunction, the diagnosis will be even more obvious [41]. If the sleep-related abnormality is linked to delta sleep, however, it will not become apparent until this sleep stage develops and lasts for at least several minutes. We had one near miss SIDS infant who lacked a sensitivity to carbon dioxide tension during delta (stage 3–4 NREM) sleep specifically, rather than NREM sleep in general [41]. Although the progressive carbon dioxide retention and hypoxia related to alveolar hypoventilation are seen clearly in this stage, they may be identified in infants between six weeks and three months of age by a long central apnea or a complete and abrupt respiratory arrest. Carbon dioxide challenges during NREM sleep as a whole or, in rare cases, only in delta sleep, will demonstrate the absence of respiratory response with worsening carbon dioxide retention and oxygen desaturation.

2. Full-term infants with long central sleep apnea usually do not have any signs of CCHS. They do not retain carbon dioxide during NREM sleep, and investigations during the day while the infants are awake eliminate the common causes of apnea, including sepsis to low hemoglobin, patent ductus arteriosus, and seizure disorders. The apneic events are discovered by polygraphic monitoring during sleep and suggest an irregularity rather than a constant abnormality in the central control of breathing during sleep.

3. Infants with Pierre Robin syndrome or Crouzon's syndrome also may have long central apneas during sleep. Le Drouarin's research demonstrated that, at least in birds, nearly all the anterior facial structures

derive from neuro-ectodermal crests [42]. Applying these investigations to humans enables one to follow the embryologic development of the human cervicocephalic region. Most neurocristopathies, including Pierre Robin syndrome, involve both neurologic and facial malformations [43]. Prognosis for these infants is often poor; one-quarter, for example, die in infancy [44], often abruptly during sleep without any obvious cause of death. In our patients, long central apneas during sleep occurred several weeks or months before the appearance of mixed and obstructive apnea, which were more common after six months of age [29].

Regardless of the cause, long central apneas during sleep occurred with secondary oxygen desaturation, bradycardia, and asystoles. These postneonatal central apneas rarely have been associated with any other type of cardiac arrhythmia during polygraphic recordings.

Mixed and Obstructive Apneas. Both mixed and obstructive events ranging between three and twenty seconds or more in duration have been observed in near miss SIDS infants [16, 38, 45–48]; they have been noted in infants who have had short central apneas at earlier recordings [48, 49]. We cannot always explain the mechanisms that are responsible for their appearance. A subgroup of near miss SIDS infants had a vague history of a "runny nose" or symptoms of a mild "cold" prior to the near miss event. Polygraphic recordings revealed clusters of central and/or mixed apneas, usually of short duration. The clusters lasted for ten or fifteen minutes, often including a long, mixed apneic event that induced oxygen desaturation as indicated by a $tcPO_2$ electrode or ear oximeter. When present, cardiac arrhythmias were always seen with the obstructive component of the mixed event (Figure 5.7) [50]. The most common cardiac arrhythmia we recorded in several infants was a sinus arrest that lasted from two to five seconds. Although cultures obtained from this subgroup were negative, these infants had muscle hypotonia, particularly shoulder hypotonia, at a developmental neurologic evaluation [51]. They had abnormal breathing events of varied severity during sleep for the following two to three months, but breathing patterns during sleep were completely normal between six to nine months of age. Despite the negative cultures, we hypothesized that these infants had a semi-acute illness with a neurotropic factor [50].

Kelly and Shannon reported on a group of infants who also had severe, long obstructive events and long central events that were documented by polygraphic recording [45]. The obstructive events generally were noted after six months of age. One infant's symptoms improved temporarily with atropine sulfate. The authors suspected that a laryngospasm initiated the obstructive apnea.

Mixed and obstructive sleep apnea were observed in near miss infants

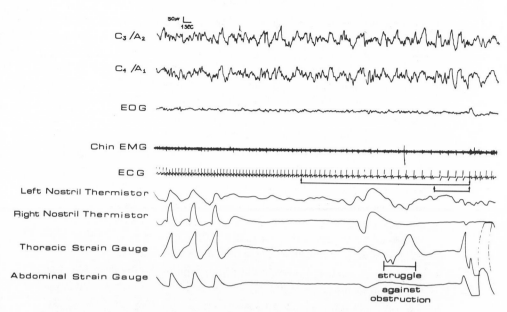

FIGURE 5.7. Polygraphic recording of a mixed apnea during NREM sleep in a male six-week-old, full-term, near miss SIDS infant. Thoracic swings during the second half of the apnea were observed during the struggle against a closed airway. Bradycardia occurs during the obstructive segment of the apnea; note the negative T waves, the switch from a sinusal to a nodal rhythm, and the broadening of the QRS complex (Channel 5 from top, underlined segment)[30].

who later developed a typical obstructive sleep apnea syndrome [52]. These infants did not have long mixed and obstructive events, but more frequent short events than seen normally during twenty-four-hour monitoring. At successive polygraphic monitorings, these infants continued to have frequent mixed and obstructive apneic events and began to snore. By the time the children were two years of age, symptoms of obstructive sleep apnea syndrome had developed. Findings in this sub-group of infants raise the possibility of discrete malformation of the oropharynx and the mandible as a contributing factor in mixed and obstructive sleep apnea in infancy. Further studies revealed that the relationship between the lower mandible, the hyoid bone, and the length of the soft palate is important in the development of mixed and obstructive events during sleep [53]. It is difficult to appreciate the mild-to-moderate anatomical abnormalities in these infants because they do not have typical retro or micrognathia. At a later age, however, it is apparent that their posterior airway space is very small, particulary behind the base of the tongue [54]. The computed tomographic (CT) scanner permits more thorough evaluation tof the hypopharynx during awake periods and the two sleep states in these cases and demonstrates an abnormal reduction of the hypopharynx.

Finally, central, mixed, and obstructive events during sleep may be related to esophageal reflux [55–59]. The relationship between reflux and apneic events is not always clear, and a certain amount of reflux is normal during infancy. Nevertheless, specific correlations between apneas and reflux have been made in some infants [55–59] (Figure 5.8).

In summary, during sleep some infants have long central or mixed and obstructive apnea that can be related to a number of factors, some of which are clearly identified:

1. rarely, a congenital central alveolar hypoventilation syndrome;
2. an obvious or discrete malformation or malposition of the mandible and the hyoid bone leading to an abnormal positioning of the soft tissues of the upper airway, particularly the tongue and soft palate. As a result, the posterior airway space is abnormally small;
3. a semi-acute illness, probably viral in origin despite the negative cultures, that involves a neurotrophic component that transitorily disturbs the control of ventilation during sleep (i.e., respiratory syncytial virus, which is known to induce severe apnea during sleep? Other viruses?);
4. a laryngospasm of unclear origin that could be associated with esophageal reflux [60]. The relationship between esophageal reflux and central, mixed, and obstructive sleep apnea is unknown. Although reflux during sleep apnea has been monitored objectively, it is possible that an obstructive event triggered the reflux [61]. Without simultaneous measurement of airflow, however, this possibility cannot be investigated.

Obviously, a combination of the factors outlined above may induce long sleep apneas that eventually become mixed or obstructive events. A mild occlusion, in conjunction with a cold, viral infection, and swelling of the mucous membranes, for example, may cause an obstructive apnea that in turn induces esophageal reflux [61].

It is important to emphasize that apneic events of similar duration can have different effects. Central apneic events often induce milder oxygen desaturation than mixed or obstructive events of equal duration [49]. We also have noted that bradycardia and other cardiac arrhythmias appear more quickly with obstructive than with central apnea. This may be related to major changes in the autonomic nervous system induced by the repetitive Muller and Valsalva maneuvers in the obstructive portion of an apnea.

Siblings of SIDS Victims

In systematic longitudinal studies of respiration in subsequent siblings of SIDS victims, Hoppenbrouwers et al. [62] found that, unlike near miss

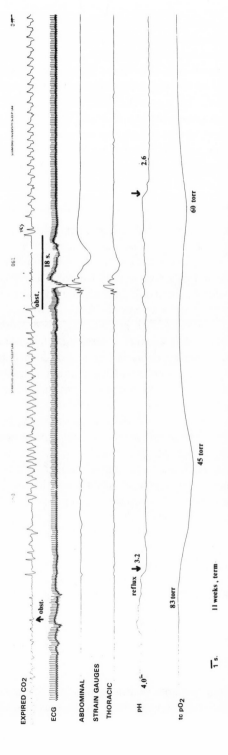

FIGURE 5.8. Polygraphic monitoring performed during NREM sleep in a male nine-week-old, near miss SIDS infant. During the obstructive event, which develops first, the struggle to clear the obstruction increases transdiaphragmatic pressure sufficient to force open the lower esophageal sphincter and induce a reflux.

SIDS infants, these subjects had a higher respiratory rate in early infancy along with fewer short breathing pauses, similar to normal controls. On the basis of this finding, the authors hypothesized that the mild tachypnea noted indicated a relative lack of oxygen. Kelly et al., [63] on the other hand, found an increase in periodic breathing and short central apnea. Neither team found very long apneic events, regardless of their type, or severe cardiac arrhythmias with post neonatal apnea. Perhaps the small number of siblings considered and the analysis performed, which combined only individuals without focusing on subgroups and specific outlayers, precluded any very significant findings.

Termination of the Apnea and the Arousal Response

From normative data, it appears that apneas during sleep are common but that these events are short and terminate quickly. If apneas are prolonged, specific defense mechanisms must be triggered to enhance ventilation. Arousal is, as Phillipson and Sullivan emphasized, a strong ventilatory defense mechanism during sleep [64]. It enables the vital organs under the control of the autonomic nervous system to adapt when they are challenged by abnormal conditions. Phillipson et al. [65–67] showed in dogs that the arousal response to hypoxia, hypercapnia, nasal occlusion, and laryngeal stimulation is more depressed in REM sleep than in NREM sleep, and that a depressed arousal response, which is easily induced by nonventilatory manipulations such as sleep fragmentation, leads to abnormal ventilatory responses. It has been suggested that there is an impaired or depressed arousal response during sleep in infants with long apneic events. In an analysis of the distribution of apneas during sleep, we found that apneas tended to cluster before a final arousal in near miss SIDS infants (Figure 5.9). Apneas were also more frequent during longer sleep periods [16]. When one considers indices of arousal (Figure 5.10), such as body movements and number of sleep stage changes [68], near miss SIDS infants have fewer, although they often have more instances of apnea. Challamel et al. [69] and Hoppenbrouwers et al. [70] also noted this phenomenon in near miss SIDS infants. Ariagno et al. [71], studying the arousal response to ventilatory challenges during sleep, found that some near miss infants had delayed arousal without periodic breathing when presented with a hypoxia challenge, particulary during NREM sleep whereas controls had a shorter arousal response frequently preceded by periodic breathing. Shannon et al. [72] demonstrated that near miss SIDS infants had a diminished hypercarbic ventilatory response; Hunt et al. [73, 74] not only confirmed their results but also found that near miss SIDS infants have a deficient hypoxic ventilatory sensitivity.

It appears, then, that infants with long apneic episodes during sleep have a decrease in arousal response during sleep. This could be a factor in the persistence of apnea once it has begun. This decrease in arousal response could be secondary to external challenges. As indicated earlier, sleep fragmentation in dogs [75] and sleep deprivation in humans [76] can increase the duration of apnea and decrease the arousal response. Minor "colds" in infants with polygraphically-documented long apneas during sleep may induce sleep fragmentation and deprivation, and some near miss infants are reported to have a "cold" or runny nose just prior to their near miss event. An abnormally small hypopharynx also may have an impact on the ventilatory response to hypoxia, hypercapnia, and arousal; this can be seen in adult subjects with obstructive sleep apnea syndrome who have had tracheostomy [77] or in subjects with mandibular malformation who have had maxillomandibular surgery (Guilleminault, unpublished observation 1985). From these observations, it follows that postnatal apneas may lengthen in duration in the presence of a mild anatomical abnormality of the hypopharynx and a progressive decrease in arousal response. The condition could develop because a mild upper airway anatomical abnormality required increased diaphragmatic effort to maintain airway patency. Airway patency would be further compromised during sleep, particularly during REM sleep because of the atonia of the genioglossus and other muscles of the pharyngeal region. The change of air flow in the upper airway and the various stimulations induced by the respiratory load (which was created by the mild anatomical abnormality) would feed back to the central control of breathing, resulting in a decreased response to hypoxia and hypercapnia. (This occurs in adult patients with obstructive sleep apnea who have a mandibular malformation or a small oropharynx [77].) The decreased response can be accentuated by genetically determined ventilatory responses to hypoxia and hypercapnia so that the apneas will lengthen. Apneas also can be increased by external factors such as a cold that fragments sleep and modifies the apnea by enlarging upper airway mucosa or lymphoid tissues. Some of these speculations are supported by observations made on infants, children, and adults with Obstructive Sleep Apnea Syndrome (OSAS) before and after treatment. In summary, regardless of the factors involved, infants may have a decreased arousal response that prolongs the duration of apneas during sleep.

Are Postnatal Apneas Involved in SIDS?

Whether postnatal apneas are involved in SIDS is a controversial issue. Currently, one may say that long apneic events have occurred during sleep in infants who eventually became SIDS victims. These long apneas are associated with hypoxia, which may further decrease the arousal response and the control of ventilation. Mixed and obstructive events have been observed with bradycardia and cardiac arrhythmias, particularly sinus arrest.

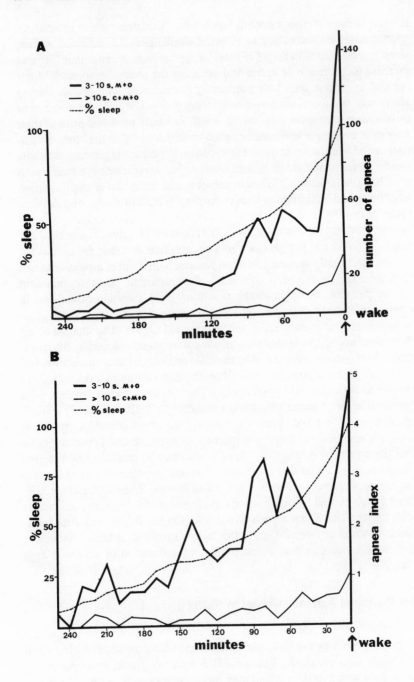

FIGURE 5.9. *(opposite page)* Apnea frequency and arousals. (A) Number of mixed and obstructive apneic events lasting from three to ten seconds and pauses of any type lasting for more than ten seconds for each ten-minute segment of sleep before wake are presented. Percent sleep time in each segment is plotted for reference. Sleep in 194 sleep periods recorded for twenty-three infants within two weeks of a near miss event is presented with respect to terminating wake. Scale on left refers to percent sleep, scale on right refers to number of apneic events, and scale at base of figure refers to time in ten-minute intervals. (B) To correct for difference in amount of sleep time in each segment, the apnea index ([total apnea divided by total sleep time in minutes] multiplied by 60) calculated from data presented in A, with sleep as a function of time before awakenings is presented. Apnea index for mixed and obstructive events lasting longer than ten seconds is calculated for ten-minute intervals before waking. Scales are same as in A. As seen clearly in A and B, mixed and obstructive pauses and pauses lasting longer than ten seconds are not distributed evenly with respect to sleep, and they increase sharply in the last ten minutes before awakening. As a test for significance, each infant's apnea index for pauses of both types within ten seconds of any scored wake was compared to his or her index for remaining sleep, using matched pairs t test. Difference is significant at P = 0.01 level [38].

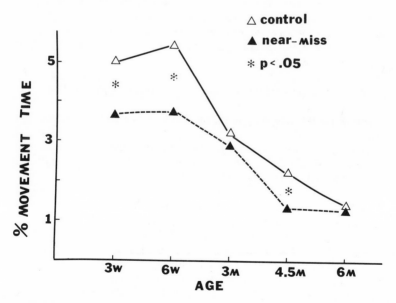

FIGURE 5.10.
Movement time, defined as an abrupt increase in tonic muscle tone with artifacts appearing in other polygraphic channels, is an index of arousal during sleep. Near miss SIDS infants have less movement time than normals, regardless of the age at which the near miss SIDS event occurs [68].

Long postnatal apneas thus represent a risk factor. The combination of elements that contribute to the appearance of apnea during sleep also may dampen the arousal response, the defense mechanism against this risk factor. Postnatal apnea induces desaturation, which further depresses the control of breathing. Theoretically, therefore, the presence of long postnatal apnea, which indicates an existing dysfunction of air exchange during sleep, also could indicate the possibility of further abrupt cardiorespiratory decompensation, but the studies performed to date have only identified risk factors.

References

1. Steinschneider, A. 1972. Prolonged sleep apnea and the SIDS: Clinical and laboratory observation. *Pediatrics* 50:646–654.
2. Guilleminault, C., W.C. Dement, R. Wilson, and V. Zarcone. 1972. "Respiration problems and sleep disorders." (abstract) In *Sleep Research,* ed. M.H. Chase, W.C. Stern, and P.L. Walter.
3. Guilleminault, C., W.C. Dement, and N. Monod. 1973. Syndrome mort subite du nourrisson: apnees au cours du sommeil. *Nouvelle Presse Medicale* 2:1355–1358.
4. Beckwith, J.B. 1970. "Observations of the pathological anatomy of the sudden infant death syndrome." In *Sudden Infant Death Syndrome: Proceedings of the Second International Conference on Causes of Sudden Death of Infants,* ed. A.B. Bergman, J.B. Beckwith, and C.G. Ray. Seattle: University of Washington Press.
5. Naeye, R.L. 1974. SIDS: "Evidences of antecedent chronic hypoxia and hypoxemia." In *SIDS 1972,* ed. R.R. Robinson. Toronto: Canadian Foundation for the Study of Infant Deaths.
6. Naeye, R.L. 1974. Hypoxemia and the Sudden Infant Death Syndrome. *Science* 186:837–838.
7. Beckwith, J.B. 1983. "Chronic hypoxemia in the sudden infant death syndrome." In *Sudden Infant Death Syndrome,* ed. J.T. Tildon, L.M. Roeder, and A. Steinschneider. New York: Academic Press.
8. Cole, S., L.B. Lindenberg, F.M. Galioto, Jr., P.E. Howe, A.C. DeGraff, J.M. Davis, R. Lubka, and E.M. Gross. 1979. Ultrastructural abnormalities of the carotid body in sudden infant death syndrome. *Pediatrics* 63: 13–17.
9. Naeye, R.L., R. Fisher, M. Ryser, and P. Whalen. 1976. Carotid body in sudden infant death syndrome. *Science* 191:567–569.
10. Guntheroth, W.G. 1963. Comments in *Sudden Death in Infants,* ed. by R.J. Wedgwood and E.P. Benditt. Bethesda, Md.: U.S. Department of Health, Education and Welfare.
11. Bergman, A.B., C.G. Ray, M.A. Pomeroy, P.W. Wahl, and J.B. Beckwith. 1972. Studies of the sudden infant death syndrome in King County, Washington. III. Epidemiology. *Pediatrics* 49:860–870.
12. Guilleminault, C., R.L. Ariagno, L.S. Forno, L. Nagel, R. Baldwin, and

M. Owen. 1979. Obstructive sleep and near miss for SIDS. I. Report of an infant with sudden death. *Pediatrics* 63:837–843.

13. Thoman, E.B., M.P. Feese, P.T. Becker, C. Acedbo, V.N. Morin, and W.D. Tynan. 1978. Sex differences in the ontogeny of sleep apnea during the first year of life. *Physiolog Behav* 20:699–707.

14. Hoppenbrouwers, T., J.E. Hodgman, R.M. Harper, and M.B. Sterman. 1980. Respiration during the first six months of life in normal infants. IV. Gender differences. *Early Hum Dev* 4:167–177.

15. Hoppenbrouwers, T. 1982. "Electronic monitoring in the newborn and young infant: Theoretical consideration." In *Sleeping and Waking Disorders: Indications and Techniques*, ed. C. Guilleminault. Menlo Park: Addison-Wesley Publishing Co.

16. Guilleminault, C., R. Ariagno, R. Korobkin, L. Nagel, R. Baldwin, S. Coons, and M. Owen. 1979. Mixed and obstructive sleep apnea and near miss for sudden infant death syndrome: 2. Comparison of near miss and normal control infants by age. *Pediatrics* 64:882–891.

17. Hoppenbrouwers, T., J.E. Hodgman, R.M. Harper, E. Hofmann, M.B. Sterman, and D.J. McGinty. 1977. Polygraphic studies of normal infants during the first six months of life. III. Incidence of apnea and periodic breathing. *Pediatrics* 60:418–425.

18. Hoppenbrouwers, T., J.E. Hodgman, K. Arakawa, R. Harper, and M.B. Sterman. 1980. Respiration during the first six months of life in normal infants. III. Computer identification of breathing pauses. *Pediatr Res* 14:1230–1233.

19. Kelly, D.H., and D.C. Shannon. 1979. Periodic breathing in infants with near-miss sudden infant death syndrome. *Pediatrics* 63:355–358.

20. Coup, A., D. Coup, S.T. Wealthall, and S. Withy. 1983 "The development and abnormalities of breathing patterns." In *Sudden Infant Death Syndrome*, ed. J.T. Tildon, L.M Roeder, and A. Steinschneider. New York: Academic Press.

21. Beal, S. 1984. In *Summary and Recommendations of a Workshop on Post-Neonatal Mortality and Cot Death*, ed. P.D. Gluckman. Auckland, New Zealand: Public Health Service.

22. Orr, W.C., M.L. Stahl, J. Duke, M.A. McCaffree, P. Toubas, C. Mattice, and H.F. Krous. 1985. The effect of sleep state and position on the incidence of apnea in infants. *Pediatrics* 75:832–835.

23. Martin, R.J., A. Okken, and D. Rubin. 1979. Arterial oxygen tension during active and quiet sleep in the normal neonate. *Pediatrics* 94: 271–274.

24. Martin, R.J., N. Herrell, and M. Pultusker. 1981. Transcutaneous measurement of carbon dioxide tension: Effect of sleep state in term infants. *Pediatrics* 67:622–625.

25. Hanson, N., and A. Okken. 1980. Transcutaneous oxygen tension of newborn infants in different behavioral states. *Pediatr Res* 14:911–915.

26. Gould, J.B., A.F.S. Lee, O. James, L. Sander, H. Teger, and N. Fineberg. 1976. The sleep state characteristics of apnea during infancy. *Pediatrics* 59: 182–194.

27. Guilleminault, C., M.W. Hill, F.B. Simmons, and W.C. Dement. 1978.

Obstructive sleep apnea: Electromyographic and fiberoptic studies. *Exp Neurol* 62:48–67.

28. Onal, E., M. Lopata, and T.D. O'Connor. 1982. Pathogenesis of apneas in hypersomnia-sleep apnea syndrome. *Am Rev Respir Dis* 125:167–174.

29. Guilleminault, C. 1984. Diagnosis, pathogenesis, and treatment of the sleep apnea syndromes. *Review of Internal Medicine and Pediatrics*. Berlin: Springer-Verlag.

30. Guilleminault, C., and R.L. Ariagno. 1978. Why should we study the infant "near-miss for sudden infant death?" *Early Hum Dev* 2(3):207–218.

31. Thach, B.T., and A.R. Stark. 1979. Spontaneous neck flexion and airway obstruction during apneic spells in preterm infants. *J Pediatr* 94:275–281.

32. Parmelee, A.H., E. Stern, and M.A. Harris. 1972. Maturation of respiration in prematures and young infants. *Neuropaediatrie* 3:294–304.

33. Waggener, T.B., I.D. Frantz, A.R. Stark, and R.E. Kronauer. 1982. Oscillatory breathing patterns leading to apneic spells in infants. *J Appl Physiol: Respir, Environ Exercise Physiol* 52:1288–1295.

34. Steinschneider, A., and D.D. Rabrizzi. 1976. Apnea and airway obstruction during feeding and sleep. *Laryngoscope* 86:1359–1366.

35. Steinschneider, A., S.L. Weinstein, and E. Diamond. 1982. The sudden infant death syndrome and apnea/obstruction during neonatal sleep and feeding. *Pediatrics* 70:858–863.

36. Johnson, P., and D.M. Salisbury. 1975. "Sucking and breathing during artificial feeding in the human neonate." In *Symposium on Development of Upper Respiratory Anatomy and Function*, ed. J.F. Bosma and J. Showacre. Washington, D.C.: U.S. Government Printing Office.

37. Mathew, O.P., M.L. Clark, M.H. Pronske, H.G. Luna-Solarzano, and M.D. Peterson. 1985. Breathing pattern and ventilation during feeding in term infants. *J Pediatr* 106:810–813.

38. Guilleminault, C., R. Ariagno, R. Korobkin, S. Coons, M. Owen-Boeddiker, and R. Baldwin. 1981. Sleep parameters and respiratory variables in "near-miss" sudden infant death syndrome infants. *Pediatrics* 68:354–360.

39. Shannon, D.C., D.W. Marsland, J.B. Gould, B. Callahan, I.D. Todres, and J. Dennis. 1976. Central hypoventilation during quiet sleep in two infants. *Pediatrics* 57:342–346.

40. Armstrong, D., P. Sachis, C. Bryan, and L. Becker. 1982. Pathological features of persistent infantile sleep apnea with reference to the pathology of sudden infant death syndrome. *Ann Neurol* 12:169–174.

41. Guilleminault, C., J. McQuitty, R.L. Ariagno, M.J. Challamel, and R. Korobkin. 1982. Six infants with congenital alveolar hypoventilation syndrome. *Pediatrics* 70:684–694.

42. Le Drouarin, N. 1978. "The neural crest in the neck and other parts of the body. Morphogenesis and malformations of face and brain." In *Birth Defects*, ed. D. Bergsma. New York: National Foundation of the March of Dimes.

43. Bolande, R.P. 1974. The neurocristopathies. *Hum Pathol* 5(4):409–429.

44. Couly, G., and C. Le Lievre-Ayer. 1983. La crete neurale cephalique et les malformations cervico-faciales humaines. *La Revue De Pediatrie* 9:5–20.

45. Kelly, D.H., and D.C. Shannon. 1981. Episodic complete airway obstruction in infants. *Pediatrics* 67:823–827.

46. Kahn, A., D. Blum, P. Waterschoot, E. Engelman, and P. Smets. 1982. Effects of obstructive sleep apneas on transcutaneous oxygen pressure in control infants, siblings of sudden infant death syndrome victims, and near miss infants: Comparison with the effects of central sleep apneas. *Pediatrics* 70:852–857.

47. Tonkin, S.L., J. Partridge, D. Beach, and S. Whiteney. 1979. The pharyngeal effect of partial nasal obstruction. *Pediatrics* 63:261–271.

48. Steinschneider, A. 1975. Nasopharyngitis and prolonged sleep apnea. *Pediatrics* 56:967–971.

49. Guilleminault, C., R. Peraita, M. Souquet, and W.C. Dement. 1975. Apneas during sleep in infants: Possible relationship with sudden infant death syndrome. *Science* 190:677–679.

50. Guilleminault, C., R. Ariagno, S. Coons, R. Winkle, R. Korobkin, and M. Souquet. 1985. Long-term follow up of eight near miss SIDS infants with cardiac arrhythmias during sleep. *Pediatrics* 76:236–242.

51. Korobkin, R., and C. Guilleminault. 1979. Neurologic abnormalities in near miss for sudden infant death syndrome infants. *Pediatrics* 64:369–374.

52. Guilleminault, C., M. Souquet, R.L Ariagno, R. Korobkin, and F.B. Simmons. 1984. Five cases of near miss sudden infant death syndrome and development of obstructive sleep apnea syndrome. *Pediatrics* 73:71–78.

53. Riley, R., C. Guilleminault, J. Herran, and N. Powell. 1983. Cephalometric analyses and flow volume loops in obstructive sleep apnea patients. *Sleep* 6:304–317.

54. Guilleminault, C., G. Heldt, N. Powell, and R. Riley. 1986. Small upper airway in near-miss sudden infant death syndrome infants and their families. *Lancet* 1:402–407.

55. Herbst, J.J., L.S. Book, and P.T. Bray. 1978. Gastroesophageal reflux in near miss sudden infant death syndrome. *J Pediatr* 92:73–75.

56. Leape, L.L., T.M. Holder, J.D. Franklin, R.A. Amoury, and R.W. Ashcraft, 1977. Respiratory arrest in infants secondary to gastroesophageal reflux. *Pediatrics* 60:924–927.

57. Jeffrey, H.E., I. Reid, P. Rohilly, and D.J.C. Read. 1980. Gastroesophageal reflux in near miss sudden infant death infants in active but not quiet sleep. *Sleep* 3:393–399.

58. Walsh, J.K., M.L. Farrell, W.G. Keenan, M. Lucas, and M. Dramer. 1981. Gastroesophageal reflux in infants: Relation to apnea. *J Pediatr* 99:197–201.

59. Ariagno, R.L., C. Guilleminault, R. Baldwin, and M. Owen-Boeddiker. 1982. Gastroesophageal reflux and apnea in full term "near miss" SIDS infants. *J Pediatr* 100:894–897.

60. Downing, S.E., and J.C. Lee. 1975. Laryngeal chemosensitivity. A possible mechanism for sudden infant death. *Pediatrics* 55:640–646.

61. Guilleminault, C. 1984. The uvula and sudden infant death syndrome. *Pediatrics* 71:319–320.

62. Hoppenbrouwers, T., J.E. Hodgman, D. McGinty, R.M. Harper, and M.B. Sterman. 1980. Sudden infant death syndrome: Sleep apnea and respiration in subsequent siblings. *Pediatrics* 66:205–214.

63. Kelly, D.H., A.M. Walker, L. Cahen, and D.C. Shannon. 1980. Periodic

breathing in siblings of sudden infant death syndrome victims. *Pediatrics* 66:515–520.

64. Phillipson, E.A., and C.E. Sullivan. 1978. Arousal: The forgotten response to respiratory stimuli. *Am Rev Respir Dis* 118:807–809.

65. Phillipson, E.A., C.E. Sullivan, D.J.C. Read, E. Murphy, and L.F. Kozar. 1978. Ventilatory and waking responses to hypoxia in sleeping dogs. *J Appl Physiol* 44:512–520.

66. Phillipson, E.A., L.F. Kozar, A.S. Rebuck, and E. Murphy. 1977. Ventilatory and waking responses to CO_2 in sleeping dogs. *Am Rev Respir Dis* 115:251–259.

67. Sullivan, C.E., E. Murphy, L.F. Kozar, and E.A. Phillipson. 1978. Waking and ventilatory responses to laryngeal stimulation in sleeping dogs. *J Appl Physiol* 45:681–689.

68. Coons, S., and C. Guilleminault. 1985. Motility and arousal in near-miss for SIDS infants. *J Pediatr* 107:725–732.

69. Challamel, M.J., M. Revol, C. Leszczynski, and G. Debilly. 1981. In *Progres en Neonatologies,* ed. A. Minkowski and J.P. Ralier. Basel: S. Karger.

70. Hoppenbrouwers, T., J.E. Hodgman, K. Arakawa, D.J. McGinty, J. Mason, R.M. Harper, and M.B. Sterman. 1978. Sleep apnea as part of a sequence of events: A comparison of three months old infants at low and increased risk for sudden infant death syndrome (SIDS). *Neuropaediatrie* 9:320–337.

71. Ariagno, R., L. Nagel, and C. Guilleminault. 1980. Waking and ventilatory responses in near-miss for SIDS infants during sleep. *Sleep* 3:351–359.

72. Shannon, D., D.H. Kelly, and K. O'Connel. 1977. Abnormal regulation of ventilations in infants at risk for sudden infant death syndrome. *N Engl J Med* 297:747–750.

73. Hunt, C.E., K. McCulloch, and R.T. Brouillette. 1981. Diminished hypoxic ventilatory responses in near-miss sudden infant death syndrome. *American Physiological Society* 50:1313–1317.

74. McCulloch, K., R.T. Brouillette, A.J. Guzzetta, and C.E. Hunt. 1982. Arousal responses in near-miss sudden infant death syndrome and in normal infants. *J Pediatr* 101(6):911–917.

75. Bowes, G., G.M. Woolf, and C.E. Sullivan. 1980. Effect of sleep fragmentation on ventilatory and arousal responses of sleeping dogs to respiratory stimuli. *Am Rev Respir Dis* 122:899–908.

76. Guilleminault, C., and M. Rosekind. 1981. The arousal threshold: Control of ventilation and sleep apnea. *Clin Respir Physiol* 17:341–349.

77. Guilleminault, C., and J. Cummiskey. 1982. Progressive improvement of apnea and ventilatory response to CO_2 following tracheostomy in obstructive apnea syndrome. *Am Rev Respir Dis* 126:14–20.

6

The Cardiac Theory and Sudden Infant Death Syndrome

PETER J. SCHWARTZ, M.D.

The interest in the role of a cardiac mechanism in sudden infant death syndrome (SIDS) has been kept alive more because of the repeated disillusionment with other theories than because of an actual widespread belief in this possibility. Among the many intriguing aspects of the tragic and puzzling problem of SIDS is the amazing mixture of hard and soft science as evidenced by any critical review of the published studies. This may be due partially to the involvement of investigators with diverse backgrounds so that the interested audience often does not have the expertise necessary to recognize a study's potential weaknesses and to identify its erroneous conclusions. This generalization is particularly valid regarding the role of cardiac mechanisms in SIDS, largely because there are few cardiologists and cardiovascular physiologists involved in SIDS research.

This chapter (1) reviews the cardiac theory and, in more detail, the specific hypothesis proposed years ago [1]; (2) presents data from the related and ongoing Milan prospective study; and (3) analyzes the various arguments generally used against this hypothesis.

The Cardiac Theory

The cardiac theory had its origin in the late sixties [2] in connection with an after dinner conversation between Froggatt and Ward [3], a letter to *The Lancet* by Fraser and Froggatt [4], and an article by James in 1968 [5]. What Froggatt and Ward realized, considering the variety of more or less extravagant theories of causation of SIDS, was that no one had addressed the possibility that the heart would simply stop beating. Subsequently, Fraser and Froggatt suggested that disorders of cardiac conduction might be involved in some sudden unexplained deaths in infancy. James proposed that malignant arrhythmias or conduction disturbances might represent the final common pathway for SIDS. This suggestion was based largely on his finding that reabsorptive degeneration was present in the conduction system of SIDS infants and infants who died of known causes, but was not present in stillborn infants at term or in adults. James' conclusions have been questioned by Valdes-Dapena et al. [6], Anderson et al. [7], and Lie et al. [8].

Recently Marino and Kane [9] reported on abnormalities found in the conduction system of some infants who died suddenly. Among seven victims, two had an accessory pathway and four had persistent fetal dispersion of the atrioventricular (AV) node. In an editorial comment on this article, James noted that "since the evidence of Marino and Kane strongly supports the cardiac hypothesis, it is surprising for them to state in their discussion that the majority of crib deaths are from primary apnea" [10].

Marino and Kane's findings support the cardiac theory, but only up to a point. The presence of accessory pathways (which they considered the strongest finding) provides one possibility, but a postmortem study cannot reveal whether that accessory pathway was functionally active and, moreover, there can be no evidence that an arrhythmia dependent on pre-excitation was the cause of death. The lack of adequate numbers of pathologic studies in controls (age-matched infants who died of known causes) severely limits the inferences that can be made by sporadic observations in infants who died suddenly. On the other hand, the most serious criticism of these studies is the fact that the absence of abnormalities in the conduction system does not argue necessarily against sudden cardiac death. Indeed, if ventricular fibrillation is the cause of death, no abnormalities will be found at postmortem examination, as is the case with the long QT syndrome and with the majority of deaths due to a sudden and documented arrhythmia.

Several years elapsed before the cardiac theory was proposed on more solid grounds [1, 11, 12]. In their paper, outstanding for its lucid and cogent analysis, Froggatt and James examined, as a general theory of causation, the possibility that SIDS victims die of lethal arrhythmias produced by a disturbance in the normal electrical activity of the heart [11]. They concluded that the cardiac hypothesis is no less likely than others that ascribed SIDS to respiratory causes. It is fair to note that sudden cardiac death is the single leading cause of mortality in the western world [13]. The emphasis in the Froggatt and James Paper [11] was that a primary cardiac death is possible in SIDS; my work stressed how developmental abnormalities in the cardiac sympathetic innervation may favor the onset of lethal arrhythmias and may become manifest before any symptom, thus allowing early identification of some of the babies at risk [1, 2, 14]. These concepts are based on the understanding of the pathogenetic mechanisms of the congenital long QT syndrome, the most intriguing example of neurally mediated non-coronary sudden death occurring in apparently healthy individuals [15]. The current knowledge on the long QT syndrome is summarized in the following paragraphs.

The Long QT Syndrome

The idiopathic long QT syndrome (LQTS) [16, 17] is characterized by prolongation of the QT interval, sporadic alternation of the T wave [18], and syncopal episodes due to "torsades-de-pointe," a type of ventricular tachyarrhythmia with a high tendency to deteriorate into fibrillation. These syncopal episodes eventually result in the sudden death of quite a large portion of affected individuals. In a few cases, death occurs during the first attack, but more often it is preceded by several syncopal episodes. It is important to know that "torsades-de-pointe" is often self-terminating; the manifestations of these episodes depend on their duration and on their hemodynamic consequences. If the patient is not standing and can therefore better cope with the transient fall in arterial blood pressure without ECG monitoring, some of these episodes will be completely unnoticed, and yet they all are very close to sudden death (Figure 6.1).

Initially, LQTS was considered a typical hereditary disease but, with time, this notion has changed. Data on almost 800 patients show that a large portion of these cases have no familial involvement; most cases are sporadic. These data further imply that if a patient with the sporadic type of LQTS dies suddenly and does not have a prior ECG, the correct diagnosis may never be made because the QT interval of parents and siblings may be normal.

In LQTS, the syncopal episodes usually are induced by emotional or physical stress, conditions in which sympathetic activity increases suddenly. On the basis of clinical and experimental evidence, Schwartz et al. proposed that the basic defect in LQTS is a congenital lower-than-normal right cardiac sympathetic activity, which results reflexly in an imbalance with dominant sympathetic nerves on the left side [16]. They also proposed that the syncopal episodes were the consequence of bursts of sympathetic activity mostly dependent on the dominant left stellate ganglion [16]. In support of this view, separate studies found that ablation of the right stellate ganglion (right stellectomy) or stimulation of the left stellate ganglion reproduced the electrocardiographic characteristics of LQTS— lengthening of the QT interval [19] and alternation of the T wave [18]. Right stellectomy, which reflexly augments left-sided cardiac sympathetic activity [20], increases the incidence of life-threatening arrhythmias during acute myocardial ischemia [21], exercise [22, 23], and emotional stress [24], and increases ventricular excitability [25]. Furthermore, right stellectomy lowers the threshold for ventricular fibrillation, (i.e., increases the ventricular vulnerability to fibrillation [26]. LQTS patients often have a lower-than-normal heart rate and a decreased capability to increase it during exercise. These observations can be explained by lower-than-normal right cardiac sympathetic activity because sympathetic control of the heart rate is exerted primarily through the right stellate ganglion

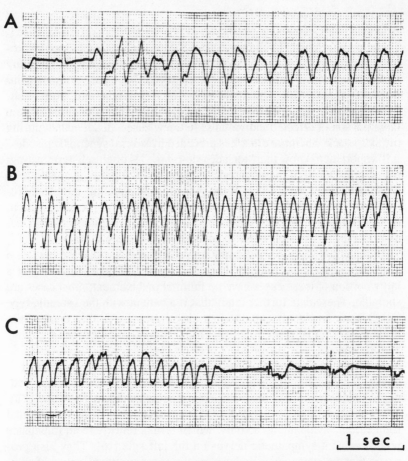

FIGURE 6.1. R.C. five years. Patient affected by the idiopathic long QT Syndrome. The three tracings show the beginning, the intermediate phase and the spontaneous termination of an episode of "torsades-de-pointe" which lasted more than 30 seconds. The episode occurred while the patient was lying in her bed, and there was no obvious external sign of what was happening. This patient, who continued to have frequent syncopal attacks despite full dose beta blockers, underwent left stellectomy in 1978 and remained free from syncopal episodes until the summer of 1982.

[22, 27, 28]. Finally, analysis of body surface isopotential maps in LQTS patients also provided findings that fit with a lower-than-normal right cardiac sympathetic activity [29]. The tight relationship between the autonomic nervous system and sudden cardiac death and the high arrhythmogenic potential of sympathetic imbalance is reviewed in detail elsewhere [20, 30].

The pathogenetic hypothesis of a congenital sympathetic imbalance with left-sided dominance implies a protective effect of either beta adrenergic blocking agents or left stellectomy. The major antiarrhythmic and antifibrillatory effect of left stellectomy has been demonstrated [31, 32]. Updated information on almost 800 LQTS patients indicates that the extremely high mortality (71 percent) of untreated patients was dramatically reduced by either beta-blocking agents (6 percent) or by left stellectomy (6 percent) [17]. Furthermore, the two therapies combined provide additional protection [33]. Thus, understanding the pathogenetic mechanism of LQTS has guided a therapeutic approach that has radically changed the prognosis of the affected patients.

The "Sympathetic Imbalance" Hypothesis

In 1976, I suggested that some developmental aspects of cardiac innervation were related to sudden death during infancy [1]. Subsequently, one aspect of this hypothesis was taken to represent the entire proposal, and it became known as the "QT hypothesis" [2].

The background of this hypothesis lies in the pathogenetic mechanisms of the long QT syndrome, as discussed earlier, and in the strong relationship between the autonomic nervous system and sudden death [30]. Basically, the proposal was that *some* SIDS deaths depend on ventricular fibrillation that is induced by a sudden increase in sympathetic activity affecting a heart with a decreased electrical stability. The specific mechanism proposed was an imbalance between right and left cardiac sympathetic nerves, resulting in a left-sided dominance. This type of imbalance is quite arrhythmogenic and often manifests with a prolongation of the QT interval [18]. The latter has been recognized as being associated with a particularly high risk for sudden death under a variety of circumstances [34, 35].

The cardiac sympathetic imbalance may occur either as a congenital event, in which case it would remain unmodified over time, or as a developmental phenomenon, in which case it would be modified by the progression of time. The latter would be a transient sympathetic imbalance.

Some SIDS cases may represent the hereditary type of the long QT syndrome. This has indeed occurred a number of times, but I have never thought nor proposed that this possibility might account for more than a few SIDS cases. Nonetheless, it has been almost exclusively in this diminutive way that this hypothesis has been discussed in the literature.

The distribution of right and left cardiac sympathetic nerves is likely to be symmetrical and homogeneous in most infants; however, as is true for most biological phenomena, this distribution probably will follow the Gaussian, or normal, curve. This implies that a few infants will have to be at the extremes of the curve. Those with the lowest level of right-sided sympathetic activity would be the infants at the greatest risk for life-threatening arrhythmias and sudden death. They are likely to show either a constant prolongation of the QT interval or a paroxysmal prolongation during increases in sympathetic activity. Some of these infants who escape SIDS may later be identified as affected by the sporadic type of the long QT syndrome. This condition also may result in a number of stillbirths and/or late abortions.

The sympathetic innervation of the heart becomes functionally complete by approximately the sixth month of life [2]. The right and left sympathetic neural pathways occasionally may develop at different rates. When this occurs, a delay in the right side or an acceleration in the left may lead to a *temporary* imbalance of the harmful type described earlier. A sudden increase in sympathetic activity, elicited by whatever cause, may easily trigger ventricular tachyarrhythmias in these electrically unstable hearts and precipitate sudden death. The possibility of a *time-limited* imbalance in the cardiac sympathetic innervation implies that these infants would be at high risk for SIDS, but for a limited period of time. Therefore, if they survive the high risk period, they may have a completely normal life.

Of these three possible mechanisms of imbalance in the cardiac sympathetic innervation, the latter two have several intriguing implications. The more obvious marker for this type of imbalance would be a prolongation of the QT interval in the standard ECG, evident sometimes after birth. Other markers may be a lower-than-normal heart rate or unusually long pauses in sinus rhythm. If the sympathetic imbalance hypothesis is correct, these markers would allow the early identification of some future SIDS victims. The practical implications are self evident; because these infants would be at risk of dying because of a sympathetic discharge affecting their electrically unstable hearts, effective protection could be conferred by administering a beta adrenergic blocking agent for a 7- to 8-month period.

In the "sympathetic imbalance" hypothesis, an important role is played by the trigger event: the sudden increase in sympathetic activity. It is interesting to note that most of the conditions that have been associated with SIDS by the epidemiologic studies also are associated with increased sympathetic activity. Among these conditions the following are briefly considered: sleep, winter months, lower socioeconomic class, apnea, and upper respiratory infections. During REM sleep there are bursts of sympathetic and vagal activity; furthermore, QT interval is longer during sleep than during wakefulness [36–38]. Exposure to cold and sudden noises increases sympathetic activity. These conditions are more often found in low-income families where heating is frequently inadequate and when overcrowded rooms facilitate high-pitched interactions and spread of infections. Abrupt transition between sleep and wakefulness may impair the electrical stability of the heart and favor even ventricular fibrillation in individuals prone to arrhythmias [39]. Also, sleep disruption causes dangerous rebounds in REM sleep. Apnea, thought by many to be an important cause for SIDS, induces hypoxia and elicits a chemoreceptive reflex by which *both* vagal and sympathetic activity are greatly increased. Upper respiratory infections often are associated with the common cold and attendant mucous formation, which may easily induce temporary yet total obstruction of airflow through the nostrils. This requires switching from nasal to oral respiration, a maneuver that newborns often are unable to perform, with resultant hypoxia [40, 41].

There is experimental evidence for developmental imbalance in the cardiac sympathetic innervation. Kralios and Millar [42] studied puppies of different age groups using electrical stimulation of the various cardiac nerves and measuring changes in ventricular refractoriness. They found a nonuniform maturation of cardiac nerves and, more specifically, observed that at the third week of life there is a predominance of left-sided nerves. This finding may provide the physiologic substrate for a time-limited decrease in cardiac electrical stability and may explain the temporary prolongation of the QT interval observed in normal infants [43].

The "sympathetic imbalance" hypothesis represents one specific aspect of a wider concept, that which implies a critical role *in some SIDS cases* for developmental abnormalities in cardiac innervation. These abnormalities may reduce the electrical stability of the heart, thus predisposing some infants to ventricular fibrillation. As an example, insufficient or delayed development of the vagal efferent activity with a lack of its protective effects may accentuate the arrhythmogenic potential of increases in sympathetic activity [44–46]. In this case, the markers of this kind of developmental sympathetic-parasympathetic imbalance may be a higher-than-normal heart rate or a reduced beat-to-beat variability.

The value of a scientific hypothesis is stimulation of research in new directions to provide confirmation or dismissal. The only way to test the "sympathetic imbalance" hypothesis is to organize a large prospective study in an *unselected population* of infants, with the goal of analyzing the QT interval and heart rate during the neonatal period and following all of these infants for the possible occurrence of SIDS.

The Milan Prospective Study

In 1976, we began to test the "sympathetic imbalance" hypothesis by obtaining electrocardiograms in an unselected population of newborns on the fourth day after birth and at the second, fourth, and sixth months of age [43]. All of these infants were followed prospectively for possible SIDS and, from 1982, those showing either cardiac arrhythmias or prolongation of the QT interval have entered a special program involving frequent examinations with 24-hour Holter monitoring. As of June 30, 1987, 13,500 nonconsecutive newborns were enrolled. The one-year survival data and QT measurements are now available for 10,000 infants; among them, there have been 10 SIDS cases. Four other infants born at the two participating hospitals died of SIDS; unfortunately, they were among infants not enrolled in the study for a variety of organizational reasons (holidays, etc.).

When infants are four days old, the QTc (QT interval corrected for heart rate) is 397 ± 18 msec (mean ± 1 SD). It increases significantly ($p < 0.0001$) to 409 ± 15 msec at the second month; at four months it is still at 406 ± 15 msec, and it returns to 400 ± 14 msec at six months of age (Figure 6.2). Whenever there is a trend, some individuals overshoot; in 3.6% of infants, QTc increased by more than 40 msec.

In addition to the 10 infants who died of SIDS, four infants died due to different causes. Whereas the four non-SIDS victims had a QTc well within the normal limits, six of ten SIDS victims had a prolonged QTc (defined as prolongation of the QTc by more than two standard deviations from the mean). If one considers the number of newborns with a prolonged QT interval, our data suggest that for these infants the risk for SIDS is approximately 30/1,000 live births [47]. If confirmed, this would become the single most important risk factor for SIDS.

Our data on the incidence and evolution of cardiac arrhythmias in infancy were reported elsewhere [48]. That study, together with the one by Southall et al., provided the largest data base on cardiac arrhythmias in an unselected population of newborns [49]. However, these studies do not illuminate the potential relationship between cardiac arrhythmias and SIDS. It is essential to realize that this relationship cannot be dismissed by the absence of arrhythmias in the ECG recordings of future SIDS victims because, as an example, most patients affected by the long QT syndrome are in regular sinus rhythm until the very moment of their syncopal episode due to an unheralded ventricular fibrillation.

The Milan prospective study demonstrated conclusively that QT interval lengthens *physiologically* and *temporarily* during the first few months of life. This indicates a trend, that in some infants may become excessive, toward a reduction of cardiac electrical stability that is simultaneous with the peak incidence of SIDS. Any viable hypothesis for SIDS must account for its characteristic age distribution, and our results prove that the sympathetic imbalance hypothesis is not in conflict with this epidemiologic characteristic. The small but growing number of SIDS victims in our prospective study for whom electrocardiographic data are available shows a remarkable finding. The presence of a clearly prolonged QT interval in six SIDS victims cannot be viewed as a chance event; on the other hand, it is too early to speculate on the percentage of SIDS victims in whom a QT prolongation can be expected. While more data are being accumulated, it seems fair to say that these results indicate that an unknown percentage (probably not less than 30 percent) of infants who subsequently become SIDS victims can be expected to have a prolonged QT interval on the

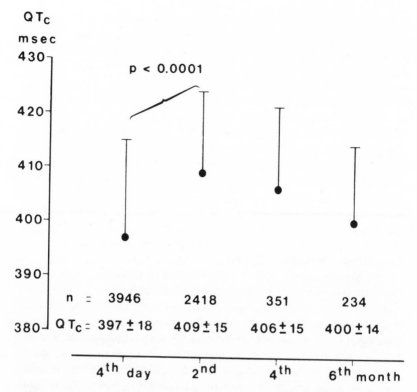

FIGURE 6.2. QT interval in healthy infants, corrected for heart rate, at age four days and two, four, and six months. The number of infants studied at each stage is shown. The bar represents 1 SD.

fourth day of life. Should this be confirmed, we would have a marker for truly high risk infants at last, and preventive measures could be implemented.

The QT Controversy

The hypothesis [1] that a number of SIDS cases may be due to a primary cardiac death favored by a developmental imbalance in the cardiac innervation (likely to be manifested by a prolongation of the QT interval) and precipitated by a sudden increase in sympathetic activity rapidly generated an unresolved controversy [50–59]. Many aspects of this controversy, and particularly the pathophysiologic aspects, have been analyzed in detail elsewhere [2, 14]. The more general points are discussed in the following paragraphs.

The sympathetic imbalance hypothesis has been interpreted as stating that SIDS victims are affected by the long QT syndrome. Moreover, it has been incorrectly assumed that LQTS is always hereditary. This has led some investigators to analyze the electrocardiograms of parents or siblings of SIDS victims with the incorrect implication that they would have found prolonged QT intervals if the sympathetic imbalance hypothesis were correct [50, 51]. Two studies of this kind have yielded opposite results; however, neither is very relevant to the hypothesis under discussion. Kukolich et al. found normal QT intervals among relatives of twenty-six SIDS victims [51]. The only legitimate conclusion from this study seems to be that these victims were unlikely to be affected by the hereditary type of LQTS, which leaves entirely unchallenged the other possibilities discussed earlier. One must remember that the number of sporadic cases of LQTS exceeds that of familial cases and no experienced cardiologist would rule out the diagnosis of LQTS because of a normal QT interval among the relatives of the patient. Therefore, negative findings in electrocardiographic studies performed in relatives of SIDS victims are not relevant to the "sympathetic imbalance" hypothesis.

The second major problem originates from the use of infants at "high risk" for SIDS to address the role of LQTS in SIDS. The most important category is, of course, that of the near miss infants. The subsequent occurrence of a sudden death in some of these infants (1.4 percent according to the largest review) [60] has led prematurely to the equation that near miss equals SIDS. Several caveats are appropriate. It is generally accepted that the near miss infants represent a mixed population, only part of which really had an unexplained episode of near death [61]. Moreover, a respiratory death is rather slow and allows time for struggle and cyanosis, whereas death by ventricular fibrillation is instantaneous and silent. A mother is more likely to observe her child dying a respiratory rather than a cardiac death, thereby allowing her to intervene and revive the infant with the end result of having created a new near miss case [62]. If indeed most true near miss infants would have died a respiratory death, it is not surprising that most studies of these infants found some respiratory abnormality. As a matter of fact, with the acceptance of the near miss infants as an integral part of SIDS, apnea became the focus of research. The near miss infants represent a subgroup at a somewhat higher risk for SIDS who may provide information highly relevant to the role of respiratory abnormalities in the genesis of some cases of SIDS, but they also may constitute a source of quite misleading information if acritically extrapolated to the entire SIDS problem [62]. More precisely, the examination of the near miss infants is unlikely to provide any information on those SIDS victims who die because of a primary cardiac death, and these findings should not be used to argue either against or in favor of the possibility of a cardiac mechanism in SIDS. Unfortunately, this has been done a number of times [52–55], providing little benefit and adding confusion to an already complex matter.

The criticism of *this use* of data collected in near miss infants applies also to studies performed in other high risk infants, such as the siblings of SIDS victims and premature infants. The main question is the real meaning of high risk. These groups seem to have an incidence of SIDS close to 0.5 percent [63], which, although double that for normal infants, is relatively low. Moreover, this implies that, with a 99 percent or 99.5 percent false positive rate, only five of every 1,000 infants studied actually would become SIDS victims. To study only thirty or fifty of these infants and then draw conclusions from the absence of a given variable is not scientifically sound. Such conclusions may mislead a gullible audience, but they have no bearing on the SIDS problem.

A couple of examples may clarify this point. In an article by the rather definitive title, "The role of the QT interval in the sudden infant death syndrome," Kelley et al. concluded that QT interval prolongation does not play a major role in SIDS [52]. They examined twenty-one near miss infants three of whom subsequently died of SIDS. The QT intervals of these infants were compared to those of forty-six controls and no differences were found. As discussed earlier, the normality of the ECG findings in eighteen near miss infants is not surprising because, given the low incidence of SIDS in this group, one would need four times as many infants (approximately seventy) to have a potential SIDS victim in that group. The only acceptable conclusion of that study is that three SIDS victims, who were likely to belong to the group with a respiratory death, had a seemingly normal QT interval.

More recently Montague et al. concluded that "marked cardiac dysrhythm and QT prolongation are not primary causes of SIDS" [55]. These investigators studied seventeen infants "at risk for SIDS" based upon their having an episode of unexplained apnea [13], being a subsequent sibling of a SIDS victim [5], or being a near miss infant [1]. Analysis of the QT interval and of body surface potential maps, when compared with seventeen control subjects, revealed that the QT interval was shorter in the at risk group. (This finding, which probably reflects augmented sympathetic tone, is likely to be the result of the greater stress generated in these infants by the very unusual handling most survivors of a near miss episode receive.) A negative finding in such a small group of infants with an average risk for SIDS of 1 percent (99 percent false positives) is of no value in assessing any hypothesis. There seems to be confusion on the issue of the totally different importance of positive and negative findings. The presence of a given factor or variable demonstrates that a given possibility is real and the question left is the rate of occurrence. The absence of such a variable indicates only that it is not present *in the population under study*, but no extrapolation can be made to a more general population, particularly when the event to be predicted (i.e., SIDS death) has a low incidence (0.2 percent). From the analysis just made, it should be clear that the only way to test the cardiac theory correctly and, specifically the sympathetic imbalance hypothesis, is, as indicated ten years ago [1], to perform a large prospective study on normal infants, wait for some SIDS deaths to occur, and then determine whether the victims were showing markers of cardiac electrical instability before death.

I am aware of only two attempts of this kind; one is the Milan prospective study already discussed, and the other is the study performed by Southall et al. in England [58, 59]. In one of these studies, the QT interval was measured from Holter recordings. Data interpretation is difficult with this type assessment because of the different frequency responses of the electrocardiographic amplifiers in the tape recorder; this tends to produce a lengthening of the QT interval that may obscure inter-subject differences [58], and often precludes the exact recognition of the return of the T wave to the baseline because the high-pass filters selectively affect the slower part of ventricular repolarization. Nonetheless, some of the longest QTc values did belong to SIDS victims. To overcome this technical limitation, Southall et al. repeated the study with a standard ECG and accumulated data on over 7,000 infants, among whom were fifteen SIDS victims [59]. Six of the fifteen victims (40 percent) had a QTc in the upper ninetieth percentile. In other words, there were four times more SIDS victims with a long QT interval than would have been expected by chance. Southall's conclusion, based on lack of significant difference between the average QTc of the survivors and that of the victims, was that QT interval measurement cannot be used to predict infants at risk of SIDS. My interpretation is different, because I do not think it reasonable biologically to combine the QTc values of several victims, some of whom may have died because of a non-cardiac mechanism and have normal ventricular repolarization. The significant point seems to be that forty percent of the victims had a QTc value in the upper portion of the normal distribution. What remains to be determined is how many SIDS victims were among the group of infants with a prolonged QT interval; this ratio will provide an indication of the risk for these infants. Unfortunately, despite the continuous and meritorious effort by Southall to provide sufficient data collected prospectively, this study also has an important limitation. Due to the social and logistic organization of the British hospitals, newborns are discharged on the third day of life; as a result, the vast majority of ECG recordings in Southall's study are performed on either the first or second day of life. Walsh showed (Table 6.1) that the variability of the QT interval is extreme during the first two days of life with 16 to 20 percent of infants showing marked QT prolongation, while by the fourth day of life the variability has almost disappeared and only 1.5 percent of infants has a prolonged QT interval [64]. The reasons for so many infants with prolonged QT interval in the first forty-eight hours may relate to transient electrolyte imbalance. The main point is that during the first two days, one may find a number of

TABLE 6.1 Distribution of Cases according to QTc Interval during the First Week of Life

QTc (msec)	340–420	430–480	490–540
1st day	20	33	13 (20%)
2nd day	14	42	11 (16%)
3rd day	16	48	3+ (4%)
5th–6th day	29	38	1* (1.5%)

+ Maximum 510 msec
* 490 msec
Source: Modified from Walsh, Z.S. 1963. Electrocardiographic intervals during the first week of life. *American Heart Journal* 66:36[64].

"spurious" prolonged QT intervals that would disappear in the next few days. This is bound to obscure the presence of a truly prolonged QT interval; in other words the "noise" level is too high during the first two days of life to allow the current identification of those few infants who really have a non-transient long QT interval. As with the old saying "at night all cats look alike," one has to wait for a reduction in the spontaneous QT variability and then make the measurements. This is why we obtained all our initial ECG studies on the fourth day of life in the Milan prospective study.

I hope this discussion clarifies why even unbiased investigators had some difficulty in placing the "QT controversy" in the proper light. It is encouraging to see some of the changes in the commentaries by an expert and independent observer such as Valdes-Dapena [61, 65].

Conclusions

The year 1985 marked an important transition in SIDS research. For more than a decade the leading hypothesis was the "apnea hypothesis" with a number of theoretical and practical (i.e., home monitors) implications. Yet the pendulum swings. The Task Force on Prolonged Infantile Apnea stated, "The vast majority of infants with prolonged apnea are not victims of SIDS; most SIDS victims were never observed to have had prolonged apnea prior to the terminal event and a causal relationship between prolonged apnea and SIDS has not been established" [66]. In a review entitled "Are some crib deaths sudden cardiac deaths?" [65], Valdes-Dapena, after indicating that most of the so-called tissue markers of hypoxia and hypoxemia [67] have not been verified in subsequent, better-controlled studies [68], stated, "we are now experiencing a counterwave of skepticism concerning the validity of the apnea hypothesis." She further wrote, "spontaneous idiopathic pathologic apnea may be responsible for 5 percent to 7 percent of crib deaths."

As to the cardiac hypothesis, progress has been made as clearly indicated by the preliminary results of the ongoing Milan prospective study. As discussed earlier, the cardiac hypothesis cannot be tested in small selected groups; as generally true in scientific research, shortcuts are, in the long run, seldom rewarding and often misleading. Valuable information can come only from long and tedious prospective studies in unselected populations. Nonetheless, we begin to see some light at the end of the tunnel. More markers of cardiac electrical instability, such as level of heart rate and beat-to-beat variability, need to be looked at in addition to the QT interval. Our findings already indicate that in a percentage yet to be defined (but conservatively estimated now at probably not less than 30 percent), SIDS victims may be expected to have had, on the electrocardiogram, abnormalities that would allow identification of a subgroup at very high risk.

These concepts and the data presented here indicate that the "sympathetic imbalance" hypothesis, although not yet proven beyond doubt, can less and less be dismissed on the basis of current knowledge. The potential for early identification of some future SIDS victims and the extreme likelihood, if the hypothesis is correct, of having available an effective and safe preventive strategy (temporary use of beta adrenergic blocking agents) demand an accurate and unbiased evaluation of the cardiac hypothesis [69].

References

1. Schwartz, P.J. 1976. Cardiac sympathetic innervation and the sudden infant death syndrome: A possible pathogenetic link. *Am J Med* 60:167–172.
2. Schwartz, P.J. 1981. "The sudden infant death syndrome." In *Review in Perinatal Medicine,* ed. E.M. Scarpelli and E.V. Cosmi. New York: Raven Press.
3. Froggatt, P. 1977. A cardiac cause in cot death: A discarded hypothesis? *J Ir Med Assoc* 70:408–414.
4. Fraser, G.R., and P. Froggatt. 1966. Unexpected cot deaths. *Lancet* 2:56–57.
5. James, T.N. 1968. Sudden death in babies. *Am J Cardiol* 22:479–506.
6. Valdes-Dapena, M.A., M. Greene, N. Basavanad, R. Catherman, and R.C. Truex. 1973. The myocardial conduction system in sudden death in infancy. *N Engl J Med* 289:1179–1183.
7. Anderson, R.H., J. Bourton, C.T. Burrow, and A. Smith. 1974. Sudden death in infancy: A study of cardiac specialized tissue. *B Med J* 2:135–139.
8. Lie, J.T., H.S. Rosenberg, and E.E. Erickson. 1976. Histopathology of the conduction system in the sudden infant death syndrome. *Circulation* 53:3–8.
9. Marino, T.A., and B.M. Kane. 1985. Cardiac atrioventricular junctional tissues in hearts from infants who died suddenly. *J Am Coll Cardiol* 5:1178–1184.
10. James, T.N. 1985. Crib death. *J Am Coll Cardiol* 5:1185–1187.
11. Froggatt, P., and T.N. James. 1973. Sudden unexpected death in infants: Evidence on a lethal cardiac arrhythmia. *Ulster Medical Journal* 42:136–152.
12. Schwartz, P.J. 1974. Experimental reproduction of long QT syndrome and SIDS. NIH Grant Application No. 1 R01HD 08796–01.
13. Lown, B. 1979. Sudden cardiac death: The major challenge confronting contemporary cardiology. *Am J Cardiol* 43:313–328.

14. Schwartz, P.J. 1983. "Autonomic nervous system, ventricular fibrillation and SIDS." In *The Sudden Infant Death Syndrome,* ed. J.T. Tildon, L.M. Roeder, and A. Steinschneider. New York: Academic Press.

15. Crampton, R.S., and P.J. Schwartz. 1978. "Some aspects of sudden cardiac death." In *Neural Mechanisms in Cardiac Arrhythmias,* ed. P.J. Schwartz, A.M. Brown, A. Malliani, and A. Zanchetti. New York: Raven Press.

16. Schwartz, P.J., M. Periti, and A. Malliani. 1975. The long QT syndrome. *Am Heart J* 89:378–390.

17. Schwartz, P.J. 1985. The idiopathic long QT syndrome: Progress and questions. *Am Heart J* 109:399–411.

18. Schwartz, P.J., and A. Malliani. 1975. Electrical alternation of the T wave: Clinical and experimental evidence of its relationship with the sympathetic nervous system and with the long QT syndrome. *Am Heart J* 89:45–50.

19. Yanowitz, R., J.B. Preston, and J.A. Abildskow. 1966. Functional distribution of right and left stellate innervation to the ventricles: Production of neurogenic electrocardiographic changes by unilateral alteration of sympathetic tone. *Circ Res* 18:416–428.

20. Schwartz, P.J. 1984. "Sympathetic imbalance and cardiac arrhythmias." In *Nervous Control of Cardiovascular Functions,* ed. W.C. Randall. New York: Oxford University Press.

21. Schwartz, P.J., H.L. Stone, and A.M. Brown. 1976. Effects of unilateral stellate ganglion blockade on the arrhythmias associated with coronary occlusion. *Am Heart J* 92:589–599.

22. Schwartz, P.J., and H.L. Stone. 1979. Effects of unilateral stellectomy upon cardiac performance during exercise in dogs. *Circ Res* 44:637–645.

23. Austoni, P., R. Rosati, L. Gregorini, E. Bianchi, E. Bortolani, and P.J. Schwartz. 1979. Stellectomy and exercise in man (abstract). *Am J Cardiol* 43:399.

24. Schwartz, P.J. 1978. Experimental reproduction of the long QT syndrome (abstract). *Am J Cardiol* 41:374.

25. Schwartz, P.J., R.L. Verrier, and B. Lown. 1977. Effect of stellectomy and vagotomy on ventricular refractoriness in dogs. *Circ Res* 40:536–540.

26. Schwartz, P.J., N.G. Snebold, and A.M. Brown. 1976. Effects of unilateral cardiac sympathetic denervation in the ventricular fibrillation threshold. *Am J Cardiol* 37:1034–1040.

27. Langley, J.N. 1892. On the origin from the spinal cord of the cervical and upper thoracic sympathetic fibres, with some observations on white and grey rami communicantes. *Philosophical Transactions of the Royal Society of London* 183(B)107:85–124.

28. Schwartz, P.J., and H.L. Stone. 1976. Role of right stellate ganglion during exercise. *European J Clin Invest* 6:328.

29. Bertoni, T., L. De Ambroggi, E. Locati, M. Stramba-Badiale, and P.J. Schwartz. 1984. Time integral analysis of surface recovery potentials in the long QT syndrome (abstract). *Circulation* 70(II):221.

30. Schwartz, P.J., and H.L. Stone. 1982. The role of the autonomic nervous system in sudden coronary death. *Ann NY Acad Sci* 382:162–181.

31. Schwartz, P.J., and H.L. Stone. 1980. Left stellectomy in the prevention of ventricular fibrillation caused by acute myocardial ischemia in conscious

dogs with anterior myocardial infarction. *Circulation* 62:1256–1265.

32. Schwartz, P.J. 1984. "The rationale and the role of left stellectomy for the prevention of malignant arrhythmias." In *Clinical Aspects of Life-Threatening Arrhythmias,* ed H.M. Greenberger, H.E. Kulbertus, A.J. Moss, and P.J. Schwartz. *Annals of the New York Academy of Sciences* 427: 199–221.

33. Moss, A.J., P.J. Schwartz, R.S. Crampton, E. Locati, and E. Carleen. 1985. Heritable malignant arrhythmias: A prospective study of the long QT syndrome. *Circulation* 71:17–21.

34. Schwartz, P.J., and S. Wolf. 1978. QT interval prolongation as predictor of sudden death in patients with myocardial infarction. *Circulation* 57:1074–1077.

35. Moss, A.J., and P.J. Schwartz. 1982. Delayed repolarization (QT or QT prolongation) and malignant arrhythmias. *Mod Concepts Cardiovasc Dis* 51:85–90.

36. Ferrer, P.L., and M.J. Jesse. 1977. Prolonged QT index in "near miss" sudden death in infancy. *Clin Res* 25:64a.

37. Ferrer, P.L., and N.S. Talner. 1974. Changes in the QT index with sleep in young mammals. *Pediatr Res* 8:349.

38. Browne, K.F., E. Prystowsky, J.J. Heger, D.A. Chilson, and D.P. Zipes. 1983. Prolongation of the QT interval in man during sleep. *Am J Cardiol* 52:55–59.

39. Wellens, H.J.J., A. Vermeulen, and D. Durrer. 1972. Ventricular fibrillation occurring on arousal from sleep by auditory stimuli. *Circulation* 46:661–665.

40. Moss, M.L. 1965. The veloepiglottic sphincter and obligate nose breathing in the neonate. *J Pediatr* 67:330–331.

41. Swift, P.J.F., and J.L. Emery. 1973. Clinical observations on response to nasal occlusion in infancy. *Arch Dis Child* 48:947–951.

42. Kralios, F.A., and C.K. Millar. 1978. Functional development of cardiac sympathetic nerves in newborn dogs: Evidence for asymmetrical development. *Cardiovasc Res* 12:547–554.

43. Schwartz, P.J., M. Montemerlo, M. Facchini, P. Salice, D. Rosti, G. Poggio, and R. Giorgetti. 1982. The QT interval throughout the first six months of life: A prospective study. *Circulation* 66:496–501.

44. Verrier, R.L., and B. Lown. 1978. "Sympathetic–parasympathetic interactions and ventricular electrical stability." In *Neural Mechanisms in Cardiac Arrhythmias,* ed. P.J. Schwartz, A.M. Brown, A. Malliani, and A. Zanchetti. New York: Raven Press.

45. Billman, G.E., P.J. Schwartz, and H.L. Stone. 1982. Baroreceptor reflex control of heart rate: A predictor of sudden cardiac death. *Circulation* 66:874–880.

46. Schwartz, P.J., and H.L. Stone. 1985. "The analysis and modulation of autonomic reflexes in the prediction and prevention of sudden death." In *Cardiac Electrophysiology and Arrhythmias,* ed. D.P. Zipes and J. Jalife. Orlando, Fla.: Academic Press.

47. Segantini, A., T. Varisco, E. Monza, V. Songa, M. Montemerlo, P. Salice, G.L. Poggio, D. Rosti, and P.J. Schwartz. 1986. QT interval and the sudden

infant death syndrome: A prospective study. *J Am. Coll. Cardiol.* 7:118A.

48. Schwartz, P.J., and P. Salice. 1984. Cardiac arrhythmias in infancy: Prevalence, significance and need for treatment. *Eur Heart J* 5:43–50.

49. Southall, D. P., A.M. Johnson, E.A. Shinebourne, P.G.B. Johnston, and D.G. Vulliamy. 1981. Frequency and outcome of disorders of cardiac rhythm and conduction in a population of newborn infants. *Pediatrics* 68:58–66.

50. Maron, B. J., C. E. Clark, R.E. Goldstein, and S.E. Epstein. 1976. Potential role of QT interval prolongation in sudden infant death syndrome. *Circulation* 54:423–430.

51. Kukolich, M.K., A. Telsey, J. Ott, and A.G. Motulsky. 1977. Sudden infant death syndrome: Normal QT interval on ECGs of relatives. *Pediatrics* 60:51–54.

52. Kelly, D.H., D.C. Shannon, and R.R. Liberthson. 1977. The role of the QT interval in the sudden infant death syndrome. *Circulation* 55:633–635.

53. Haddad, G.G., M.A.F. Epstein, R.A. Epstein, N.M. Mazza, R.B. Mellins, and E. Krongrad. 1979. The QT interval in aborted SIDS infants. *Pediatr Res* 13:136–138.

54. Steinschneider, A. 1978. Sudden infant death syndrome and prolongation of the QT interval. *Am J Dis Child* 132:688–691.

55. Montague, T.J., J.P. Finley, K. Mukelabai, S.A. Black, S.M. Rigby, C.A. Spencer, and B.M. Horacek. 1984. Cardiac rhythm, rate and ventricular repolarization properties in infants at risk for sudden infant death syndrome: Comparison with age and sex matched control infants. *Am J Cardiol* 54:301–307.

56. Guntheroth, W.G. 1982. *Crib death—Sudden infant death syndrome*. New York: Futura Publishing.

57. Guntheroth, W.G. 1982. Editorial: The QT interval and sudden infant death syndrome. *Circulation* 66:502–504.

58. Southall, D.P. 1983. Identification of infants destined to die unexpectedly during infancy: Evaluation of predictive importance of prolonged apnea and disorders of cardiac rhythm or conduction. *Br Med J* 286:1092–1096.

59. Southall, D.P., W.A. Arrowsmith, and J.R. Alexander. 1986. QT interval measurements in infants destined to suffer sudden infant death syndrome. *Arch Dis Child* 61:327–333.

60. Southall, D.P. 1983. Home monitoring and its role in the sudden infant death syndrome. *Pediatrics* 72:133–138.

61. Valdes-Dapena, M.A. 1980. Sudden infant death syndrome: A review of the medical literature 1974-1979. *Pediatrics* 66:597–612.

62. Schwartz, P.J. 1976. Near miss sudden infant death. *Lancet* 2:853.

63. Irgens, L.M., R. Skjaerven, and D.R. Peterson. 1984. Prospective assessment of recurrence risk in sudden infant death syndrome siblings. *J Pediatr* 104:349–351.

64. Walsh, Z.S. 1963. Electrocardiographic intervals during the first week of life. *Am Heart J* 66:36–41.

65. Valdes-Dapena. 1985. Are some crib deaths sudden cardiac deaths? *J Am Coll Cardiol* 5:113B–117B.

66. The Task Force on Prolonged Infantile Apnea. 1985. Prolonged infantile apnea: 1985. *Pediatrics* 76:129–131.

67. Naeye, R.L. 1977. The sudden infant death syndrome: A review of recent advances. *Arch Pathol Lab Med* 101:165–167.
68. Merritt, T.A., and M.A. Valdes-Dapena. 1984. SIDS research update. *Pediatric Annals* 13:193–207.
69. Schwartz, P.J. 1987. The quest for the mechanism of the sudden infant death syndrome. Doubts and progress. *Circulation* 75:677–683.

7

The Medical Management of Cardiorespiratory Monitoring in Infantile Apnea

DOROTHY H. KELLY, M.D. and DANIEL C. SHANNON, M.D.

Researchers have reported sudden and unexplained death in infants with increased incidence of both prolonged apnea [1, 2] and short apnea [3, 4]. Because of these reports, infants with a history of prolonged apnea are being identified, evaluated, and treated. Prolonged apnea is defined by the American Academy of Pediatrics as an unexplained and frightening episode of cessation of breathing for twenty seconds or longer or of shorter duration if associated with bradycardia, cyanosis, or pallor [5]. If, after a thorough evaluation, the episode remains unexplained and therefore untreated, the infant must be continually observed for a recurrence of prolonged apnea. Electronic monitoring can assist the caretakers in the constant surveillance of the infant [5, 6]. The Academy of Pediatrics cautioned that if electronic monitoring is used in the home, it should be done only after thorough training of the parents in cardiopulmonary resuscitation and in the use of the monitor. They also suggested that parents should have psychosocial support available to them [5].

The concept of monitoring respiration is not new. The earliest report of monitoring breathing movements that we are aware of describes the custom in New England graveyards in the late 1700s. A string was tied around the chest of a buried corpse because of the fear of suspended animation and brought through a tube to the surface where it was attached to a bell. The graveyard sexton was expected to monitor the ringing of these bells, which would indicate that the corpse had revived and that the sexton should exhume the body to enable the person to survive. Another early report documented the monitoring of respiration of the rear gunner of World War I pilots with an oscilloscope; if the breathing movements ceased, the pilot no longer had protection from the rear. Newer devices to monitor breathing movements have been developed since then and have been applied in medicine to detect respiration in infants, children, and adults in the hospital and, most recently, in the home. This chapter discusses the use of electronic monitoring of respiration and heart rate of infants in the home.

Current Understanding

Whom to Monitor

Home monitoring is considered for two major groups of infants (1) infants who have had an unexplained episode of prolonged apnea, and (2) infants with a positive family history of apnea of infancy (AOI) or sudden infant death syndrome (SIDS).

Infants with Clinical Apnea. In infants with clinical apnea, monitoring would be recommended at home for (1) infants who have an *unexplained* episode of apnea associated with a change in tone and color and who do not respond to gentle stimulation but do respond to vigorous stimulation or resuscitation; (2) infants who have an episode of sleep onset apnea that responds to gentle stimulation if they have either repeat episodes requiring gentle stimulation or abnormalities on a sleep polygraph or pneumogram; and (3) infants whose awake onset episode is explained by gastroesophageal reflux but who either have abnormalities on a sleep polygraph or pneumogram or continue to have episodes despite antireflux measures. Home monitoring also is recommended for thriving preterm infants ready for discharge and full-term infants less than one month of age who (1) have abnormalities on recordings, (2) have clinical apnea and bradycardia that is incompletely controlled with methylxanthines, or (3) cannot tolerate methylxanthines as treatment for the clinical apnea/bradycardia that is documented by sleep polygraph or pneumogram.

Infants with Family History. Siblings of SIDS victims reportedly are at an increased risk of SIDS [6]. Although some controversy exists about this [7, 8], since 1976 according to the protocol at the Massachusetts General Hospital (MGH), subsequent siblings have been examined by (1) physical and neurologic examination, (2) a pneumogram to evaluate for central apnea, bradycardia, and periodic breathing, and (3) a nap study to evaluate for hypoxemia and hypercarbia and determine if the infant has easily identifiable abnormalities in control of ventilation. Home monitoring is recommended for siblings of SIDS victims with unexplained abnormalities (approximately 12 percent of those seen in the MGH program). For the infant who has had two or more siblings with SIDS, home monitoring is recommended regardless of testing since 18.5 percent of these infants die and 29.6 percent have at least one episode of sleep apnea requiring vigorous stimulation or resuscitation to restore breathing during the course of home monitoring [9]. In addition, monitoring is recommended for all siblings who have had an unexplained episode of apnea and/or bradycardia. Those whose presenting apneic episode occurred during sleep and required resuscitation to terminate are at greatest risk: two out of eight of these siblings in the MGH program died, and an additional four required either resuscitation or vigorous stimulation to terminate a subsequent episode of sleep apnea during home monitoring [10]. Finally, because of the increased incidence of SIDS in the surviving twin [11], monitoring is also recommended for these infants.

How to Evaluate

Evaluation of the Symptomatic Infant

Any infant who has had an episode of prolonged apnea should be hospitalized for evaluation. During the evaluation, the infant should be maintained on cardiopulmonary monitoring and cared for by a staff trained in infant resuscitation. Initial evaluation should consist of a complete history of the episode taken from the observer(s), so that the state, position, color, tone, breathing movements, and the presence or absence of cough, stridor, or fluid in the mouth can be evaluated. In addition, the amount of stimulation that was necessary to terminate the episode, the duration of the episode, and presence and duration of any abnormality when breathing resumed should be ascertained. A careful history may be helpful in making the diagnosis of gastroesophageal reflux, seizures, or airway obstruction. Evaluation also should include a careful physical and neurologic assessment. Laboratory tests should be performed to determine if there is a treatable cause for the apneic episode. Etiologies to consider include (1) congenital abnormalities such as heart disease, especially patent ductus arteriosis and cardiac arrhythmias; (2) craniofacial and airway abnormalities such as choanal atresia, choanal stenosis, laryngeal cord paralysis, subglottic stenosis, and vascular ring; (3) infectious processes such as sepsis, meningitis, encephalitis, pneumonia, pertussis, RSV, and infant botulism; (4) metabolic abnormalities such as hypoglycemia, hypocalcemia, hyponatremia, and hypothermia; (5) hematologic abnormalities such as anemia; (6) neoplastic abnormalities such as a CNS or tracheal tumor; (7) neurologic abnormalities such as intracranial hemorrhage and seizures; (8) and other abnormalities such as gastroesophageal reflux, anomalies in control of ventilation, excessive amounts of medication that suppress ventilation, and, rarely, pyloric stenosus. Laboratory tests should include complete blood count, urinalysis, serum concentrations of sodium, potassium, chloride, calcium, and phosphorous, arterial blood gases, chest radiographs, electrocardiogram, barium swallow, electroencephalogram, and, when appropriate, urine culture, blood culture, and culture of the cerebrospinal fluid, bronchoscopy, CAT scan, Tuttle test or 24-hour esophageal pH probe monitoring. Infants in whom a cause is found should be tested after treatment is completed to determine if there are any persistent abnormalities on polygraphic or pneumographic recordings. If such abnormalities are detected, home monitoring is recommended for the infant. In addition, if seizures are diagnosed based on history or the observations of the event in an infant who has had an episode of sleep apnea requiring either vigorous stimulation or resuscitation, and the infant has a normal EEG, home monitoring is recommended until complete control of the seizure disorder has been achieved with anticonvulsant therapy.

Finally, infants whose episode of prolonged apnea remains unexplained should be evaluated to determine if there are abnormalities in control of ventilation. If on pneumogram and/or polygraphic testing, prolonged apnea, bradycardia, or marked hypoventilation (mean $P_ACO_2 \geq 50$ mmHg) is demonstrated, treatment with methylxanthines should be started in addition to home monitoring. If the only abnormality found is excessive periodic breathing, treatment with methylxanthines is not necessary unless the infant has a repeat episode of apnea, bradycardia and/or hypoxemia.

Evaluation of the Infant with a Family History of SIDS and/or Apnea

Currently, subsequent infants born to parents who have had one or more previous children with apnea and/or SIDS are evaluated through the MGH program. This evaluation at one to three weeks of age consists of a thorough physical and neurologic evaluation, home nocturnal pneumogram, and assessment of hypoxia or hypercarbia (mean $P_ACO_2 \geq 46$ mmHg) while awake, feeding, and in quiet and active sleep during daytime nap. If results of the evaluation are normal, a second home nocturnal pneumogram at six to eight weeks of age is recommended. If abnormalities are detected, the infant is evaluated in an attempt to determine a treatable cause. If none is found, home monitoring is recommended with the addition of methylxanthines if (1) symptomatic apnea and/or bradycardia develops or (2) the infant has prolonged apnea, bradycardia, or marked hypoventilation (mean $P_ACO_2 \geq 50$ mmHg). Treatment with methylxanthines is not recommended if the only abnormality found is an increased percentage of sleep time spent in periodic breathing.

For infants with two or more previous siblings who died of SIDS and/or had AOI, the above evaluation and criteria for treatment with methylxanthine apply. In addition, because of a high incidence of death, significant apnea, and/or bradycardia [9], home monitoring is recommended for all these infants.

How to Monitor

Type of Monitor

Once a decision has been made to monitor an infant at home, the type of monitor necessary to monitor adequately certain physiologic parameters for the infant must be determined. Usually, a device that monitors both respiration and heart rate will be most appropriate. Because it has been documented that many infants with apnea of infancy have both central and

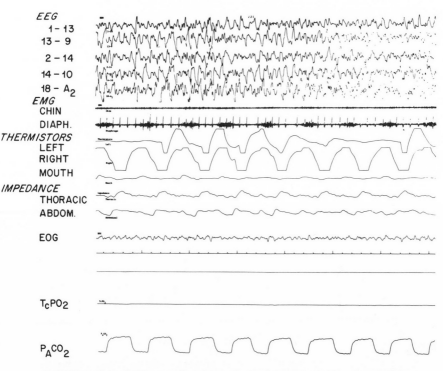

FIGURE 7.1. Polygraphic recording demonstrating intermittent airflow through left nostril. If a thermistor had been placed only in this nostril, the lack of flow could generate a false positive alarm for obstructive apnea.

obstructive apnea [3, 4], the device used in the home must be able to monitor for both of these events as well as for isolated bradycardia. Occasionally, monitoring for desaturation also may be necessary. The typical cardiorespiratory monitor used in the home setting detects chest movement with an impedance transducer. Although an impedance transducer will not be able to identify obstructive apnea (lack of airflow with continued respiratory movements), the bradycardia, which generally accompanies this, will be identified by the cardiac rate detector in the monitor. Obstructive apnea can be identified by the use of the thermistors. However, it is extremely difficult to use thermistors in the home setting because frequently they are covered by secretions or dislodged by the infant, resulting in false positive alarms. Furthermore, during a single night, we have identified on polygraph recordings numerous episodes of infants breathing through alternate nostrils (Figure 7.1). Therefore, two thermistors are needed to avoid false positive alarms. We also have identified numerous episodes of continued airflow detected by an end tidal carbon dioxide sensor, but not detected by functioning right and left nasal as well as oral

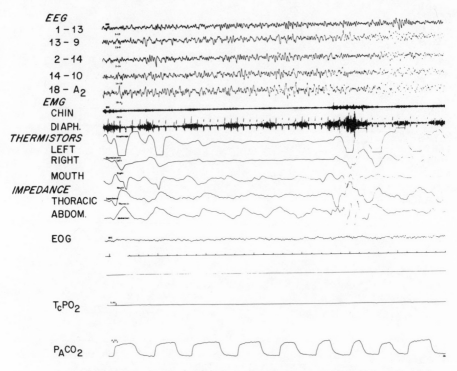

EEG
1 – 13
13 – 9
2 – 14
14 – 10
18 – A$_2$
EMG
CHIN
DIAPH.
THERMISTORS
LEFT
RIGHT
MOUTH
IMPEDANCE
THORACIC
ABDOM.

EOG

T$_c$PO$_2$

P$_A$CO$_2$

FIGURE 7.2. Polygraphic recording demonstrating lack of airflow as indicated by right, left, and mouth thermistors with good airflow detection by end tidal carbon dioxide canula placed in the mouth. There is no hypercarbia or hypoxemia associated with this.

thermistors (Figure 7.2). If the thermistor is set for maximum amplitude at the usual size breaths, there will be unapparent fluctuation in the signal generated by these small breaths. Because of these technical problems, we believe that the current thermistors are impractical devices for monitoring respirations in the home setting. For similar reasons, devices for measuring end tidal carbon dioxide are impractical. Also, instruments that transcutaneously measure partial pressure of oxygen are technically difficult to use in long-term monitoring because the electrode must be changed frequently. Devices for monitoring airflow and oxygen saturation are being developed to eliminate these limitations.

Finally, when an infant with AOI also has a pacemaker, one must realize that the currently available infant home cardiorespiratory monitors are heart *rate* detectors and not *qRS* detectors. They will detect the pacemaker spike as well as the qRS complex and thus will detect the physiologic signal (heart rate) at a rate higher than the actual rate. Also, in our experience, the pacemaker signal at times has contaminated the impedance channel, essentially making it impossible to detect apnea during the

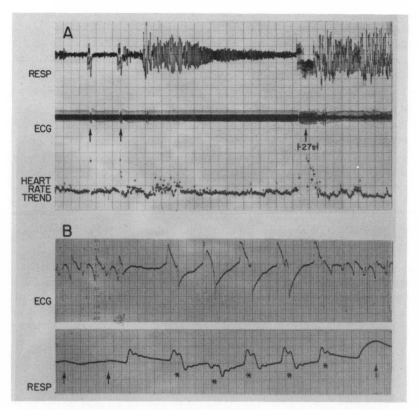

FIGURE 7.3. Pneumogram tracing showing three episodes of brief (one beat) periods of bradycardia followed by paced qRS complexes (arrows) at sixty-eight BPM lasting up to twenty-seven seconds. This signal also is seen on the impedance (respiratory) channel, as seen best in 3B and indicated by *. The normal impedance signal is indicated by an arrow. No alarms were associated with these events despite monitoring with an infant cardiorespiratory monitor set to alarm after 20 seconds of apnea and with a heart rate less than eighty BPM.

period of time that the pacemaker is firing (Figure 7.3) and, therefore, no alarm is sounded. Thus, such an infant will require a cardiac monitor capable of differentiating a pacer spike from a qRS complex at a minimum. We also suggest monitoring the respiratory status of such an infant with an infant oximeter.

Because prolonged central apnea (lack of airflow and lack of breathing movements) can occur in the absence of bradycardia (Figure 7.4), a cardiac monitor alone is not sufficient to monitor adequately an infant for prolonged apnea. Monitoring of breathing movements is necessary to detect such an occurrence. Two types of instruments currently are available for monitoring breathing movements of the infant at home: mattress monitors and impedance transducers. In general, mattress devices have a large

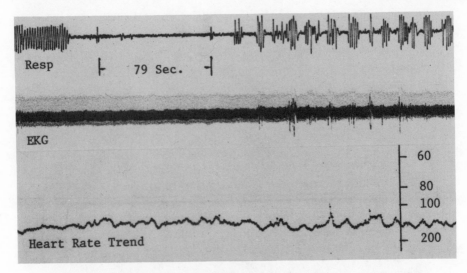

FIGURE 7.4. Prolonged apnea lasting seventy-nine seconds with only minimal cardiac deceleration and no bradycardia.

number of false positive alarms secondary to position changes that occur as the infant grows. Although impedance devices also have false positive alarms, usually careful instruction to the parents and attention to appropriate placement of electrodes and the electrode belt, result in infrequent false positive alarms (one false positive alarm per infant per two weeks in the MGH program). Thus, we believe that the best device presently available for monitoring AOI infants in their home is a cardiorespiratory monitor that monitors respiration by impedance transducers.

Monitor Settings

Normal full-term infants have many episodes of apnea of ten to twelve seconds in duration and occasionally lasting up to fourteen seconds [12, 13]. These episodes cause numerous true positive alarms and result in needless parental anxiety and fatigue if the monitor was set on a ten-second apnea delay. This setting is recommended only if the infant appears to desaturate very quickly so that cyanosis is apparent during episodes of apnea lasting ten to fifteen seconds. The rate at which an infant desaturates during apnea is based on the amount of oxygen in the lung and blood at the onset of apnea, as well as on the metabolic rate of oxygen consumption and the presence or absence of right-to-left shunting. Significant desaturation during apneas of less than twenty seconds is seldom documented. In infants with symptomatic apnea, we have documented numerous episodes of central apnea lasting fifteen to nineteen seconds, which do not cause significant desaturation and which the infant resolves spontaneously. Thus, setting the alarm for these shorter apneas would cause needless fatigue and anxiety in the caretaker. Therefore, a twenty-second apnea delay setting is recommended. However, if recordings or clinical observations indicate that bradycardia or significant desaturation occurs during apneic episodes lasting less than twenty seconds, a shorter apnea delay would be appropriate.

The heart rate threshold of the monitor is generally set at a rate of eighty BPM for full-term newborns. When the infant is two to four months of age, the setting is changed to seventy BPM, and to sixty BPM when the infant is three to six months of age. This assures that an alarm will sound in the early seconds of true bradycardia, but will not give needless true positive alarms for the brief heart rate deceleration that becomes prominent with sighs as the infant grows and his or her average heart rate decreases. Occasionally, in infants who are older than six months, the heart rate settings will have to be changed to fifty-five or fifty BPM since sinus arrhythmia may become more prominent, resulting in needless frequent brief bradycardia alarms at higher settings. If an infant continues to be monitored after twelve months of age, the heart rate setting may need to be changed to fifty BPM because of the frequently seen pattern of a prominent sinus arrhythmia with brief heart rate deceleration to fifty-five BPM. Changing the heart rate settings with age eliminates the brief cardiac alarms that are not accompanied by color or tone change.

Education of the Caretakers

Every person who will be responsible for the care of the monitored infant must be fully trained in (1) the use and troubleshooting of all the equipment, (2) specific observations of the infant, (3) graded intervention during alarms including infant cardiopulmonary resuscitation, and (4) the means of making home monitoring safer and easier. The instruction must be accomplished to the physician's satisfaction prior to the discharge of the infant. Several handbooks [14–17] are available to assist the physician or other medical personnel in training the caretakers. It is the physician's responsibility [5] to assure that all caretakers are thoroughly versed in the following material. The parents must understand how to use and troubleshoot all the prescribed equipment; if malfunctions occur, they need to understand how to make minor repairs. They should be knowledgeable about various electrode placements, as well as usage and care of the electrode belt, lead wires, and patient cable. Methods of observing the infant to permit correct assessment at the time of the alarm must be understood as well as methods of intervening so that a graded pattern of intervention will be used (Figure 7.5). Basically, the caretakers are trained to intervene immediately if there is a color change. If there is no color change, we suggest that they wait ten seconds from the sound of the alarm before they

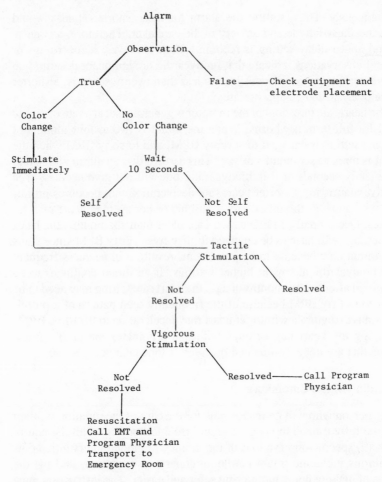

FIGURE 7.5. Stepwise response to monitor alarms.

intervene to enable them to make appropriate observations and allow time for the infant to resolve the apnea and/or bradycardia, a reassuring observation for the parents. After ten seconds, if the infant continues to be apneic or bradycardic, they should touch the baby lightly and proceed to gentle shaking in order to restore breathing or to resolve bradycardia. If this does not resolve the problem, they should shake the infant more vigorously being careful to control the head so that injury will not occur during vigorous shaking. Caretakers must be particularly cautious with this since many of the infants who do not respond to gentle stimulation are somewhat limp and probably at more risk for serious injury if the head is not adequately supported during vigorous stimulation. Finally, if vigorous stimulation fails to rectify the situation, the caretaker should begin cardiopulmonary resuscitation according to the American Heart Association guidelines. If resuscitation is necessary, the caretaker should call the local emergency medical technicians and go to the emergency room so that the infant may be evaluated and receive further intervention if necessary. If the episode resolved with intervention other than CPR, the physician should be contacted immediately so that he or she may determine if other intervention is necessary. Once the situation has resolved, the parents should keep careful accounts of exactly what occurred and what intervention was necessary to terminate the event (Figure 7.6).

Finally, before discharge from the hospital, the parents should be taught methods of living with the monitor. These include being aware of "noisy and quiet" housework so that when the infant is on a monitor, they will not engage in noisy housework that could interfere with their ability to hear the monitor alarm. When the monitor is installed in their home, they should check all areas of the house so that they will recognize the areas from which they cannot hear the monitor and should not go into those areas when the infant is being monitored by the device. There are numerous suggestions available to parents including dealing with the extended family, friends, and community members, methods of traveling with infants on a monitor, skin care, siblings' adjustments to the presence of a monitor at home, and many others. This information is available in the handbooks [14–17]. The physician must emphasize that *all* caretakers should be thoroughly versed in monitoring as well as infant cardiopulmonary resuscitation; lack of familiarity with this information resulted in one death in our program.

Support for Families during Home Monitoring

Caring for an infant with apnea in the home is anxiety provoking as well as restrictive. The introduction of electronic monitoring into the home usually can make caring for such an infant much less stressful because the monitor generally is viewed as an electronic babysitter, allowing the caretakers to be out of sight of the infant as long as they are within hearing range of the monitor alarm. Most families find the addition of the monitor provides relief and, in fact, some have difficulty giving up the monitor once there is a medical recommendation to discontinue its usage. However, if monitoring is introduced without adequate support personnel, many families find that this device is extremely difficult to use. As a result, there are many false positive alarms, which add to the stress of the already difficult task of caring for an infant with apnea at home. For this reason, we strongly encourage thorough training prior to discharge of the infant from the hospital; after discharge we recommend that the family have adequate support. Frequent telephone calls by the program nurse and home visits by the visiting nurse or the program nurse to assess the amount

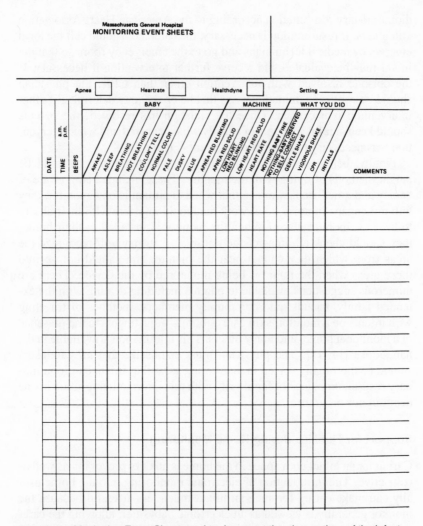

FIGURE 7.6. Monitoring Event Sheet used to document the observations of the infant and intervention used by the caretaker with monitor alarm.

of parental anxiety as well as their understanding of the teaching program are extremely helpful [18]. In addition, a physician who can respond to medical problems of the infant and a technician who can respond to technical problems with the monitor must be available to the parents twenty-four hours a day. Social workers, psychologists, and psychiatrists should be available to help families cope with financial and marital problems, as well as behavioral problems in siblings and the difficulties that extended family members and friends may have in understanding the nature and seriousness of the problem. Most families report that their anxiety, although significant during the first few weeks at home, is markedly diminished by adequate training and support [18, 19].

The Treatment of Apnea during Home Monitoring

Many infants whose initial evaluation resulted in negative findings or who had only minor abnormalities in control of ventilation will have recurrent episodes of apnea during monitoring at home. These often occur during the course of an upper respiratory infection (URI) [20, 21].

If apnea is to be recurrent, generally it occurs during the first two months of home monitoring. The highest incidence of severe episodes of sleep apnea requiring resuscitation (33 percent) and the highest mortality (13 percent) during home monitoring is in infants whose initial episode required resuscitation [10]. Rarely, these severe repeat episodes will be so frequent and so severe during an intercurrent stress such as a URI that mechanical ventilation will be necessary. If apnea occurs during home monitoring, we recommend that the infant be reevaluated especially for reflux, seizures, and abnormalities in control of ventilation; if an abnormality is found, it should be treated vigorously. If the infant shows abnormalities in the control of ventilation, we recommend that (1) methylxanthines be started in a dose sufficient to produce a serum trough level above 10 mcg/ml, and (2) the infant be retested to determine if the abnormalities have resolved. If treatment is successful, we suggest that the medication be continued for approximately six to eight weeks and then tapered. If symptoms develop during the tapering of the medication, it should be reinstituted for an additional eight weeks. After the methylxanthine is discontinued, the infant should be retested to determine if the abnormality has resolved. If gastroesophageal reflux is found and the infant continues to have episodes of prolonged apnea despite antireflux positioning and thickening, we recommend the addition of metaclopramide at 0.5 mg to 1 mg/kg/day in four doses. Antireflux measures include positioning prone or supine at $\geq 30°$ and thickening of the formula with cereal (one to three teaspoons/ounce of formula). If significant episodes of apnea requiring resuscitation continue despite this treatment and a definite relationship between reflux and apnea and/or bradycardia can be confirmed with polygraphic recordings including pH probe, a fundoplication is recommended.

If, on reassessment of the infant with recurrent prolonged apnea, no abnormality is found, and the infant continues to have well-documented episodes of apnea requiring resuscitation, continual recording of respiration and heart rate during alarms should be instituted to clarify the nature of the events and permit more effective therapy. In addition, for this small group of infants with recurrent severe idiopathic AOI, prolonged hospitalization should be considered because mortality is extremely high (28 percent [10]).

Discontinuance of the Home Monitor

Home monitoring may be discontinued when the following criteria are met: The infant has had (1) no apnea requiring vigorous stimulation or resuscitation for three months (4 months if the infant is twelve to eighteen months and six months if the infant is older than eighteen months); (2) no twenty-second apneas for at least two months; (3) at least two normal consecutive recordings in the home with a minimum of two weeks between recordings; (4) no symptoms during the stress of an upper respiratory illness or an immunization; (5) resolution of the abnormalities present on testing and on physical examination such as lack of oral breathing or bradycardia to nasal obstruction. The longer symptom-free periods in the older infants are recommended because we have found that the frequency of apnea decreases with increased age.

Because discontinuance usually is stressful for the families, the frequency of contact with the family by support personnel should be increased during this period. In addition, during monitoring, the family should generally understand the criteria for discontinuance so that they will anticipate with the physician the time when he or she will recommend that monitoring be discontinued. With these techniques, families usually need only a brief period for weaning themselves from the monitor. If increased support is given to the family during the time of this discontinuance, psychological or psychiatric help rarely is needed. In the MGH program, approximately 95 percent of families have stopped monitoring the infant within one to two weeks of the medical recommendation to do so, and the average infant is monitored 5.5 months. When monitoring has been discontinued, continued follow up of these infants at regular intervals for physical, neurologic, and developmental assessments is important. Follow-up studies have demonstrated mild developmental delays in some of these infants as well as occasionally persistent mild hypercapnea or the occurrence of typical obstructive sleep apnea syndrome [22, 23].

In summary, most infants referred for evaluation of a frightening spell do not need to be monitored at home. With careful evaluation, a cause for the event can be found in approximately one-third of infants referred. An additional one-third require no treatment because careful evaluation reveals no abnormality, and they have been referred for what is concluded to be a minor event, or because of a family history of SIDS and/or AOI. Finally, the remaining one-third have idiopathic AOI or apnea of prematurity (AOP) and are treated with methylxanthine and/or home monitoring. If the home monitoring is used, careful instruction of all caretakers is necessary so that the outcome of monitoring will be successful (72 percent of the deaths in our program occur due to noncompliance). Most deaths occur in a small subset of infants with AOI (initial event of sleep onset apnea requiring resuscitation and/or vigorous stimulation) or with a family history of SIDS (two or more previous siblings have died of SIDS). Thus, in these high risk monitor populations it is necessary to be extremely vigilant in monitoring techniques to decrease these apparently unnecessary deaths.

References

1. Steinschneider, A. 1972. Prolonged apnea and the sudden infant death syndrome: Clinical and laboratory observations. *Pediatrics* 50:646–654.
2. Kelly, D.H., and D.C. Shannon. 1981. Episodic complete airway obstruction in infants. *Pediatrics* 67:823–827.
3. Guilleminault, C., R.L. Ariagno, L.S. Forno, L. Nagel, R. Baldwin, and M. Owen. 1979. Obstructive sleep apnea and near miss for SIDS: 1. Report of an infant with sudden death. *Pediatrics* 63:837–843.
4. Steinschneider, A., S.L. Weinstein, and E. Diamond. 1982. The sudden infant death syndrome and apnea/obstruction during neonatal sleep and feedings. *Pediatrics* 70:858–863.
5. Task Force on Prolonged Apnea: Prolonged apnea. 1978. American Academy of Pediatrics. *Pediatrics* 61:651–652.
6. Peterson, D.R., N.M. Chinn, and L.D. Fisher. 1980. The sudden infant death syndrome: Repetitions in families. *J Pediatr* 97:265–267.
7. Irgens, L.M., R. Skjaerven, and D.R. Peterson. 1984. Prospective assessment of recurrent risk in sudden infant death syndrome siblings. *J Pediatr* 104:349–351.
8. Peterson, D.R., E.E. Sabotta, and J.R. Daling. 1986. Infant mortality among subsequent siblings of infants who died of sudden infant death syndrome. *J Pediatr* 108:911–914.
9. Oren, J., D.H. Kelly, and D.C. Shannon. 1987. Familial occurrence of sudden infant death syndrome and apnea of infancy. *Pediatrics* 80:355–358.
10. Oren, J., D.H. Kelly, and D.C. Shannon. 1986. Identification of a high-risk group for sudden infant death syndrome among infants who were resuscitated for sleep apnea. *Pediatrics* 77:495–499.
11. Spiers, P.S. 1974. Estimated rates of concordancy for the sudden infant death syndrome in twins. *Am J Epidemiol* 100:1–7.
12. Kelly, D.H., L.M. Stellwagen, E. Kaitz, and D.C. Shannon. 1984. Apnea and periodic breathing in normal infants during the first twelve months. *Am Rev Respir Dis* 129:A208.
13. Hunt, C.E., R.T. Brouillette, D. Hanson, R.J. David, I.M. Stein, and M. Weissbluth. 1985. Home pneumograms in normal infants. *J Pediatr* 106:551–555.
14. Haight, B.F., D. Kelly, and K.C. McCabe. 1983. *A Manual for Home Monitoring* 2nd ed. Landover, Md.: National SIDS Foundation.
15. Barr, A. 1979. *At Home with a Monitor: A Guide for New Parents*. Landover, Md.: National SIDS Foundation.
16. Ad Hoc Committee, National SIDS Foundation. 1982. *A Handbook for Infant Monitoring: A Training and Reference Source for the Parents of Infants who are being Monitored due to Cardiorespiratory Abnormalities*. Marietta, Ga.: Healthdyne.

17. Kelly, D.H., R.L. Ariagno, and T.A. Merritt. 1982. *Guidelines for Evaluating and Monitoring Infants with Cardiorespiratory Abnormalities.* Landover, Md.: National SIDS Foundation.
18. Cain, L.P., D.H. Kelly, and D.C. Shannon. 1980. Parents' perceptions of the psychological and social impact of home monitoring. *Pediatrics* 66:37–41.
19. Kelly, D.H., D.C. Shannon, and K. O'Connell. 1978. Care of infants with near-miss sudden infant death syndrome. *Pediatrics* 61:511–514.
20. Steinschneider, A. 1975. Nasopharyngitis and prolonged sleep apnea. *Pediatrics* 56:967–971.
21. Keens, T.G., P.C. Dennies, C.D. Lew, and A.C.G. Platzker. 1982. Risk of subsequent apnea in infants surviving near-miss sudden infant death syndrome. *Clin Res* 30:151A.
22. Deykin, E., M.L. Bauman, D.H. Kelly, C. Hsieh, and D.C. Shannon. 1984. Infancy apnea and neurologic cognitive and behavioral status. *Pediatrics* 73:638–645.
23. Guilleminault, C., M. Souquet, R.L. Ariagno, R. Korobkin, and F.B. Simmons. 1984. Five cases of near-miss sudden infant death syndrome and development of obstructive sleep apnea syndrome. *Pediatrics* 73:71–78.

PART II

The Psychological Impact and Management of Sudden Infant Death Syndrome

8

Acute Loss and Grieving Reactions: Treatment Issues

JAN L. CULBERTSON, PH.D., and DIANE J. WILLIS, PH.D.

The loss of an infant to sudden infant death syndrome (SIDS) constitutes a crisis for the parents, siblings, and extended family of the infant. Much has been written about the need for crisis intervention for families of SIDS victims and about the potential for prolonged or pathologic reactions in the survivors [1–8]. However, there is a need for a detailed review of the nature of grieving responses in parents and children, with an emphasis on the process of normal grieving, the "tasks" to be accomplished during the period of mourning, descriptions of pathologic grieving responses, and suggestions both to facilitate normal grieving and to provide treatment for complicated grieving.

This chapter focuses on the clinical features of grieving reactions, with a particular emphasis on the specific responses of parents and the developmental trends in children's response to loss. Treatment suggestions are made for clinical intervention and facilitation.

The Nature of Grieving

Grieving—is it a physical illness, a psychiatric disorder, or a normal reaction to loss of a loved one? The fact that grieving results in acute somatic and psychological pain is unquestionable. Although most mental health professionals consider grieving to be a normal response to the loss of a person to whom one has close affectional bonds [9], unresolved or pathologic expressions of grief may underlie a variety of psychiatric disorders [10, 11]. Bowlby stated that "clinical experience and a reading of the evidence leave little doubt of the truth of the main proposition—that much psychiatric illness is an expression of pathological mourning—or that such illness includes many cases of anxiety state, depressive illness, and hysteria, and also more than one kind of character disorder" [11]. A number of studies also link grieving to morbidity and mortality, particularly in the loss of a spouse [11–15]. Engel argued that intense bereavement is as psychologically traumatic as serious physical illness and that it is a departure from a state of health and well-being [16]. Just as healing is necessary in cases of physical illness, healing also is necessary to restore the bereaved to a state of equilibrium psychologically. He saw mourning as a process that takes time before one can achieve full restoration of function [16].

It is evident that bereavement is an extremely complex process that can be experienced in a variety of ways. For everyone, the process entails mental and somatic distress. However, some may undergo this process and subsequently return to their original state of health, whereas others may need intervention; some may reach a higher level of growth and renewal by virtue of their grieving, whereas others may experience prolonged depression, illness, or even death. What accounts for the differences in the way individuals experience bereavement? What are the characteristics of normal grieving? When does grieving become pathologic? How does the sudden loss of an infant differ from other types of loss? How do adults and children differ in their response to loss? Finally, how may grieving parents and children be treated to avoid the pathologic ramifications of bereavement? These are the questions addressed in this chapter.

Symptomatology of Normal Grieving

Lindemann, in his classic 1944 article, described acute grief as a "definite syndrome," with both somatic and psychologic symptomatology [9]. Lindemann conducted a series of psychiatric interviews with 101 patients who had recently lost loved ones. Whether the death was expected or tragically sudden, whether the symptoms appeared immediately after the crisis or were delayed, were exaggerated or hardly apparent, there was an amazing similarity in the symptoms described by Lindemann's patients. Common to all were "sensations of somatic distress occurring in waves lasting from twenty minutes to an hour at a time, a feeling of tightness in the throat, choking with shortness of breath, need for sighing, an empty feeling in the abdomen, lack of muscular power, and an intense subjective distress described as tension or mental pain." [9] Lindemann summarized the symptoms of the bereaved into five primary categories. First, somatic distress was common, including a feeling of exhaustion and lack of strength. Digestive symptoms included lack of appetite, poor sensation of taste, and feelings of hollowness in the abdomen. The second cluster of symptoms related to altered sensorium, with most patients reporting a preoccupation with the image of the deceased, a slight sense of unreality and a feeling of increased emotional distance from other persons. Many of Lindemann's patients reported concern about this aspect of their grief response because they worried that they may be approaching insanity. A third constellation of symptoms revolved around feelings of guilt. The bereaved repeatedly searched their actions prior to the death for evidence of failure to do the "right thing" or for signs of negligence, or they experienced remorse over an argument with the deceased just prior to the death. Fourth, the patients often reported feelings of hostility or disturbance in relationships with others following the death of a loved one. These feelings included increased irritability, a distancing in the relationship, and a wish not to be bothered by others. Finally, the bereaved reported a loss of patterns of conduct or an inability to function as they had before the loss. There was restlessness, an inability to sit still, and a moving about in aimless fashion. Yet, at the same time, there was also a lack of ability to initiate and maintain organized patterns of activity. Patients reported a sense of mechanically going through the motions of their daily routines. The customary activities of living that were meaningful with the deceased often lost their significance to the bereaved. Lindemann also described a sixth characteristic shown by many, which involved the bereaved person's assuming the traits of the deceased. This sometimes involved adopting mannerisms of the deceased or showing a sudden interest in former activities of the deceased [9].

In his excellent book on grief counseling, Worden elaborated on the symptoms described by Lindemann [17]. He discussed the manifestations of normal grief as falling into four main categories: feelings, physical sensations, cognitions, and behaviors.

1. *Feelings.* As reported by Worden, the most common feeling experienced by the bereaved is that of intense sadness. Although sadness is an expected emotion, the survivor often is surprised to find that he or she feels angry, as well. Worden suggested that anger may come from two sources—a sense of frustration resulting from being unable to prevent the death, and from "a kind of regressive experience" occurring after the loss of a loved one [17]. In the loss of someone close, regression may be associated with a sense of helplessness, anxiety about being unable to exist without the deceased, and anger that accompanies feelings of anxiety. Because it is often difficult to acknowledge anger toward the deceased, it is common for the anger to be displaced upon someone else (e.g., the physician, other family members, the funeral director, friends, or God). Turning the anger inward upon oneself is an unhealthy adaptation to the loss of someone close, and can lead to severe depressive or even suicidal behavior at its most maladaptive stage. Guilt, or self reproach, may be experienced, although often the guilt feelings are irrational. The survivor may focus on events that happened or failed to happen around the time of the death, and project blame onto himself or herself relating to the death. Anxiety may be reported as a result of the survivor's feeling unable to survive without the deceased, or because the death of someone close may increase awareness of one's own mortality. Feelings of helplessness may be closely correlated with anxiety, especially in the early stages of a loss. With a sudden death,

shock often is the initial predominant emotion, and many survivors report feeling "numb" after learning of the death. A sense of loneliness and yearning for the deceased may follow, especially as the feelings of shock and numbness recede. At this point, the survivor focuses on the day-to-day experiences that once were shared with the deceased and must face the void left by the death. Feelings of fatigue and listlessness are common. If the loved one died after a prolonged illness, the survivor may report a feeling of emancipation or relief. None of the feelings described in this section represent pathologic reactions to grief, but they may become pathologic if they persist for a long time or are of excessive intensity [17].

2. *Physical Sensations.* The most commonly reported physical sensations include hollowness in the stomach, tightness in the chest, tightness in the throat, oversensitivity to noise, a sense of depersonalization (e.g., a sense of "unreality"), breathlessness, weakness in the muscles, lack of energy, and a dry mouth. These symptoms may be reported to a physician if they cause sufficient concern, but usually they represent normal responses and resolve without medical intervention [17].

3. *Cognitions.* The thought patterns common to grieving are believed by some researchers and clinicians to trigger emotional reactions, particularly reactions that persist over time. Thoughts such as disbelief or confusion may be most apparent in the early stages of grieving and usually accompany feelings of shock. Especially in the death of an apparently healthy child, as in the case of sudden infant death syndrome, young parents may have had little previous experience with death and may believe that it cannot happen to them. Confusion can accompany a sense of "unreality," causing the bereaved to be forgetful and to have difficulty organizing thoughts or concentrating. Other cognitive patterns include preoccupation or obsession with thoughts of the deceased. Often accompanying a feeling of yearning is a "sense of presence" of the deceased or thoughts about the deceased's being a part of one's daily life. Auditory and visual hallucinations, usually transient, frequently are reported by the bereaved and typically occur during the first weeks after the death. These hallucinations do not signify a severe emotional disorder, and do not necessarily indicate that the person is developing a pathologic grief reaction; they may actually facilitate the grieving process [17].

4. *Behaviors.* Numerous behaviors are commonly reported as part of the grieving process. Sleep disturbances may involve either difficulty going to sleep at night or disruption of sleep in the middle of the night. If fatigue persists, medical intervention sometimes is necessary; however, sleep disturbances usually correct themselves without medical involvement. Appetite disturbances also can accompany grieving, either in the form of overeating or undereating; however, loss of appetite is the more common manifestation and significant weight changes may occur. Absent-minded behavior often is reported, as is restless overactivity or aim-

lessness. Reports of dreaming about the deceased are common; these dreams may be helpful to the mental health professional in understanding the course of the grieving process. Dreams may suggest preoccupation with guilt, or conversely, a resolution of intense guilt. Some dreams may be reminders of pleasant times with the deceased. Whatever form they take, they may provide useful diagnostic and treatment information in working with the bereaved. Some survivors may be intent on avoiding reminders of the deceased, and thus may withdraw socially. They may quickly discard all things associated with the loved one, or even arrange for a quick disposal of the body. In the extreme, this avoidance reaction could lead to a complicated grief reaction that persists beyond the normal period. The opposite type of behavior consists of treasuring objects that belonged to the deceased, or visiting places or carrying objects that remind the survivor of the deceased. Searching or "calling out" for the deceased may occur either aloud or subvocally. Sighing and crying also are frequent behaviors of the bereaved.

Frey and others have examined the presence of catecholamines (mood-altering chemicals produced by the brain) in tears that result from emotional stress [18]. Because stress causes chemical imbalance in the body, there is speculation that tears remove toxic substances and help reestablish homeostasis. Although it is not yet clear how tears function to help, it is apparent that they do relieve emotional stress [17].

This review of the various feelings, physical sensations, thoughts, and behaviors associated with normal grieving demonstrates the diversity of possible reactions—all of which may be a part of the normal, or nonpathologic, process of bereavement. However, it is important to examine the special circumstances surrounding the death of an infant, and how parental responses may differ from those discussed.

Parental Reactions to the Death of an Infant

The reactions of parents to the loss of an infant can best be understood in the context of attachment theory, or the origins and development of early parent-infant bonds. Ainsworth defined attachment as "an affectional tie that one person forms to another specific person, binding them together in space and enduring over time. Attachment is discriminating and specific. One may be attached to more than one person, but one cannot be attached to many people. Attachment implies affect. Although the affects may be complex and may vary from time to time, positive affects predominate, and we usually think of attachment as implying affection or love" [19].

Bowlby theorized that attachment between humans occurs out of a need for security and safety and is developed to ensure survival [20]. Because of the extended period of helplessness for the human infant, Bowlby feels that the infant must have relatively stable behavioral systems that elicit maternal caregiving and thus ensure his or her survival through the long period of immaturity. Bowlby described an interactional model of attachment in which the infant, even at birth, possesses the behavioral capabilities to respond differentially to environmental stimuli and is an active participant in the reciprocal process of attachment with his or her caregiver. During the period of later infancy and early childhood, the child's attachment becomes more goal directed and the emphasis is placed on the maintenance of attachment. When loss of the attachment figure is threatened, the child experiences intense anxiety and emotional distress. Bowlby postulates that this early attachment relationship with a significant person(s) early in life determines the child's ability to form attachments later in life. In fact, the literature abounds with both animal and cross-cultural human models for attachment, and for the grieving responses apparent after the loss of an attachment figure. Bowlby stated that when loss or threat of loss occurs, "all the most powerful forms of attachment behavior become activated—clinging, crying, and perhaps angry coercion" [20]. These behaviors are followed by withdrawal, apathy, and despair [17].

The implications of Bowlby's theory for grieving parents are twofold—relating to their emotional responses to loss of an attachment figure (i.e., their infant), and also relating to the intensity of their attachment to their infant. The parents' intense emotional distress—anxiety, yearning, anger, withdrawal, apathy, and despair—would be expected reactions to separation from their loved one, or "the love object" to use Freud's term [21]. The task of mourning is seen as the gradual surrender of attachment to the deceased.

Some parents who lose an infant to SIDS relate that relatives and friends often imply that it is "easier" to lose a young infant than an older child, since strong attachments with the infant have not "had time" to form. This notion is refuted by several researchers.

Bowlby's interactional model for attachment is founded on the idea that the infant is born with certain species-specific behavioral systems that elicit parental caretaking and attachment behaviors [20]. However, others suggest that the process of attachment for the *parent* begins long before the birth of the infant [22]. Klaus and Kennell pointed out that many cultural and familial factors help prepare the mother and father for becoming attached to their young, such as the parents' own childhood experiences, their attitude toward parenthood, and the support systems available to them as they assume parenthood [23]. Caplan [24] described two primary adaptive tasks of pregnancy that are important in the development of attachment: (1) acceptance of the pregnancy, which Bibring et al. [25] described as the mother's identification of the growing fetus as an "integral part of herself," and (2) perception of the fetus as a separate individual [23]. The sensation of fetal movement may coincide with the sense of the fetus as an individual and may intensify the feelings of attachment. Although parents may vary in their readiness for parenthood, and indeed may vary in the degree of attachment they form with their offspring, it is apparent that the psychological mechanism for development of a strong attachment is present even prior to the infant's birth.

Additional evidence for the early development of attachment to an infant comes from a study by Kennell and colleagues [22]. They studied the mourning responses of mothers who lost infants at various times after birth. Using the degree of mourning as a measure of affectional bonding, they noted that mothers displayed intense bereavement whether their infant lived one hour or many days, whether the infant was full-term or an unviable preterm, whether the pregnancy was planned or unplanned. The presence of mourning responses in all mothers, regardless of the age or condition of their infant, was felt to suggest that significant affectional ties had been formed by the time of or soon after the birth of the infant [22].

Thus, parents who lose an infant to SIDS would be expected to display intense grieving responses, regardless of the age of their infant at the time of death. There is ample evidence to suggest that strong parent-infant attachment may exist at the time of the infant's death, and that the ensuing emotional distress of the parents is to be expected and is very logical in terms of attachment theory.

The Process of Mourning

Worden refers to the term "mourning" as the process that occurs after a loss, whereas "grief" is the personal experience of the loss [17]. Mourning, or the adaptation to loss, appears to be an essential process that must be completed before equilibrium can be reestablished. Freud described the process as doing "grief work." There have been numerous conceptualizations of the stages or phases involved in mourning. Elizabeth Kubler-Ross first suggested "stages of dying," which have been applied to the mourning process, as well. These include emotional and behavioral reactions of denial, rage and anger, bargaining, depression, and acceptance [26]. The misinterpretation of these stages as occurring in a rigid sequence, and always occurring in every person, has resulted in the formulation of concepts to explain the process of mourning.

Rubin described the primary process in bereavement as "loosening of the affective bond to the deceased" [27]. This process of detachment is thought to follow a predictable course, with three predictable stages. The first stage is the acute grief period, which typically lasts from three to twelve weeks. The second stage is the mourning period, usually less disruptive than the acute grief period. According to Rubin, the mourning period may last from one to two years. Whereas the acute grief period is characterized by dramatic changes in behavior, the mourning period is characterized by a more subdued process of detachment from the deceased. The final stage occurs when the detachment process has reached its conclusion and a resolution has been achieved. At this point, homeostasis has been accomplished and personality or behavioral changes accompanying the mourning period have stabilized [27].

Worden preferred to conceptualize mourning in terms of the "tasks" that must be accomplished by the bereaved in order to reestablish equilibrium [17]. He stated that it is essential for the bereaved to accomplish these tasks before mourning can be completed. The lack of completion of the tasks can lead to impaired growth and development. The four tasks of mourning are as follows:

Task 1: To Accept the Reality of the Loss. The first task of mourning involves the acceptance of the finality of the loss, the fact that the loved one is dead and will not return. Although searching for the deceased is common, this task of mourning involves accepting the fact that a reunion is not possible. The opposite of believing the loss is real is denying the loss, either through denying the facts of the death, denying that the loss has much meaning to the bereaved, blocking the reality of the loss from one's mind, or denying that death is irreversible. Although a brief period of searching for the deceased is expected, this reaction usually is short-lived and the bereaved will move on to the second task of mourning [17].

Task 2: To Experience the Pain of Grief. The second task involves the experience of emotional, behavioral, and physical pain. Although the type and intensity of pain may vary from person to person, it appears necessary for the bereaved to experience the pain of grief in order to get the "grief work" done [12]. It may be tempting to suppress the pain through medication, denial, or distraction, but Parkes stated that "anything that continually allows the person to avoid or suppress the pain can be expected to prolong the course of mourning" [12]. Completion of this task of mourning may be made more difficult because of society's discomfort with feelings of pain, and the subtle or not-so-subtle messages sent to mourners that they should deny or avoid expressing their feelings. It is important for the bereaved to work through this difficult stage of mourning so that they do not carry their pain with them for years [17].

Task 3: To Adjust to an Environment in Which the Deceased is Missing. The degree of adjustment required depends on the relationship between the mourner and the deceased and on the roles played by the deceased. The mourner often must develop new skills or change the roles he or she formerly played in order to adapt to life without the loved one. For parents who lose an infant to SIDS, this may entail a major readjustment of their roles as parents to return to a stronger focus on their roles as husband and wife. The tendency to conceive again quickly, before completion of tasks 2 and 3, is common [17]. The "replacement child" may be seen by parents as a way of easing their intense pain and helping themselves adjust to the loss of their infant to SIDS. However, the attempt to replace the lost child is often problematic for both the parents and the subsequent child, as the sibling may be constantly compared with the dead child [8, 28, 29]. It is essential for the bereaved, in this case the parents, to resolve the previous tasks of mourning before moving on to the fourth and final task.

Task 4: To Withdraw Emotional Energy and Reinvest It in Another Relationship. This task involves an emotional withdrawal from the deceased so that emotional energy can be reinvested in another relationship. Some persons have difficulty with this task because of anticipatory grieving—fear of investing in a new relationship and then facing another loss. Others find it difficult to deinvest in the deceased, as if to do so would mean dishonoring the memory of the deceased. To move through this task of mourning is to realize that loving other persons does not negate the love one had for the deceased [17].

Although there is no definite timetable for the completion of mourning, Worden suggested that mourning is complete when the tasks of mourning are accomplished [17]. Some would suggest that mourning never ends entirely, but that, over time, the bereaved can come to think of the deceased without pain. Grieving is a very individual process, with the timetable varying widely. However, most would agree that mourning rarely is completed in less than one year, and that even two years is not too long to expect grieving reactions.

Determinants of Grief

A number of factors determine the intensity and duration of grieving responses; the most important of these is the developmental stage and conflict issues of the individual involved. Although the developmental trends in grieving are discussed in another section of this chapter, the most important determinants of grief for adults were summarized by Worden as follows [17]:

1. *Who the Person Was.* Differences in grieving responses will relate to whether the deceased is a spouse or child, a distant relative, or an immediate family member [17].

2. *The Nature of the Attachment.* As stated, the intensity of grieving responses is believed to be related to the strength of the attachment. However, the security of the attachment is important, as well. Whether the survivor depended upon the deceased for his or her own sense of well being or self esteem can affect the intensity of grieving. The presence of ambivalent feelings toward the loved one is not uncommon, but if the negative feelings are equal to or exceed the positive, grieving may be more difficult. Strong feelings of guilt or anger at being left may occur [17].

3. *Mode of Death.* The expected death of a loved one likely will be responded to differently than an accidental or sudden death. The death of a

child will be grieved differently than that of an older person. Several studies indicated that survivors of sudden death have a more difficult time one to two years later than those who have some warning of the approaching death [17]. In his study of the bereavement of mothers who lost an infant to SIDS, Rubin found that the passage of several years alleviated but did not heal the feelings of loss. The attachment to the deceased child continued to be a significant component of these women's lives [27].

4. *Historical Antecedents*. It is important to understand whether the bereaved has a history of grieving adequately over previous losses or whether there was incomplete grieving previously. The person with an unresolved grief likely will have a more difficult time dealing with the recent loss, as will persons with a history of mental health problems such as depression [17].

5. *Personality Variables*. Worden suggested that variables such as the age and sex of the person, how well they express their feelings, how well they handle anxiety, and how they cope with stressful situations may determine their grieving responses. Persons with certain personality disorders, such as Borderline or Narcissistic personality, may have a more difficult time coping with a loss [17].

6. *Social Variables*. Knowing something about the ethnic, social, and religious background of the survivor will be helpful in understanding how a person is likely to grieve, although it is not entirely clear how participation in rituals affects bereavement [17].

Examination of these variables may help the mental health professional better predict how the bereaved is likely to react and better facilitate the grieving process through counseling. However, the reactions of children to loss of a loved one require further discussion within the context of their developmental stages and levels of cognitive/emotional awareness. The reactions of children who lose a sibling to SIDS are reviewed in the next section.

Developmental Trends in the Concept of Death

A child's concept of death does not necessarily fall into discrete ages and stages. It is generally understood, however, that very young children under age four or five years do not view death as permanent and that children in late childhood or early adolescence develop an understanding of the concept of death. The exception to these developmental trends has been found in young children who are dying of cancer, in that they seem to understand beyond their expected level of cognitive functioning that they are dying [30] (Spinetta et al., 1983. Unpublished manuscript). The age at which this accurate understanding of death occurs for most children varies, and the transition in conceptual reasoning of death can vary [31].

First and foremost, numerous studies demonstrate that a child's mental or intellectual development generally takes precedence over chronological age in the understanding of death [32–37]. Early developmental studies demonstrated the child's transition in thinking relative to the concept of death. Nagy [38] and Anthony [39] were two of the early investigators who described three approximate age levels for a child's developmental concept of death. Nagy studied three to ten-year-old children and collected her information in three ways: (1) children seven to ten years of age were asked to "write down everything that comes to your mind about death"; (2) children six to ten years of age were asked to draw pictures of death— many of the older children included explanations with their drawings; (3) discussions of compositions and drawings were held with all children to clarify and amplify each child's meanings. The last approach was designed to get the child talking about death in an effort to understand his or her ideas and feelings about the concept [38]. Nagy categorized her results into three developmental stages:

1. The child who is less than five years of age usually does not recognize death as an irreversible fact; in death the child sees life.
2. Between the ages of five and nine, death is most often personified and thought of as a contingency.
3. Only at the age of nine and later does the child begin to view death as a process that happens to us according to certain laws [38].

Children Five Years of Age and Under

Children less than five years of age basically feel there is no definitive death and that death is merely a departure or sleep. They believe that the deceased may be altered but continues to exist. The major fears or concerns of a child this age involve separation from a loved one rather than concerns over the permanency of death. It is in this earlier stage of development that children may misinterpret a prolonged absence of their mother or father as death. It is not as if the mother or father did not continue to exist, but that they exist in a different form [38]. Another example of this form of reasoning may be seen with the child whose sibling dies of SIDS and is buried. The child might view the sibling as now living in a cemetery under conditions of reduced mobility.

In viewing developmental trends, Piaget's observations and writings teach us a great deal about the cognitive capacity of children. The child from one and one-half years to five years of age (and even up to seven years) is in the preoperational stage of cognitive development according to Piaget [40]. At this stage, the child has developed language and the capacity for representational thought. That is, he or she has the ability to treat objects as symbolic of something else (e.g., the child plays with blocks as though they are cars, or uses a broom to represent a horse which he or she may ride through the house). During this stage of development, the child is egocentric in his or her thinking and has difficulty seeing events from the perspective of someone else. Everything is viewed from his or her personal perspective or experience [40]. Thus, when death occurs, the child relates it to his or her own experience, such as when a favorite animal died.

Children four to six years of age, being egocentric in their thinking, react to death in a manner consistent with their own experiences, perhaps based upon what they have seen on television or have been told by adults or have experienced. They usually are not capable of "cognitive reciprocity" (i.e., learning outside the realm of their experiences). In this young age group, children are highly imaginative and often resort to magical thinking [40]. Because they tend to be egocentric and think magically, they may attribute the death of a sibling to something they have done. For example, the child may have been resentful or jealous of the sibling, may have taken the sibling's toy, or accidentally hit the sibling and therefore may attribute the loss to something he or she did or thought. When asked about death in general and what dying means, children at this age level usually attribute it to doing something bad, being bad, or disobeying mother. As a result of personalizing the loss, the young child may feel guilty and be fearful of retribution.

The lack of overt grief displayed by the five-year-old or younger child may be misinterpreted by the parents as cold and unfeeling when it is a normal reaction for a child this age. Perhaps the most distressing observations made by the child at this age involve the parents' reaction to the loss. Since the death of a child to SIDS can have a dramatic impact on the parents, the family system is disrupted and parental grief often affects the surviving sibling's efforts to cope and adapt to the altered family system [41]. The child may feel sad and anxious and worry that something he or she did has upset the parents. The parents' sadness over the deceased also can cause the child to feel responsible for the disappearance of his or her sibling. Additionally, parents may increase their closeness to surviving children and may begin to overprotect or cling to younger children. It is as if the parent is trying to be closer to the deceased child through closeness to the remaining siblings [41]. Young children also may develop somatic symptoms in the form of stomach aches, or they may be overly concerned about potential "abandonment" by other family members. Consistent and patient reassurance is often sufficient to enable the child to resolve his or her anxieties [42]. With adequate support, love, and understanding the child can emerge from this tragic family crisis relatively unscathed. This is not to say that children will not present behavioral symptoms as the result of a sibling loss. The symptoms may vary and may manifest in the form of enuresis, nightmares, school phobias, crying, clinging, anorexia, somatic complaints, and other regressive behaviors [43]. Above all, guilt appears to be a major symptom that must be dealt with in the surviving child [44].

As children develop, there seems to be a gradual change in the concept of death between ages five and six years, depending upon the mental capacity of the child. Death is still viewed as a temporary or gradual notion, but the idea of death itself is not denied [38].

Children Five Years to Nine Years of Age

Children in stage two of Nagy's study (five to nine years of age) most often personified death (i.e., equated death with a person) [38]. In Koocher's study of children's conception of death, none of the children in the five to nine year age range personified death [45]. Koocher speculated that the difference between his and Nagy's study in the way children view death may be cultural, because Nagy's subjects were Hungarian children. Koocher [45] and Kubler-Ross [46] found that slightly older children (ages seven to twelve) are more concrete in their thinking and usually attribute death to a catastrophic event (e.g., someone or something, such as guns, cancer, God, drugs, or poison). This age group is still immature in their cognitive development and they may not mourn as adults mourn. Again, Piaget's observations and writing on child development are instructive. The child in the middle years seems to be very interested in "why" things happen. Piaget [47] found that children in the concrete-operational stage of cognitive development are bewildered by death and ask questions about the cause of death, as though death could not happen by "chance" as in SIDS. When the child's sibling dies as a result of SIDS, the child will want to ask many questions. The open and communicative family should recognize the child's need to know "why" and explain as well as they can the cause of death. The health professional also may offer to talk with the child, especially when the parents are too overwhelmed by grief to do so.

Behaviorally, the seven- to twelve-year-old child understands the uniqueness of death and even fears death. This age group also may experience anger and guilt over the loss of a baby to SIDS. Some will feel that death is a form of punishment for wrongdoing [37]. The child at this age may become moody, withdrawn, and stop talking, or the parents may be the recipients of temper tantrums or other regressive behavior. Children of all ages may probe for more information about the cause of the baby's death, but the middle aged child wants to know "why."

It must be remembered that the surviving children from preschool age through middle childhood may develop a transient fear of being left alone or a fear that their parents might also die and leave them [48]. To prevent this fear from developing into a chronic, lifelong fear, parents and other family or health personnel will need to reassure the child and take the time to offer explanations. Explanations need to be brief and geared toward the child's level of understanding. Cliches and deceptions must be avoided, such as telling the child that the sibling was taken to live with God or went to sleep and died, without an explanation of why. Going to sleep may be equated with dying and could arouse nighttime fears in the surviving child.

Children Nine to Twelve Years of Age and Older

Stage three (nine years and older) children are capable of understanding death [38]. The child twelve years and older is capable of more abstract formal reasoning and recognizes that death can be caused by illness or accidents and not necessarily by catastrophic events, as their younger siblings believe. A child this age may grieve the loss of the baby in relation to the role the lost baby played in the child's life, and he or she will be concerned about the parents. Depending upon the openness of communication in the family and the availability of the parents, the child this age may suffer in silence [38].

Children and adolescents in this age range do grieve and do feel a sense of guilt. Children of all ages may attempt to cope with their grief by focusing on schoolwork or school related activities, crying when alone, keeping an object that belonged to the deceased, looking at pictures of the deceased, seeking solace through religion, and/or maintaining their normal routine [44].

It is important that the family maintain open communication with the surviving children and be supportive of each other. The health professional may want to speak with all members of the family subsequent to the loss of a child to SIDS and continue to be available to all members of the family. Another parent who previously lost a child to SIDS also can provide support and could be called upon to aid the family.

In summary, the effect of SIDS upon siblings and the reactions they exhibit as a function of the loss are dependent upon (1) the developmental stage of the child's psychological growth; (2) whether or not the child has the age-appropriate cognitive capacity to deal with the loss; (3) the nature of the role the deceased baby played in the child's life; (4) the coping mechanisms and support systems available to the siblings; and (5) the nature of the circumstances surrounding the death.

Pathologic Grieving

Pathologic grief was defined by Horowitz et al. as "the intensification of grief to the level where the person is overwhelmed, resorts to maladaptive behavior, or remains interminably in the state of grief without progression of the mourning process toward completion. . . . [It] involves processes that do not move progressively toward assimilation or accommodation but, instead, lead to stereotyped repetitions or extensive interruptions of healing" [49]. Freud [21] and Abraham [50] differentiated normal from pathologic grief, with normal grieving characterized by painful dejection, loss of interest, and inhibition of activities and pathologic grieving characterized by episodes of panic, hostility toward the self, regression to a preoccupation with the self, and other signs of poor self-esteem. Horowitz noted that whereas the distinctions between normal and pathological grieving described by Freud and Horowitz suggest an "excessive cleavage," field studies of bereavement suggest that some of the reactions originally considered to be pathologic are fairly common [49]. Therefore, it is believed that normal and pathologic grieving probably fall along a continuum rather than being distinct reactions, and that pathology is related more to the intensity and duration of a reaction than to the presence or absence of specific behaviors [49].

Worden described four types of complicated grief reactions: chronic grief, delayed grief, exaggerated grief, and masked grief reactions [17]. *Chronic* grief is prolonged, is excessive in duration, and never reaches a satisfactory end. The bereaved person usually is quite aware that he or she has not resolved the grieving process, and is "marking time" rather than getting on with living. *Delayed* grief reactions refer to a partial, suppressed, or incomplete reaction at the time of the original loss, with the more intense grieving reactions surfacing later, perhaps in response to only a minor loss. These delayed reactions may even occur as one vicariously observes another person experiencing a loss. If the grieving is not adequately completed at the time of the original loss, it is carried forward and experienced at the time of a later loss. *Exaggerated* grief reactions involve the "intensification of a normal grief reaction to the extent that the person feels overwhelmed and resorts to maladaptive behavior" [17]. Examples of problems developing from this type of complicated grief reaction include phobias and irrational despair. Most people suffering this type of grief reaction seek therapy because their excessive despair interferes significantly with their functioning. *Masked* grief reactions may manifest as physical symptoms or some type of aberrant or maladaptive behavior. Often, those with masked grief reactions do not see the relationship between their symptoms and the loss [17].

Failure to grieve may result from a number of factors, including the type of relationship the person had with the deceased (e.g., whether ambivalent or overly dependent); circumstantial factors surrounding the loss (e.g., factors such as the cause of death and how clearly the cause is understood); historical factors involving previous loss and separations and how they were handled; personality style of the bereaved (e.g., whether one is able to express feelings openly or tends to withdraw and withhold expression of painful emotions, or whether one's self-concept is that of being "strong" or "helpless"); and social factors, such as the absence of a social network or the social negation of a death (as in the case of abortion or suicide) [17]. Some parents of SIDS infants report being socially ostracized by family members, professionals, and friends, as if their infant's death was caused by their own negligence or even abuse.

Diagnosis of pathologic grieving may be difficult, particularly when the patient presents with behavioral or somatic complaints and no mention of a significant loss. The astute clinician will carefully obtain a detailed history, including a history of loss, in order to diagnose an unresolved grief reaction. Lazare offers a number of clues to aid in diagnosis of complicated grief reactions [10].

1. Inability of the patient to speak about the deceased without intense, fresh sadness and grief

2. Triggering of an intense grief reaction or overreaction by relatively minor events

3. Frequent references to themes of loss.

4. Unwillingness to surrender or even move the belongings of the deceased

5. Presence of physical symptoms similar to those of the deceased just before death

6. Drastic changes in life style following a loss

7. A long history of either mild depression (with guilt or lowered self-esteem) or false euphoria following the death

8. Overidentification with the deceased by imitating actions or personality characteristics

9. Self-destructive impulses

10. Prolonged, unaccountable sadness occurring at special times that were meaningful with the deceased

11. Phobia related to the symptoms of illness or circumstances that lead to the death

12. History of avoiding the funeral or other rituals related to the death, or lack of a social support network at the time of the loss.

Although none of these clues individually would be sufficient to support a diagnosis of a complicated grief reaction, such indications should be taken seriously and considered when making the diagnosis [10].

Facilitating Normal Grieving in Adults

Many persons experiencing normal or uncomplicated grieving reactions will not request or need professional guidance. However, some believe that loss of a child places parents at greater risk for complicated grieving and that they may need help to work through their acute grief and long-term reactions to a resolution. In a study of fifty parents of SIDS infants, DeFrain and Ernst found that SIDS was considered the most severe crisis these parents had ever experienced [1]. The families studied took an average of 8.3 months to regain the level of family organization they had had prior to the death, and individual parents took an average of 15.9 months to regain their prior level of personal happiness. There were reports of intense guilt and numerous other psychological and physical difficulties. One of the most striking findings was that 60 percent of the parents who had lost an infant to SIDS moved within two and one-half years of the death. It is possible that these parents felt that only by leaving their homes could they recover from the shock of the death [1]. Mandell and Wolfe reported fertility problems among the thirty-two women they studied who had lost an infant to SIDS. Thirty-one percent had spontaneous abortions and 34 percent could not conceive for one year after the death; these mothers all reported harsh grief reactions and a feeling of failure as a mother [8]. Likewise, Booher and Little reported that 10 percent of previously fertile mothers of SIDS infants will have fertility problems and that spontaneous abortions will occur in 12 to 15 percent of subsequent pregnancies [51]. Rowe et al. found that six of twenty-six mothers who had suffered a perinatal death of their infant experienced a prolonged grief reaction (twelve to twenty months). Those mothers with a surviving twin or a subsequent pregnancy less than five months after the death were at a higher risk for prolonged grieving reactions [7]. Drotar and Irvin reported that mothers whose infant dies may find that their relationship with surviving or subsequent children is profoundly influenced [2]. Thus, infant death particularly seems to pose special problems for the survivors. Families who survive infant death, and particularly sudden infant death, warrant careful follow-up and support during the grieving process.

Worden stated that the general goal in grief counseling is to help the survivor complete the four tasks of mourning described [17]. He outlined several principles and procedures to facilitate the process of normal grieving.

1. *Help the Survivor Actualize the Loss.* This task involves helping the bereaved come to a greater awareness that the loss really has occurred. Encouraging persons to talk about the loss, the circumstances of the death, the funeral or other rituals associated with the death, and memories of the deceased can be helpful [17].

2. *Help the Survivor to Identify and Express Feelings.* Worden suggested that many survivors have difficulty with feelings of anger, guilt, anxiety, and/or helplessness. The anger may stem from a sense of frustration or from the intense pain experienced during the bereavement. At other times, the anger may result from a sense of regressive helplessness. The anger may be turned inward upon oneself or displaced upon someone else, such as the physician, hospital staff, funeral director, or clergy. The

grief counselor may help the bereaved by exploring the source of this anger and developing a better balance between the negative and positive feelings that exist. If the anger is turned inward, the counselor must be alert for signs of possible suicidal behavior, either in thought or action. When feelings of guilt are apparent, the counselor may help the bereaved distinguish between irrational guilt and real guilt. Irrational guilt may lessen through the counselor's help with "reality testing" and reassurance that the bereaved did not actually cause the death of the loved one. Working through real guilt is more difficult, but the bereaved can be helped to come to accept themselves and their actions and to put the strong feelings of guilt behind them.

Anxiety may stem from feelings of helplessness, and a concern that it is not possible to survive alone. The counselor may be helpful to the bereaved in pointing out internal and external resources that will help them manage on their own. With others, the anxiety results from a sense of their own mortality. The heightened awareness of one's own mortality may require open discussion or may fade with time if not discussed. The counselor will need to decide how best to approach this type of anxiety in each case. Sadness, and the expression of that sadness through crying, may be denied or suppressed until the bereaved are given "permission" to express their feelings. The counselor may help override society's reaction to expression of emotion by allowing the bereaved a time to express their feelings openly [17].

3. *Help the Survivor Face Living without the Deceased.* The bereaved may need counseling to facilitate the assumption of new responsibilities and improvement of decision-making ability after the loss of the loved one. The loss may require the survivor to act more independently and to develop new skills and roles that were previously handled by the deceased. The counselor also may be helpful in discouraging major life-changing decisions, such as moving, selling one's property, changing jobs or careers, or becoming pregnant again too soon after a death [17].

4. *Facilitate Emotional Withdrawal from the Deceased.* The counselor may need to encourage some survivors to form new relationships after a death while counseling other survivors to avoid jumping into relationships too soon after the death. Either extreme in behavior may hinder adequate resolution of grief. The counselor may provide feedback as to the progress through the tasks of mourning and suggest to the survivor when he or she is ready to move into new relationships [17].

5. *Provide Time to Grieve.* Some survivors need "permission" from others to grieve. The grief counselor may help survivors realize that it takes time to adjust to a loss and all the ramifications of that loss. Special holidays or anniversaries related to the deceased may be particularly difficult, and the survivor may need time to experience and work through these difficult periods [17].

6. *Interpret "Normal" Behavior.* A common reaction to a significant loss may be the feeling that one is going "crazy," and the grief counselor may be very helpful in interpreting mourning behavior as normal. The counselor also should be aware of the past emotional functioning of the bereaved in order to determine if a person is at risk for developing severe pathology secondary to the loss. However, severe emotional reactions are rare, and most emotional reactions to grieving do fall within the range of normal [17].

7. *Allow for Individual Differences.* The wide range of behavioral responses to grieving should be recognized in order to avoid inappropriate expectations among family members. Rigid expectations of how one "should" respond to a loss frequently are damaging [17].

8. *Provide Continuing Support.* In grief counseling, it is important to be available not only during the acute grief period but also during the much longer period of mourning as the bereaved attempt to work through the various tasks of mourning. Most counselors make themselves available to the survivor and family for at least the first year after a death, and sometimes longer [17].

9. *Examine Defenses and Coping Styles.* If the survivor uses coping styles that are destructive or prevent an effective adjustment to the loss, a counselor may help explore other possible coping strategies that would be more effective in lowering distress and resolving problems [17].

10. *Identify Pathology and Refer.* The grief counselor should be able to identify pathology that is secondary to the loss and understand when it is appropriate to refer the bereaver for more specialized psychotherapy. When pathologic grieving occurs, the difficulties typically require special techniques developed with an understanding of psychodynamics, and this may or may not be within the training and expertise of the grief counselor. Counselors must recognize their limitations and know when to refer the patient to a person who is trained in psychopathology and psychotherapy, such as a clinical psychologist or a psychiatrist.

Helping Children Adjust to Loss: Guidelines for Parents and Professionals

Parents may feel a great deal of anxiety and helplessness when faced with questions about death from their children [52, 53]. Parents who lose an infant to SIDS are faced not only with their own grieving but also with the grieving responses of their surviving children. Although the parents may be able to reach beyond the immediate family for their support network, children typically rely upon their parents to provide both information and emotional support in a time of crisis. A number of authors have suggested guidelines for helping children work through their tasks of mourning.

1. It is important for parents to be aware of the child's developmental

level and capacity for understanding the significance of the loss. The developmental stages of both cognitive and emotional functioning have an impact on the child's understanding.

2. Children have the right to be included in family discussions and explanations about a sibling's death [54]. Children tend to let their imaginations run wild when adults do not take the time to explain what has happened, and they may blame themselves for the death. Explanations can be modified according to the child's cognitive level; the very young child needs only brief, sensitive, but matter-of-fact answers to his or her questions. Very young children may not understand the loss of a sibling to SIDS, but the fact that the parents talked with them could make death less frightening. One of the most valuable methods parents and health professionals can learn is to allow children to talk freely and ask their own questions after a brief explanation of SIDS is made to them [55–57].

3. Parents may feel so overwhelmed and emotional that they cannot talk to their children. Parents can be honest about their grief and sadness but they will need to do so in a mature manner that does not overwhelm or confuse the child. Open communication is important, and children will need to be allowed to ventilate emotions or ask questions they may have. As Jackson so eloquently wrote:

This, then, is of primary importance. Share feelings at the child's level of functioning and at the same time protect him from the full impact of emotional breakdown among the adults he depends on for emotional security. He can understand sadness better than deception. He can build his approach to the future better on trust than on a lie [55].

4. It is important to avoid philosophical or unhealthy explanations about the deceased infant. For example, stating that "God took ——— to heaven" is a tempting explanation but not accurate. An honest explanation can avoid misperceptions and confusion on the part of the child [56]. Prohibiting the child from attending the funeral excludes him or her from an important family function; children need to be included in the funeral process.

5. Children need activity; curtailing their activities because "they should be mourning" prohibits a child's normal outlet for emotional energy. Permitting the child to behave and act in his or her normal manner is important [42, 58]. This is not to say that the child will not grieve, but merely that children need rest from grief so that at times they are playful and carrying out daily routines and at other times they may exhibit sadness [59].

The child who exhibits grieving behavior needs parental support and patience. Reassurance that the child is loved and will not be abandoned is important.

Koocher also offered suggestions that parents and other professionals might use for discussing death with the young child whose sibling died of

SIDS [45]. Koocher's study suggested that children are ready and capable of talking about death and are pleased by the attention given to them by adults. Koocher stated that "silence teaches them only that the topic is taboo; it cannot help them to cope with their feelings of loss" [45]. He suggested that explanations of death to children under age seven or eight be simple and direct, and "draw as much as possible from the child's own experiences. In this way the relative concreteness of the younger child will produce the least possible distortion" [45]. The young child also might be asked to talk about what he or she thinks happened to the deceased sibling, and in this manner distortions in thinking can be corrected.

Guidelines for telling children about death have been summarized by Lonetto [32] as follows:

1. Children are ready and capable of talking about anything within their own experiences.
2. Use the language of the child, not the sentimental symbols we find so easy to utter.
3. Do not expect an immediate and obvious response from the child.
4. Be a good listener and observer.
5. Don't try to do it all in one discussion; that is, be available.
6. Make certain that your child knows that he or she is part of the family, especially when a death has occurred.
7. One of the most valuable methods of teaching children about death is to allow them to talk freely and ask their own questions.

Treatment of Pathologic Grieving

The goal in grief therapy is to identify and resolve the conflicts relating to separation from the deceased that prevent the resolution of the tasks of mourning [17]. Therapy is most useful in persons whose grief is absent, delayed, excessive, or prolonged. When prolonged grief occurs, the primary goal of therapy is to determine which of the tasks of mourning is incomplete, what is preventing the resolution, and then help the bereaved to move forward on these issues. When grief is masked as somatic or behavioral symptoms, the reason usually involves unresolved grief of a much earlier loss. The grief response to the earlier loss may have been absent or suppressed, but surfaces later in the form of other symptoms. Exaggerated grief may involve excessive depression, excessive anger, or other emotional features manifested in an exaggerated fashion [17]. Whatever the type of grieving response, the goal of grief therapy is to facilitate the completion of the grief task [17].

Worden suggested several procedures that should be considered along with the therapist's own theoretical framework when providing grief therapy [17]. These include ruling out physical disease in the patient and then setting up a contract and establishing an alliance. According to Worden, the patient must agree to re-explore his or her relationship with the person or persons involved in a previous loss. Reviving both positive and negative memories of the deceased is necessary to help reach a balance so that the patient can begin to work through the negative memories. Another component of grief therapy involves assessing which of the four grief tasks is uncompleted and working toward a resolution. Dealing with the affect or lack of affect associated with the memory of the deceased is important for therapy. If affect is excessively strong, the patient may need help from the therapist to restrain the overwhelming feelings. The grief therapist also will want to identify whether the patient has any "linking objects"—symbolic objects kept by the survivor to provide a link with the deceased. More than just a keepsake, this linking object is invested with symbolism and causes great anxiety if lost [17]. The therapist will assist the patient in diffusing this linking object. Acknowledging the finality of the loss is another important component of grief therapy. Volkan described some bereaved patients as having a "chronic hope for reunion" [60]. The therapist must help the patient explore what giving up grieving would mean. Finally, the therapist must facilitate the process of saying a final "goodbye" to the deceased. The timing of this varies greatly with each individual, and the therapist must allow the patient to take the lead in the process [17].

Although these general guidelines should be helpful to anyone engaged in grief therapy, the therapist's training is important. The therapist must be able to recognize and treat underlying pathology whenever it exists and to distinguish between an unresolved grieving response and other types of emotional pathology. Conversely, therapists who engage primarily in other types of routine psychotherapy would do well to remember the clinical features of unresolved grief and to explore the possibility that issues surrounding loss may play a role in the emotional functioning or dysfunctioning of patients.

Conclusion

In this chapter, we have attempted to provide a detailed review of the nature of grieving responses in adults, particularly in parents who have lost an infant suddenly and unexpectedly, and in children. The characteristics of normal grieving, the "tasks" to be accomplished during the mourning process, and descriptions of pathologic grieving responses are provided. Children's grieving reactions are discussed in the context of developmental stages of cognitive and emotional development, with the hope that this knowledge will be helpful to both parents and professionals in providing a support network for grieving children. Finally, various suggestions for facilitating normal grieving reactions and treating pathologic grieving are made. Dr. Mandell, in Chapter 10, provides additional detail specifically regarding the families of SIDS victims. However, we hope this chapter provides a theoretical framework for treatment of a variety of grieving reactions and will be particularly applicable to families who have lost an infant to SIDS.

References

1. DeFrain, J.D., and L. Ernst. 1978. The psychological effects of Sudden Infant Death Syndrome on surviving family members. *J Fam Prac* 6:985–989.
2. Drotar, D., and N. Irvin. 1979. Disturbed maternal bereavement following infant death. *Child Care Health Dev* 5:239–247.
3. Friedman, S.B. 1974. Psychological aspects of sudden unexpected death in infants and children. *Pediatr Clin North Am* 21:103–111.
4. Smialek, Z. 1978. Observations on immediate reactions of families to sudden infant death. *Pediatrics* 62:160–165.
5. Krein, N. 1979. Sudden Infant Death Syndrome: Acute loss and grief reactions. *Clin Pediatr* 18:414–423.
6. Mandell, F., E. McAnulty, and R.M. Reece. 1980. Observations of paternal response to sudden unanticipated infant death. *Pediatrics* 65:221–225.
7. Rowe, J., R. Clyman, C. Green, C. Mikkelsen, J. Haight, and L. Ataide. 1978. Follow-up of families who experience a perinatal death. *Pediatrics* 62:166–170.
8. Mandell, F., and L.C. Wolfe. 1975. Sudden Infant Death Syndrome and subsequent pregnancy. *Pediatrics* 56:774–776.
9. Lindemann, E. 1944. Symptomatology and management of acute grief. *Am J Psychiatry* 101:141–148.
10. Lazare, A. 1979. "Unresolved grief." In *Outpatient Psychiatry: Diagnosis and Treatment,* ed. A. Lazare. Baltimore: Williams and Wilkins.
11. Bowlby, J. 1980. *Attachment and Loss: Loss, Sadness, and Depression,* Vol. III. New York: Basic Books.
12. Parkes, C.M., and R.J. Brown. 1972. Health after bereavement: A controlled study of young Boston widows and widowers. *Psychosom Med* 34:449–461.
13. Clayton, P.J. 1974. Mortality and morbidity in the first year of widowhood. *Arch Gen Psychiatry* 30:747–750.
14. Heymon, D., and D. Gianturco. 1973. Long term adaptation by the elderly to bereavement. *J Gerontol* 28:359–362.
15. Clayton, P.J. 1979. The sequelae and nonsequelae of conjugal bereavement. *Psychiatry* 136:1530–1534.
16. Engel, G.L. 1961. Is grief a disease? A challenge for medical research. *Psychosom Med* 23:18–22.
17. Worden, J.W. 1982. *Grief Counseling and Grief Therapy.* New York: Springer Publishing Company.
18. Frey, W.H. 1980. Not-so-idle tears. *Psychology Today* 13:91–92.

19. Ainsworth, M.D.S. 1973. "The development of infant-mother attachment." In *Review of Child Development Research,* ed. B.M. Caldwell and H.N. Ricciuti. Chicago: University of Chicago Press.

20. Bowlby, J. 1977. The making and breaking of affectional bonds. Parts I and II. *Br J Psychiatry* 130:201–210, 421–431.

21. Freud, S. 1917. "Mourning and melancholia." In *Complete Psychological Works,* Vol. 14, trans. ed. J. Strachey. London: Hogarth Press.

22. Kennell, J.H., H. Slyter, and M.H. Klaus. 1970. The mourning response of parents to the death of a newborn infant. *N Engl J Med* 283:344–349.

23. Klaus, M.H., and J.H. Kennell. 1976. *Maternal-Infant Bonding.* St. Louis: C.V. Mosby.

24. Caplan, G. 1960. Patterns of parental response to the crisis of premature birth. *Psychiatry* 23:365–374.

25. Bibring, G.L., T.F. Dwyer, D.S. Huntington and A.F. Valenstein. 1961. A study of the psychological processes in pregnancy and of the earliest mother–child relationship. I. Some propositions and comments. *Psychoanalytic Study of the Child* 16:9–27.

26. Kubler-Ross, E. 1969. *On Death and Dying.* New York: Macmillan Publishing Company.

27. Rubin, S. 1981. A two-track model of bereavement: Theory and application in research. *Am J Orthopsychiatry* 51:101–109.

28. Cain, A., and B. Cain. 1964. On replacing a child. *American Academy of Child Psychiatry* 3:443–455.

29. Kirkley-Best, E., and K.R. Kellner. 1982. The forgotten grief. *Am J Orthopsychiatry* 52:420–429.

30. Spinetta, J., and P. Deasy-Spinetta, eds. 1981. *Living with Childhood Cancer.* St. Louis: C.V. Mosby.

31. Krupnick, J.L., and F. Solomon. 1987. "Death of a parent or sibling during childhood." In *The Psychology of Separation and Loss,* ed. J. Bloom-Feshbach and S. Bloom-Feshbach. San Francisco: Jossey-Bass.

32. Lonetto, R. 1980. *Children's Conceptions of Death.* New York: Springer Publishing.

33. Melear, J.D. 1973. Children's conceptions of death. *J Genet Psychol* 123:359–360.

34. Childers, P., and M. Wimmer. 1971. The concept of death in early childhood. *Child Dev* 42:1299–1301.

35. Hollingsworth, C.E., and R.O. Pasnau. 1977. "Response of children to death in the family." In *The Family in Mourning,* ed. C.E. Hollingsworth and R.O. Pasnau. New York: Grune and Stratton.

36. Koocher, G.P. 1975. Why isn't the gerbil moving anymore? *Children Today.* Jan-Feb., 18–21.

37. White, E., B. Elsom, and R. Prawat. 1978. Children's conceptions of death. *Child Dev* 49:307–310.

38. Nagy, M. 1959. "The child's view of death." In *The Meaning of Death,* ed. J. Feifel. New York: McGraw-Hill.

39. Anthony, S. 1940. *The Child's Discovery of Death.* New York: Harcourt, Brace & Co.

40. Piaget, J. 1960. *The Child's Conception of the World.* Paterson, N.J.: Littlefield, Adams & Co.
41. Weston, D.L., and R.C. Irwin. 1963. Preschool child's response to death of infant sibling. *Am J Dis Child* 106:74–77.
42. Mancini, M.E. 1986. "Creating and therapeutically utilizing anticipatory grief in survivors of sudden death." In *Loss & Anticipatory Grief,* ed. T.A. Rando. Toronto: Lexington Books.
43. Gyulay, J.E. 1978. *The Dying Child.* New York: McGraw-Hill.
44. Rosen, H. 1986. *Unspoken Grief: Coping with Childhood Sibling Loss.* Toronto: Lexington Books.
45. Koocher, G.P. 1974. Talking with children about death. *Am J Orthopsychiatry* 44:404–411.
46. Kubler-Ross, E. 1981. *Living with Death and Dying.* New York: Macmillan Publishing Comany.
47. Piaget, J. 1966. The Child's Conception of Physical Causality. London: Routledge & Kegen Paul.
48. Donnelly, K.F. 1982. *Recovering from the Loss of a Child.* New York: Macmillan Publishing Company.
49. Horowitz, M.J., N. Wilner, C. Marmar, and H. Krupnick. 1980. Pathological grief and the activation of latent self-images. *Am J Psychiatry* 137:1157–1162.
50. Abraham, K. 1927. "A short study on the development of the libido." In *Selected Papers on Psychoanalysis.* London: Hogarth Press.
51. Booher, D., and B. Little. 1974. Vaginal hemorrhage in pregnancy. *N Engl J Med* 290:611–613.
52. Karon, M., and J. Vernick. 1968. An approach to the emotional support of fatally ill children. *Clin Pediatr* 7:274–280.
53. Kavanaugh, R.E. 1972. *Facing death.* Baltimore: Penguin Books.
54. Koocher, G.P., and J.E. O'Malley. 1981. *The Damocles Syndrome.* New York: McGraw-Hill.
55. Jackson, E.N. 1965. *Telling a Child About Death.* New York: Channel Press.
56. Jackson, E.N. 1982. "The pastoral counselor and the child encountering death." In *Helping Children Cope with Death: Guidelines and Resources,* ed. H. Wass and C.A. Corr. New York: Hemisphere Publishing Corp.
57. Grollman, E.A., ed. 1967. *Explaining Death to Children.* Boston: Beacon Press.
58. Temes, R. 1977. *Living with an Empty Chair - A Guide Through Grief.* N.Y.: Irvington Publishing.
59. Raphael, B. 1983. *The Anatomy of Bereavement.* New York: Basic Books.
60. Volkan, V. 1972. The linking objects of pathological mourners. *Arch Gen Psychiatry* 27:215–221.

9

The Family and Sudden Infant Death Syndrome

FREDERICK MANDELL, M.D.

My first contact with a child who had died of sudden infant death syndrome (SIDS) was as an intern in a large city hospital. I responded to a call to the Emergency Room. A four-month-old infant was dead. I remember thinking that there was nothing more to be done. The emergency room was busy and I continued to see other patients, but frequently found myself staring into a small examining room where a young mother sat crying; she seemed to have been there an inordinately long time. I noticed the woman who had been cleaning the floor put down her mop; she walked into the room, put her arms around a sobbing, lonely human being and just sat with her. She did what I should have done.

Historical Overview

For hundreds of years, infants who died suddenly and unexpectedly were thought to have died of overlaying by the mother or wet nurse. Many of these tragic deaths were attributed to infants smothering in their bedding. At the end of the thirteenth century, a public notice cited the danger of suffocating infants by overlaying and forbade mothers from taking to bed with them infants who were under three years of age [1]. Although unexpected deaths did not arouse medical interest at the time, there is evidence of major concern about sudden and unexpected deaths caused by overlaying. The arcutio may be the first device used to protect infants from SIDS (Figure 9.1) [2]. The infant slept in it and the mother could breast feed by placing her breast in the notch (c). The arcutio would not allow her to roll over on the infant. The astounding infant mortality from infectious diseases and malnutrition probably conditioned parents to be more accepting of early death even if it was unexpected. Nevertheless, even in this setting, there were those whose questions implied that SIDS was a fairly frequent phenomenon prior to the nineteenth century. One such provocation appeared in the January 1855 issue of *Lancet:*

Medical Jurisprudence: Infants Found Dead in Bed

Who has not heard of cases of "overlaid" children found dead in bed? A few years since the metropolitan newspaper teemed with reports of such cases: the country journals still exhibit similar records. Yet we believe it may be stated as a fact, that not one child out of two hundred who has been found dead in bed has lost its life in consequence of having been overlaid. In Middlesex, fourteen years since, the constables, in cold weather, made incessant applications for inquests in such reputed cases. Several facts, however, soon occurred, which led to a conviction that other causes than pressure produced the death in instances where children were found dead in bed.

Had the office of coroner been generally occupied by members of the medical profession, it is impossible that the real degree of death, in these instances, would have been so long overlooked and misunderstood. But the ascertained facts lead to inferences which we believe to be irresistibly conclusive. It was due to science, to the interests of humanity, having due regard to the preservation of human life, and not less so to the feeling, and bestowed upon infantile life every possible care and attention, that the real cause of mortality, in the numerous examples of infants found dead in bed, should be thoroughly investigated. After fond and attentive parents, during weeks and months, have devoted the utmost possible attention to their helpless infant, what can be more distressing to their feelings than the imputation that the sacrifice of their offspring has arisen from their own mismanagement, carelessness, or criminal neglect? Assuredly it is the duty of coroners and medical practitioners to set the public mind right on this deeply interesting subject. Even jurors, from previously conceived erroneous notions, are often disposed to rush inconsiderately to wrong conclusions.

It must be admitted that in instances where the causes of death are precisely similar, neither externally nor internally is there a corresponding exactitude with reference to the postmortem appearances of the body. Some extraordinary examples we shall place upon record at a future period. If all postmortem examinations were to be conducted on one uniform plan, enough would doubtless soon be discovered of exact resemblance in a series of cases to enable practitioners to ascribe the causes of death to precise and adequate influences. We hope soon to be enabled to issue a tabular form for the reception of a record of all useful facts found on a scientific examination of every human body. The general use throughout the kingdom of such a form would afford an opportunity for collecting and classifying facts which would be of the utmost possible use, and within a comparatively brief period medical practitioners would be enabled to point to a portion, at least, of a code which would sustain them in their evidence against the impertinent audacity of hired bullies, who but too frequently are absurdly styled learned gentlemen.

Some of the most interesting facts connected with the discovery of infants found dead in bed are the following:

These lifeless bodies are discovered in at least ninety-five instances out of every hundred, after three o'clock in the morning. Not one out of a hundred of such bodies is discovered dead between nine and twelve at night.

The greatest number of such bodies found dead are discovered in the months of December, January, and February; the next greatest number in September, October, and November. The spring months—namely, March, April, and May, exhibit

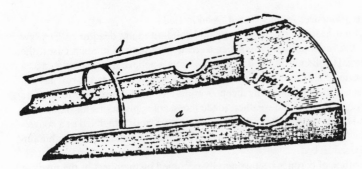

WHEN it is confidered how many are charged Over-laid in the Bills of Mortality, it is to be wonder'd that the ARCUTIO's, univerfally ufed at *Florence*, are not ufed here in *England*. The Defign above, is drawn in Perfpective, with the Dimenfions, which are larger than ufual ; and is thus defcribed :

a, *The Place where the Child lies.*
b, *The Head-Board.*
c, *The Hollows for the Nurfe's Breafts.*
d, *A Bar of Wood to lean on, when fhe fuckles the Child.*
e, *A fmall Iron Arch to fupport the faid Bar*
The Length three Feet, two Inches and a half.

Every Nurfe in *Florence* is obliged to lay the Child in it, under Pain of Excommunication. The ARCUTIO, with the Child in it, may be fafely laid entirely under the Bed-Cloaths in the Winter, without Danger of fmothering.

FIGURE 9.1. Arcutio Used to Prevent Overlaying.

When it is considered how many are charged Over-laid in the Bills of Mortality, it is to be wonder'd that the Arcutio's, universally used at Florence, are not used here in England. The Design above is drawn in Perspective with the Dimensions, which are larger than usual and is thus described:

a. The Place where the Child lies.
b. The Head-Board.
c. The Hollows for the Nurse's Breasts.
d. A Bar of Wood to lean on, when she suckles the Child.
e. A small Iron Arch to support the said Bar.
The Length three Feet, two Inches and a half.

Every Nurse in Florence is obliged to lay the Child in it, under Pain of Excommunication. The Arcutio, with the Child in it, may be safely laid entirely under the Bed-Cloaths in the Winter, without Danger of smothering.

them in the third degree; and beyond all questions, the least number are found in the summer months—June, July, and August.

Of the days of the week when such bodies are found dead, the greatest number are seen on Sunday mornings, next on Monday mornings, and the fewest on Saturday mornings.

An experience of fourteen years, in a Coroner's jurisdiction embracing between eight and nine hundred thousand souls, many portions of which are densely populated, has established the accuracy of these statements by proofs which admit of no dispute. Equally true is it that out of hundreds of examples of infants found dead in bed, only two instances have been seen in which the proof was conclusive that the little creatures had been destroyed by the pressure of persons who had been lying with them in bed. Even in one of those cases, the question might have been fairly raised, whether the signs of pressure visible on the body had not resulted from contact after death with the person who had slept with the deceased infants [3].

The first writing of sudden and unexpected death in American literature appeared in the Diary of Samuel Sewall in 1674 as, "Mr. Eyre's little son dyed, went well to bed; dyed by them in the Bed. It seems there is no symptom of Over-laying" [4].

The humanitarian approach to the problem of sudden and unexpected death was bolstered by emergence of the thymus theory; that is, that death was caused by a large thymus compressing the heart and great vessels. The acceptance of this physiologic explanation diminished the intensity of feeling that these deaths were due to neglect, accidental suffocation, or even deliberate homicide [1]. Sorrowful and guilt-ridden parents could be declared blameless when the thymus theory was demonstrated. However, in the 1850s, the thymus theory fell into disrepute when the glands of SIDS victims were compared to those of controls who had died of other causes, and it became the general attitude that suffocation was the mechanism of death.

Parents whose infants died suddenly and unexpectedly continued to live with the belief that their babies had suffocated until the 1940s and 1950s when several authors presented evidence for a natural mechanism of death and discounted suffocation. Since the 1970s, sudden infant death syndrome has been recognized as a naturally occurring entity for which parents are not responsible. Despite the academic disagreements as to cause, in the past ten years there has been a major research thrust in the area of SIDS. Federally and privately funded educational programs have reduced the amount of erroneous information that previously had subjected families to cruel and undeserved treatment and even prosecution.

Psychological Effects of SIDS on Survivors

Parents and Other Caretakers

In spite of existing programs and continued research efforts to find a cause and cure for crib death, there remains a mystique about a baby who dies suddenly from sudden infant death syndrome. The unexpected loss of a well-cared-for child evokes the harshest kind of grief reaction. Most parents talk about initial shock. One woman stated, "In the beginning, I lost all sense of being" [5]. Very few parents who have lost their infants suddenly and unexpectedly have not thought about blaming themselves. In most instances feelings of guilt are overwhelming. Parents typically recreate the events around the time of death and magnify minor omissions. Many parents talk about "if onlys;" if only I had checked the baby or hadn't changed the formula, or had taken the blanket away, or hadn't gone out that night. These parents need immediate assurance that such magnified minor omissions did not cause the baby's death. Parents feel guilty that in some way they neglected the needs of the baby. An extreme example of this was a mother who kept repeating to the Emergency Room staff that she had killed her infant. What she meant, of course, was that she must have been responsible for the baby's death.

The immediate effect on parents is overwhelming. The initial shock gives way to guilt, which often persists in spite of rational explanation. An early stage in the usual grief process is internal bargaining. When a death is sudden and due to a known cause, the concrete character of the event can be incorporated into the normal rationalization of mourning. When, however, as in SIDS, death is due to an unknown mechanism, feelings of self-condemnation and inadequacy of parenting are reinforced. This type of death is almost unique in the spectrum of pediatric disease and denies parents a prior mourning process, which in other childhood deaths may begin at the time of terminal diagnosis.

For young parents, this loss may be their first experience with family death. Uninformed relatives and friends add further remorse with innuendos of parental blame. When death involves an older person, reminiscing is a therapeutic tool in helping survivors work through their grief. In cases of SIDS, however, there is an almost universal absence of discussing any of the happy events surrounding the infant. This pattern extends beyond the limited time the infant has spent in the family and seems to relate to self-imposed restrictions on the part of family, friends, and neighbors. When visitors do come, they enforce these restrictions by avoiding talk about the infant and not allowing the parents the opportunity to reminisce or use reminiscing to help work through the grief process. Parents have stated that they would like to be able to talk about the infant, but recognize the taboo and discomfort that others have about discussing children who die. In some instances, the inability to talk about the infant delays grieving. The delayed process of grieving is more difficult, because after several days most active supports are gone.

Infants who die suddenly often are taken to an Emergency Room. Here, parents require understanding and compassion. They should be informed that their infant probably died of sudden infant death syndrome, even though this cannot be confirmed until a postmortem examination has been performed. In the emergency room, I am not afraid to tell parents that I think their child died of sudden infant death syndrome. Parents need to know why their baby died and this consideration should be given to them as soon as possible. When an adult dies, relatives are told of the possible cause of death; one may say, "I think your husband died of a cerebral vascular accident or a massive heart attack." In the case of a child, similar consideration and information should be available.

Parents advised to have an autopsy performed on their infant usually feel that this is good advice. I have never met parents who have regretted agreeing to an autopsy, but I have met many parents who have been sorry that a postmortem examination was not done. By providing information about SIDS in a sensitive manner, the physician helps parents understand that this sudden, unexplained death is a natural phenomenon even though the cause is unknown.

Not very long ago, a man woke up early in the morning to go to work. As he was leaving, he stopped to check his young infant sleeping in the crib. The baby was not breathing. He called the police to help with emergency care. After seeing that the infant was dead, the police informed the father of his rights to remain silent. In another instance a mother vividly described to me the events surrounding her baby's death, as if the death had just occurred. When her child was taken to the Emergency Room, a nurse looked at the mother in a way that insinuated somehow she was responsible for the death of the child. The mother described the nurse's innuendo vividly: "She whispered to others, she was cold and distant, and she looked at me with gleaming eyes." Then the mother told me that her baby had died fifteen years ago. In these two instances, judgment was passed on the parents by others. The lasting effect of this kind of behavior is significant. Sometimes it occurs between husband and wife. One spouse in some way blaming the other or a grandparent blaming a parent has not been an infrequent situation in cases of SIDS.

Caretakers, such as babysitters, also require information when a baby dies in their care. Caretakers may involve extended family, young adolescent sitters, or daycare centers. In cases of extended family, their closeness to the death serves as constant reminders of the tragedy. Young adolescent sitters also have feelings of guilt and responsibility for the death. They may not fully comprehend the events surrounding the death or their role as the protector of the infant. Among involved young sitters, issues of lingering or even long-term guilt and fear of caring for children in the future can become significant.

As demands for daycare increase, more and more daycare centers are facing the issue of an infant dying suddenly and unexpectedly while in their care. In some instances direct accusations of deliberate harm and neglect have been made. In other instances, the community response has been so negative that centers have been unable to continue to function. Sometimes news reports of an unexpected death in a daycare setting have created suspicion that the daycare workers have not been acting responsibly. One daycare center provider closed her facility after a second death occurred when the infant was in her care. A second daycare provider closed her home because of her perception of negative community response. In general, all caretakers need assurance that they are not responsible for these deaths. Daycare providers need counselling and information about sudden infant death syndrome. Young babysitters and extended family also require help over a longer period.

Fathers

Mothers have known the backaches of pregnancy and traditionally have been the caregivers for most infants. In fact, most research has been done on mother/infant reactions. Professional support provided to families experiencing the loss of an infant has concentrated on understanding the effects of the disruption of mother–infant bonding and its consequences on the mother's sense of self. However, expectant fathers also have hopes and fantasies for their babies. Their thoughts are filled with happy expectations and aspirations. Fathers also form significant relationships with their infants and feel the frustrating loss of hopes and dreams.

In Western society, we are only just beginning to observe the emotional importance of father–infant tenderness and loyalty. It is apparent that the behavior of the father in response to the loss of his child also requires special consideration. In a study of twenty-eight fathers who lost children to SIDS, patterns of behavior peculiar to men were identifiable [6]. For example, all but one of the fathers in the study assumed a manager-like role; they controlled their emotional expression and were preoccupied with the emotional support of the wife. These fathers became directly involved with the funeral arrangements and sought to find an explanation for the cause of death. One father stated, "Things like this happen. I don't want S. to blame herself. She was the perfect mother . . . I have to stay strong for everyone else."

This group of fathers appeared to direct their energies and attention outward whereas the mothers appeared to withdraw. The behavior of the fathers sometimes directly contrasted with that of their wives who were tearful, frequently incoherent, very much absorbed in grief, and seemed to notice very little around them. On the other hand, fathers frequently seemed almost awed by the responses from relatives, friends, and the community. "I'm telling you, this is beautiful. The whole office came to the funeral. People are just coming out of nowhere . . . I never thought they would care."

In this report, six mothers talked about the necessity to verbalize their feelings. This was generally not the pattern for fathers; their predominant coping mechanism was to keep busy. This meant taking extra courses or an additional job, accepting added work load responsibilities, or seeking energy-absorbing hobbies. Fathers also appeared to have different attitudes than their spouses in their feelings about subsequent children. Whereas many of the mothers described a sense of fear of another pregnancy, the fathers seemed to have an urgent desire to have another child as soon as possible. In the period following the SIDS death, this issue was mentioned as a frequent source of conflict.

Another difference between mothers and fathers was the fathers' lack of desire to talk about the death and their feelings about the loss. In eighteen of forty-six families, fathers seemed purposely to avoid being at home at the time of a nurse visit [6]. Mothers frequently commented that their spouses felt that talking about the baby's death would not help. In some instances mothers were secretive about their contacts with the community health nurse. One mother stated, "He doesn't want me to talk about our private problems. If I tell him that you were here, he will say, 'I don't want to know about it.' When I call you I need to wait until he is out of the house." Another father stated that he would not tell anyone about his problems because it wouldn't bring his baby back. However, when mothers did request crisis intervention, the difficulties often centered around communication with the husband or specific concerns about his behavior.

When fathers were able to discuss their involvement with the baby who had died, they frequently expressed remorse over their lack of inclusion in infant care. One father said that he kept thinking when the baby got older he would have more time. Fathers who were able to express themselves also talked about feelings of diminished self-esteem. They spoke about feeling inadequate, feeling that a part of them had died with the baby, and feeling less of a man. Special feelings of frustration and powerlessness were expressed by fathers who attempted to resuscitate their infants.

Behavioral scientists have had disproportionately little to report on the impact of the father on early childhood development. It is not surprising to note a reduction of the father's role at the time of the death of the infant. One father pointed out that when he finally broke down and cried, no one was able to hold him although they had been doing this for his wife for days [6].

In general, men seemed to be angrier and more aggressive than women, who appeared more depressed and withdrawn [6]. Sometimes fathers talked about wanting to strike out at someone. Sometimes they blamed physicians for the death or angrily magnified minor omissions. In some cases, there were thinly disguised statements of blame toward the mother who was the primary caretaker. If they were not present when the infant was found, some fathers found it difficult to accept that nothing could be done. Fathers generally have less insight into the day-to-day child rearing and child health risks, and therefore may be less equipped to accept the fragility of life and their inability to control their child's destiny.

Studies of infant attachment demonstrate that fathers interact deeply with their infant sons and daughters, and this interaction can be as sensitive to infant needs as that between mothers and infants [7–9]. A new father accommodates to the experiences of fatherhood and reshapes his world, his expectations, his images of himself, his wife, and his family. The crisis aroused by childhood death is profound.

Societal expectations for fathers are of significance. In the study by Mandell et al., the concreteness of assuming a managerial role seemed to reinforce the reality of death and provided an outlet for expression of finality [6]. Fathers indicated a need to grieve but required different outlets. Even those who sensed their own need for help either limited their requests for assistance or found that their requests were not recognized. Exposing feelings of helplessness sometimes exacerbated an already diminished feeling of self-esteem. However, if fathers are given an opportunity to express their feelings and these feelings are understood and validated in the context of their own family, their virility, and the pressures of masculine roles, fathers can utilize support constructively. Health professionals, friends, and families need to be aware of the special bondings between infants and fathers and to be sensitive to the particular effects when that bond is broken.

Surviving Siblings

New infants are quickly incorporated into family life. When infants in the home die unexpectedly, family life is suddenly changed [10–12]. Infant mortality in this country has so decreased that most children are not familiar with death by natural causes. Some children are knowledgeable of death by accidents or remote experiences such as war or natural catastrophes. In our world of television, children often think that death can be prevented if outside influences are controlled; in a sense, this gives the child a feeling of control and power over death. When death is in a remote place it has little meaning because it happens to others. Young families have not had to cope with death. Our own adult fear of death and a kind of taboo that surrounds discussions regarding the death of children does not provide an open environment in which to discuss the death of an infant with an older surviving child.

The loss of an infant in a family is particularly frightening for siblings in the home due to the catastrophic nature of the death and their inability to understand its meaning and influence on the family. The abrupt loss of an apparently healthy infant without an explainable pathologic cause intensifies family grief. In this psychological environment, surviving siblings experience loss, uncertainty, family disruption, and fear.

Readying children for the role of older sibling provides direct participation in an important family event. That place in the family is crystalized with the birth of a new infant. These new big brother and big sister roles, however, are suddenly terminated with the death of their new infant sibling. Death has entered the confines of the family and has taken another child close in age. Often children do not understand that other children can die. The role of older sibling is lost. There is a void of developmental opportunity and the child, as a survivor, immediately develops some very special qualities as a result of the loss [13].

Following the death of a sibling children feel especially vulnerable. The family entity has changed, communication and interchange between husband and wife has changed, and parental behavior and responses toward the surviving child also have changed. Parents often are able to acknowledge their overprotectiveness and permissiveness. However, the confusion and difficulties experienced by parents who are mourning often forestall the spontaneous expression of concern around surviving children. Behavioral responses in young surviving siblings may be misinterpreted by parents and health professionals. The consequences of the sibling death could become a source of distraction, dismay, and fear for the surviving child.

In a recent study of thirty-five surviving children, 80 percent of the mothers perceived changes in the child's interaction with them after the sudden and unexpected loss of a sibling [14]. Most parents described their own need to be physically closer to the surviving children. One mother stated, "We wanted and needed to hold him more . . . I don't know who needed the hugging more, him or us." Some parents remarked that they had babied a surviving child too much. This normative behavior seemed to imply the parents' need to feel once again the closeness of a parent–infant bond as well as fears for the safety of surviving children. Only a few mothers were able to express a painful need for some distance from their surviving children. There were many instances of children attempting to comfort their parents in the time of distress, but for most of the surviving children, the sight of parents crying and confused was perplexing and frightening. In some instances, this led to children's comforting parents themselves or to the older child's learning not to talk about the baby.

The changes in parent-child interaction included newly acquired separation anxiety [14]. Some of the children were able to present, with particular clarity, the fear that their parents also would disappear. Some parents also talked about the provoking tendency of surviving children to test the limits of discipline for several months after the death of a sibling.

Almost 70 percent of the children in the study demonstrated changes in sleep patterns following the baby's death [14]. In most instances this new deportment emerged within a few days after the death, although several children did not have sleep problems until several months later. Most sleep-related difficulties were seen as resistance to going to bed and to sleep. Children often expressed fears about not waking up; "We were just not able to reassure her. When we would tell her that she would be okay, she would say, 'How do you know? [14]' " Many of the sleep disturbances were accompanied by nightmares. Older children who were able to describe the nightmare often talked about the frequent theme of pursuit by monsters. One three-year-old rebuffed sleep because of her fear that a monster would take her because she killed her brother. Typically, parents relate these nighttime ordeals to the event of the baby's death. "She was right there when it happened; I was screaming; she wakes up screaming." Most children who experienced nightmares responded to comforting and parental assurance and were able to settle back to sleep. In some families, nightmares occurred more than once in the night. Some families responded by allowing their children to sleep with them. In some instances this seemed to reassure the expressed fear that their parents would leave them and not return [14].

Changes also were noticed in some of the children's social interactions with peers. These changes ranged from a noticeable quietude and withdrawn behavior to increases in aggression, which included hitting other children. Many of the children evidenced a new reluctance to go to school and others became so aggressive toward siblings and children that parents qualified their behavior as mean [14].

Health professionals encourage adult patients to talk about crises. Children also need to express their perception of what happened through talk or play or drawings. Children respond to death with different kinds of behavior. Some children have many questions, and they question the death just as they question other things they do not understand. Other children have fears that they or their parents will die. Children think magically, and they may have wished that their new brother or sister would go away. These children need to be reassured that they are not responsible for the events that have transpired and that the same thing will not happen to them. Children readily participate in silence surrounding infant death, especially when talking about the baby causes the parents to become upset. They quickly understand that the silence is a cover for something awful. Children's fantasies of death can be more frightening than the tragedy itself. Parents need to be encouraged to use the words "death" and "died." They also need to be reminded that some euphemisms may be more confusing and frightening than comforting. Parents also need to know that although the death may be explained, it is not a closed issue among surviving children and probably will come up at the most inopportune times. Children need to know that it is all right to cry, to question, and to express feelings, and parents need to assure children that their emotions are normal. Children may avoid thinking about death. It is one of their best defense mechanisms and should not be considered disinterest [15].

Professionals need to know that children's ideas about death are quite different at different age levels [16]. To the preschooler, death represents going away, is temporary, and probably reversible; he or she is unable to accept it as final. To the five-to-nine-year-olds, death happens, but it happens to other people. After this age, children understand death and its finality and that it happens to everyone. For these issues alone, the professional needs to know the age of the child, the circumstances of the death, and what the child has been told.

The behavioral issues of surviving children are of significant concern to the parents of SIDS victims. However, many parents prefer to deny additional problems or are so overwhelmed by the loss that they do not bring up these problems with health professionals. Other parents may be unwilling to open discussions about disturbed behavior at home while they are experiencing feelings of inadequacy. With an awareness that behavioral changes can occur in surviving children, those who are involved in helping these families can alleviate parental concern over these issues by providing the necessary assurances that these kinds of family interactions are not abnormal. These kinds of assurances allow parents to know that the family process of grieving involves all family members and that there is concern about the survivors as they begin to build a new family structure.

Health Professionals

Many health professionals, even those who work with children, are uncomfortable during encounters with newly bereaved parents and find these times particularly anxiety filled. Providing adequate support at a time of bereavement can be extremely difficult even for the trained and experienced counselors who provide effective support by sharing the family grief. It is an emotionally draining experience. Grieving families need someone who is genuinely interested. Nurses who visit these families often are responsible for assessing their unique needs [17]. Zoe Smialek, Nurse Coordinator for a SIDS information and counseling project, has had experience with more than 350 families who have lost infants suddenly and unexpectedly. She wrote, "Families are entitled to assistance during this distressing time from a warm, caring professional who is able to allow free expression of grief however it is manifested, and accurately answer their disturbing questions about the death of the infant [18]."

Parents' reactions to home visits by nurses have been generally positive. In Massachusetts, the acceptance rate of a home visit is 95 percent, which indicates support for professional input. Most of these families also accept a second or third professional visit. Nurses who do this well encourage parents to express themselves freely in an accepting manner. Often these feelings are not expressed to friends or relatives because they might not understand what they are hearing or they might be frightened by the overwhelming grief. In this situation, well-meaning friends tend to cut off discussion by telling parents that everything will be all right or by telling them to talk about the future when the parents want to express how they feel. Nurses in general have felt positive about their intervention with grieving parents if they are prepared with factual knowledge about sudden infant death syndrome, knowledge of the normal and abnormal grieving response, some counseling skills, and an awareness of their own reactions to death.

There are no formal educational processes to prepare physicians for the death of a child. The suddenness of SIDS adds to the state of unpreparedness. SIDS babies are also very young and if this is a first child, the physician may not know the family well. Many physicians are devastated by the unexpected death and search for reasons why. One pediatrician stated, "You always wonder if you missed something in the exam." Another remarked, "I kept reexamining the case. I had to feel there were not circumstances I could have changed" [19]. Some pediatricians react by withdrawing and not following through; in a sense, allowing families to fend for themselves. A physician wrote, "I was sad; maybe the baby had something wrong that I missed. I was disappointed that I wasn't more involved and my own guilt was magnified." In a survey of some forty-five pediatricians who lost patients to SIDS, most felt that they were educationally unprepared for this kind of loss and most felt that they wanted to talk to someone about it [19]. In general, professionals also need support in order to cope with their own feelings in response to parents in pain. One physician said, "Most deaths I can sort out, but SIDS is different. I needed a support person to help me deal with this."

Parents need encouragement and support to cope with their baby's death. This support can be provided in a variety of ways from a professional grief counselor, individual/family counseling sessions, parent-to-parent support on an individual basis, or support from a bereavement group for SIDS families. The support group aids in the resolution of early trauma of grief experienced by parents after the sudden and unexpected death of their baby. The group provides the opportunity to meet other parents who have experienced the death of an infant and who extend their friendship and understanding to newly bereaved parents. In the group setting, parents are encouraged to talk about the baby who died and express their feelings about death in a safe environment. Gradually, parents begin to cope with their loss and are supported in the process.

Subsequent Children

For parents who have lost a child, the decision to have another is difficult. Relatively few parents have experienced the loss of an apparently healthy baby. This fact most influences a parent's decision to have another child after the loss. The death of a previous sibling also has a great influence on the new child. Parents are deeply plagued by the fear of losing another child. For this reason, it is not unusual for parents to wait a long time, even years, before they decide to have another child. There are others, however, who require a subsequent pregnancy immediately. Some parents have been encouraged by relatives, medical personnel, and friends to have another child quickly in order to take their mind off the loss. Parents who have had this experience are painfully aware of the problems for both parent and child. The parent, never having worked through the original loss, finds his or her lost infant in the replacement child. The child is constantly compared with and lives in the shadow of the dead child [20]. This has been described as a "replacement child syndrome" [21], and some of these children are incapacitated by death phobias and fears of abandonment. Becoming pregnant to resolve a loss appears to be harmful to all parties.

In other instances, under psychological conditions of mourning and guilt, women who have lost children and are attempting to conceive a "replacement" child quickly may have difficulty. Investigators have been aware for a long time of the influence of emotional factors on the menstrual cycle. It is well known that its rhythm can be disrupted by stress and personality disturbances. Transcultural studies have cited a number of non-physical techniques that can cause abortion, and these kinds of spontaneous abortions have been documented in societies older than our own. In a study of women whose children died of SIDS, thirty-two attempted to have another child [22]. The expected rate of infertility in a normal population is 10 percent. Spontaneous abortion has an incidence of 15 percent. Among the thirty-two women who attempted to conceive after the loss of their child, over 30 percent had their first spontaneous abortion and almost 35 percent could not conceive after attempts for at least one year [22].

In our society, the acute grief process is spread out over time. If parents are able to work through the mourning process, the psychological environment for the subsequent newborn will be healthier. There is no replacement for a lost child, and parents who expeditiously decide to have another child may be further frustrated by difficulty in achieving pregnancy or by spontaneous abortion [22]. When pregnancy does occur, anxiety may be high. The pregnancy is often wrought by fear of a repetition of the unexpected death. Expectant mothers require patient answers as they compare pregnancies and feelings during pregnancies.

In a sensitive and informative article for parents entitled, "The Subsequent Child," Szybist wrote, "Waiting for baby is the time to seek counsel if you need to and to be honest with yourself and others. It is also a time to prepare for a rather remarkable experience—the birth of a 'subsequent child.' " She continued, "You will probably check on your sleeping baby more frequently than you did your other child. Parents of subsequent children are the first to admit that in the past they used to check their babies to see if they were covered, but now they check respirations" [23]. The article also talks about moments of panic with the subsequent child. These moments occur with the first upper respiratory infection and at the anniversary of the death of the previous infant. Also, many decisions that were at one time easy now require much effort. Breast- and bottle-feeding decisions, where to sleep, whether to smoke, room temperature, visitors, tests, and monitors are issues that may become greatly magnified.

During the first months of the subsequent infant's life, parents fear another uncontrollable sudden loss. Family relationships may be strained. Parents continue to compare illnesses, feelings, and personalities throughout the first year of life. Usually this is done inwardly and there is great relief when the subsequent child reaches the year-old mark. Parents need reinforcement of the healthy aspects of their babies. These distinct conditions test the sensitivities and perception of the health professional. Times of crisis, episodes of overprotectiveness, and moments of panic are times when invaluable psychological support can be provided with open compassion, understanding, and familiarity of the issues facing the parents who are attempting desperately to do their best with their new subsequent child. The supportive role of an understanding human being will help mitigate the emotions of family pain and the anguish of losing a child to SIDS.

References

1. Beckwith, J.B. 1975. *The Sudden Infant Death Syndrome*. U.S. Department of Health, Education, and Welfare. DHEW Publication No. 75–5137.
2. Caulfield, E. 1930. The infant welfare movement in the eighteenth century— Part I. *Annals of Medical History* 2:480–494.
3. Medical Jurisprudence: Infants found dead in bed. 1855. *Lancet* 1:103.
4. Thomas, M.H., ed. *Diary of Samuel Sewall*. 1674-1729. New York: Farrar, Straus, Giroux, 2 volumes.
5. DeFrain, J., J. Taylor, and L. Ernst. 1982. *Coping with Sudden Infant Death Syndrome*. Lexington, Mass.: D.C. Heath and Co.
6. Mandell, F., E. McAnulty, and R.M. Reece. 1980. Observations of paternal response to sudden, unanticipated infant death. *Pediatrics* 65:221–225.
7. Greenberg, M., and N. Morris. 1974. Engrossment: The newborn's impact upon the father. *Am J Orthopsychiatry* 44:520–531.
8. Abelin, E.L. 1975. Some further observations and comments on the earliest role of the father. *Int J Psychoanal* 56:293–302.

9. Lamb, M. 1975. Fathers: Forgotten contributors to child development. *Hum Dev* 18:245–266.
10. Mandell, F., and B. Belk. 1977. Sudden infant death syndrome. *Postgrad Med* 62:193–197.
11. Bergman, A.B., M.A. Pomeroy, and J.B. Beckwith. 1969. The psychiatric toll of sudden infant death syndrome. *GP* 40:99–105.
12. Krell, R., and L. Rabkin. 1979. The effects of sibling death on the surviving child: A family perspective. *Family Process* 18:471–477.
13. Weston, D.L., and R.C. Irwin. 1963. Preschool child's response to death of infant sibling. *Am J Dis Child* 106:564–567.
14. Mandell, F., E. McAnulty, and A. Carlson. 1982. Unexpected death of an infant sibling. *Pediatrics* 72:652–657.
15. Hardgrove, C., and L.H. Warrick. 1974. How shall we tell the children? *Am J Nurs* 76:448–450.
16. Koocher, G.P. 1974. Talking with children about death. *Am J Orthopsychiatry* 44:404–411.
17. Nikolaisen, S. 1981. The impact of sudden infant death on the family: Nursing intervention. *Topics in Clin Nurs* 3:45–53.
18. Smialek, Z. 1982. Observations of immediate reactions of families to sudden infant death syndrome. *Pediatrics* 62:160–165.
19. Mandell, F., M. McClain, and R. Reece. Sudden and unexpected death: The pediatrician's response. *Am J Dis Child* 141:748–750.
20. Kirkley-Best, E., and K.R. Kellner. 1982. The forgotten grief. *Am J Orthopsychiatry* 52:420–429.
21. Cain, A., and B. Cain. 1964. On replacing a child. *American Academy of Child Psychiatry* 3:443–455.
22. Mandell, F., and L.C. Wolfe. 1975. Sudden infant death syndrome and subsequent pregnancy. *Pediatrics* 56:774–776.
23. Szybist, C. 1973. *The Subsequent Child.* Chicago: National Sudden Infant Death Syndrome Foundation.

10

Family Reactions to Home Monitoring

LOIS SIMS SLOVIK, M.D. and DOROTHY H. KELLY, M.D.

Unexpected sudden death in infancy is the most common cause of death in the first year of life, excluding congenital anomalies, neonatal asphyxia, and respiratory failure [1]. With an incidence of approximately 2/1,000 live births, SIDS claims the lives of 6,000 to 10,000 infants annually in the United States [1–3]. Some infants who die unexpectedly have had a previous episode of sleep apnea (see Chapter 5).

In 1978, the American Academy of Pediatrics Task Force on Prolonged Apnea defined prolonged apnea as "cessation of breathing for 20 seconds or longer, or as a briefer episode associated with bradycardia, cyanosis, or pallor" and mandated that "beyond specific treatment of any underlying disorder, twenty-four-hour surveillance is critical to the management of prolonged apnea" [4]. This surveillance is most commonly done through the use of an electronic monitor at home. In addition to the recommendation, the task force reminded pediatricians that there is a significant psychological impact on all members of the family of this infant, whether or not monitors at home are included in the management plan. The task force suggested that families, including siblings, be evaluated and that their strengths, weaknesses, resources, and needs be assessed before any decisions were made and implemented.

Home monitoring of infants with apnea has been increasingly adopted by pediatricians. However, some studies show that a small proportion of infants die despite mechanical surveillance [5–7]. Because there are psychological and social stresses with home monitoring [8–10], its effect on the family needs to be reexamined; although there are common stresses that families experience when their infant is being monitored, their reactions to these stresses vary greatly. Thus, it is important to (1) identify and treat the common stresses of home monitoring and their sequelae, and (2) identify those families who are at risk for developing more serious psychological complications.

Home monitoring has changed over the years. In the 1970s, monitoring was accomplished by the use of a standard impedance respiratory monitor whose alarm was triggered after twenty seconds of apnea and, once triggered, sounded at one-second intervals until the infant resumed breathing. During these early years, false alarms were common and usually were caused by inappropriate electrode placement and broken leads. In an early study done by Black et al. [8] on the impact of the apnea monitor on family life, parents were asked to rank order a series of suggestions for change. Improvements in the monitor equipment ranked as the first priority. Early monitoring was difficult for parents. In addition to monitors being "primitive," the community was uneducated about the apneic child, and psychological and physical supports were not readily available. Yet, even though these parents noted that the monitoring experience had had a significant impact on their lives, they felt "overwhelmingly grateful for having an instrument that allowed them to care for their infants at home" [8].

In 1972, the First Congressional Investigation on SIDS was formed as a result of pressures from lay groups. The findings of this investigation led to the passage of the Sudden Infant Death Syndrome Act in 1974 [11, 12]. This act established a program of biomedical research on the causes and prevention of SIDS through the National Institute of Child Health and Human Development [13], established means for counseling families of SIDS infants and disseminating educational materials to the community. A natural outgrowth has been increased identification and improved treatment of infants at risk, including infants with apnea [14].

Technical and support aspects of home monitoring are improving. Although impedance respiratory monitors continue to be used, they usually are accompanied by a cardiac monitor and can be powered by battery for short-term portability. In addition, better electrodes are available such as the electrode belt, which places less stress on the infant's skin and decreases false positive alarms [15]. Also, recorders are available that can record respiration and heart rate during an alarm, providing data that can be used to differentiate real from false alarms with more accuracy. Psychological and physical supports for home monitoring are increasingly available and are a routine aspect of the monitoring program in many centers. Moreover, the medical and lay communities are now more aware, knowledgeable, and compassionate about apnea of infancy and its treatment.

The Family as a System: Premorbid Family Style

To understand the family's response to home monitoring, one must evaluate the family's premorbid history and structure, style, and method of coping with stress. Although there are common stresses that are encountered during the monitoring experience, each family's response is unique. All stressor events, transitions, and related hardships produce tension that calls for management. When the tension is not overcome, stress emerges.

Stress is a state that arises from the actual or perceived imbalance between demand (i.e., challenge, threat) and capability (i.e., resources, coping) of family functioning [16]. The intensity of the tension and resultant stress varies depending upon the extent to which the family experiences the demands exceeding their resources (personal, family system, and social).

Physicians and mental health personnel often incorporate a system's concept in their approach to the family unit [17]. Usually, they include in their problem formulation the interdependence of parts within the social context they are observing. Each major event affects everyone in the system and in turn is affected by each person's response. Caring for a child with apnea affects everyone in the immediate and extended family, and each member's response has an effect on the child. Relationships are feedback systems, and according to Minuchin, "the family is a natural group (a feedback system of relationships) which over time has evolved patterns of interacting. These patterns make up the family structure which in turn governs the functioning of family members, delineating their range of behavior and facilitating their interaction" [18].

Spouse Subsystem

A family system is composed of three major subsystems: the spouse, parental, and sibling systems. The spouse subsystem is composed of two adults who come from their own families of origin and bring with them their own rules, histories, and expectations of how things should be. The spouses' value sets must be reconciled in order to make life together possible. According to Minuchin, the spouse system's vital task is the development of boundaries that protect the spouses, giving them an area for the satisfaction of their own psychological needs without the intrusion of others, especially in-laws and children. The spouse system is vital for the child's growth in that it models for the child how intimate relations are expressed in daily interactions, including affection, conflict resolution, and methods of handling stress. What the child perceives from this subsystem will become part of his values and expectations for those he will meet in the external world. If there is any major dysfunction within the spouse system, it will reverberate throughout the family. One way for this subsystem to handle dysfunction is to stabilize pathologically by introducing the child as a distance regulator between the two adults.

Parental Subsystem

Transactions within the parental subsystem involve child rearing and social functions including those of nurturance, guidance, and control. From this relationship the child learns what to expect from people who have greater resources and strengths. The child learns what needs will be supported, what behaviors will be rewarded, and the most effective means of communicating desires. This relationship between the parental system and the children must be flexible and change as the family develops over the course of its life cycle.

Sibling Subsystem

The sibling subsystem forms the child's first peer group. Within this context children support, enjoy, attack, scapegoat, manipulate, and generally learn from each other. They develop their own transactional patterns for negotiating, cooperating, and competing and learn how to receive recognition. In an "ideal" family the children generally take different positions in the constant give and take. As they further their sense of belonging to this group, they develop a sense of individual choices and alternatives, a perception of each other and of themselves. The patterns learned here will be very important as the children move into the extrafamilial peer group.

The development of personal identity is a result of a complex feedback process. A child is born with a unique personality and attributes (physical, emotional, medical, etc.). How these attributes are perceived by the "significant others" in the child's life (for our purposes, the family) is important, as other family members will tend to reinforce the behaviors that are consistent with their perception of the child.

Children's participation in and interaction with the major family subsystems gives them a mirror in which they can see themselves and develop their identity. In order for the subsystems to function effectively, the boundaries between them must be clear and each should contain only "appropriate" members; for example, an older sibling may help to care for the monitored child, but if the sibling assumes age inappropriate (parental) power, a pathologic family structure with resultant relationship problems will develop.

Family History

When a child is born into a family, he or she enters a group that has not only a particular structure but also a unique history and rules that operate within a cultural framework. Within this context, the meaning of the child's acute episode and need for subsequent monitoring can predispose the family either to cope effectively or experience overwhelming distress. How the family defines the seriousness of the experienced stressor (having an apneic infant and needing to monitor) has both objective and subjective meaning. The objective cultural and societal seriousness (and acceptance) of the stressor represents the collective judgement of the community, whereas the subjective definition is composed of the accompanying hardships and their effect on the family. This subjective meaning reflects the family's values and previous experience in dealing with change, meeting crises, and the particular meaning that the "near miss" episode represents to them. A family's outlook can vary from seeing life changes and transitions as challenges to be met (viewing their monitored child as special and themselves blessed) to interpreting the stressor (monitoring) as uncontrollable, an overwhelming burden, a punishment, and a prelude to family disruption.

Most family systems carry with them some residue of strain, often the result of unresolved hardships from earlier stressors or transitions. Occasionally the strain may be inherent in assuming new or ongoing roles (i.e., becoming a parent, having to take care of a sick family member, etc.). When a new stressor is experienced by the family, these strains are rekindled, amplifying the current stress.

Within the family history has been the development of family rules. These rules describe the conscious or unconscious role expectations and sequences of behaviors of family members. Within a family, rules may operate effectively until overwhelming stress causes decompensation. Additional stresses can emerge from specific behaviors (solutions) that the family may use in an effort to cope with a crisis situation. A father, in his role as primary financial provider, may attempt to deal with the increased expense of monitoring and/or his wife's decision not to return to work (in order to better care for the monitored child) by assuming another job or by working overtime in his current position. Coping by getting a second job can become an additional source of family strain if it increases the loneliness and the work of the other spouse.

The family's style of communication is an important variable in its ability to cope with stress. If communication within the family, particularly between the spouses, is open and direct, the family members are more likely to express and experience mutual support and increased family cohesion. If problems and disagreements can be addressed and solved as they arise, the family will find itself able to adapt, absorb, and better tolerate stress. In contrast, families in which communication occurs in an indirect and ambiguous manner will experience a high level of tension resulting from repeated lack of conflict resolution and inability to solve problems effectively as they arise. The result will be a rigid and inflexible family system unable to absorb and adapt to the stresses of monitoring.

The Initial Phase

The Acute Episode

The circumstances surrounding the acute apneic episode of the infant are important, including where the parents were at the time, who was with the baby, what was concurrently happening in the lives of the parents, and whether or not a previous child had been lost. At the moment of the apneic episode, time stops and life changes. As one parent stated, "On October 28, our family got their wish: a beautiful baby girl was born. On the evening of May 15, Joe and I went out to celebrate our anniversary and rejoice. Everything seemed so perfect, until later that evening, when we were en route home, an ambulance passed our car and stopped directly in front of our house. We ran into the house to find our two sons and the babysitter hysterical. Our precious baby girl was gray and her eyes were dull. We went from our local hospital to Massachusetts General Hospital. Everything happened so quickly and without warning. Soon we brought home a 'monitor baby.' I'll never forget the emotions we felt. Why and how did this happen to our baby? The frustration and fear led to panic, and both Joe and I were in a deep state of exhaustion and very depressed."

The initial affective response to discovering that your infant almost died is usually shock mixed with relief; shock of "oh no! how could this happen to me?" mixed with the relief of "thank God, she's alive!" These emotions are complicated by the frenetic activity that begins with the discovery of the apneic episode and persists through the emergency ride to the hospital, the hospitalization, and then finally the return home.

Hospitalization

During the hospitalization, which is usually short (three to seven days), medical and psychosocial evaluations are done to determine the cause of the episode [5]. When the diagnosis of apnea of infancy is made, parents are taught infant cardiopulmonary resuscitation (CPR) and cardiopulmonary monitoring. Parents are taught methods of responding to both real and false alarms, means of rearranging their household and, to some extent, their lives to make monitoring more manageable [19, 20]. "We spent our daytimes in the hospital learning about the monitor and how to do CPR," said one mother. "We read and re-read the material [20] that was given to us and tried to test each other on the resuscitation protocol. We gave each of our parents a copy of the material, too, so they would understand what monitoring was all about and the impact it would have on our lives."

In addition to medical and psychosocial evaluation, support and education should begin immediately. It is during times of crisis (disruption of equilibrium) that individuals and families are most open to intervention (external influence) [21]. According to Caplan's notions of the nature of crisis resolution, the period of disruption (discovering your child has had an apneic episode and will be monitored) is self limited and may be followed by a new adaptation, which is qualitatively different from the one that preceded it. Thus, the family's equilibrium can be effectively restored by helping them to adapt or change their modes of coping and/or by changing features of the environment. Appropriate intervention and education at this time will help families survive the crisis and restabilize in a healthy pattern [22] (Figure 10.1). Moreover, because parents will be meeting the

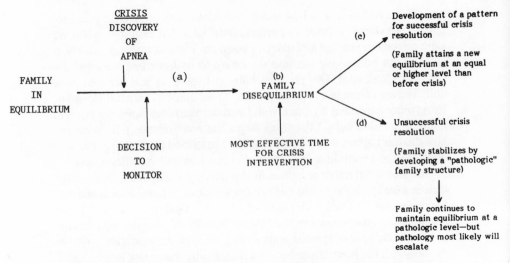

FIGURE 10.1. Process of Crisis Resolution: (a) The initial rise in tension due to the discovery of the apneic infant, followed by the decision to monitor, provokes habitual problem-solving responses and tension. (b) This increasing tension can act as a powerful stimulus to the mobilization of internal and external resources characterized by the family's utilization of novel problem-solving methods (trial and error). (c) The family attains a new equilibrium at an equal or higher level. (d) An alternative is that tension mounts leading to major disorganization, which may manifest itself either in family dysfunction or the dysfunction of one of the family members [37]. (Reprinted with permission of the authors.)

psychosocial support staff at a time when they are receptive and grateful for help, a positive alliance will be formed, making it easier for them to ask for assistance in the future.

During the hospitalization, it is common for the family's sense of relief to change to anxiety, confusion, fear, doubt, and/or denial. Denial is a normal defense mechanism that can be very useful, especially when circumstances seem overwhelming. Denial to a mild or moderate degree can be beneficial, but complete denial, especially when it involves a potentially life-threatening illness, can be disastrous. In our experience, denial appears to be a defense more often used by fathers, especially those who did not observe the acute episode. If the father's denial becomes fixed, the mother may compensate by becoming hypervigilant and overinvolved with her infant.

While the child is hospitalized, parents frequently begin to question their capability of dealing with monitoring and are faced with the realization of the enormity of their responsibility for the life of their infant. "During our stay in Boston," said one father, "I thought the monitor was the answer to our problems. I soon realized how wrong I was. I began to realize that the monitor was only there to tell us something was wrong, and that everything else was up to us. I also realized how much her life depended on us." The Wasserman study reported that initially all the parents doubted their ability to care for their infant [10]. During this early phase, some parents may begin to experience a "grief (or mourning) reaction" [23]. This "grieving" is related to the loss of the idealized expectations of being a parent with a "perfect" child. Although each family member (including grandparents) may experience it, and may react in different ways or at different times, the initial stage is usually one of emotional numbness and disbelief. Gradually the numbness will give way to a period of sadness, irritability and/or anger. These feelings are apt to intensify if the child continues to have repeated apneic episodes. For mothers, these emotions also may be complicated by post-partum physiologic and emotional changes. In contrast, other parents may view their child as special and themselves as blessed. It is important for parents to know that the myriad of emotions they are feeling is normal. As one parent stated, "By the end of the first week (referring to the hospitalization) we went home with the monitor. We were shaky, fragile, exhausted, depressed, and disorganized, as well as totally off any kind of schedule. But we were home. It was so very important for us to be told that our 'emotional state' was not unusual!"

The Adjustment Phase

Monitoring at Home

The transition home is filled with many tense moments. It is important for the medical community to provide intensive support at this time through frequent telephone calls and perhaps home visits. The pediatric pulmonary team provides twenty-four-hour availability of medical and psychological personnel.

Parents report that they are most anxious during their first week of monitoring [9, 10], often not trusting the monitor to function properly, or fearing that they would not hear the alarm [9]. Frequently, both parents respond to each alarm and tend to keep the infants close to them, with many sleeping in the parents' bedroom. Fathers are more likely to minimize the extent of anxiety and to express more concrete concerns such as potential power failures, whereas mothers are more likely to express greater anxiety and often are unable to sleep at night fearing that they will sleep through an alarm [9]. Although this anxiety is most likely secondary to the child's illness and treatment [8], at present it is difficult to determine the magnitude of each of these factors compared with those due to the normal transition to parenthood. Despite the presence of anxiety, most parents view the monitor in positive terms, as a "help" or "blessing" and a "reducer of anxiety" [9]. In uncomplicated cases with no further apnea, most parents report less anxiety after the first month of monitoring [9–10], although 27.4 percent of parents in one study still described themselves as being "very anxious" [9].

Parents soon learn to depend on the monitoring equipment. Some parents do this by making a conscious decision; others do it out of necessity. "For some reason I didn't trust the monitor, and I wouldn't admit it. I had the constant fear that Joni might not be there in the morning. I went six days with only five hours of sleep. My other children hated the monitor and probably hated me too. I couldn't blame them. Naturally, with no sleep I couldn't function at all. My family was falling apart. The experienced nurses at the lab quickly picked this up through our phone conversation and sent me to see the team psychologist, Dr. K. She told my husband and myself to trust the monitor and to alternate nights being "aware" of alarms (if we felt we had to). A week later we were sleeping through the night and things were back to normal. We couldn't even remember whose night it was to 'sleep light'!"

Some parents dislike the limitations that monitoring places on them [10], whereas others report that having a baby on a monitor at home is not difficult and in many cases (30.2 percent) makes things easier for them [9]. Moreover, most parents (72.9 percent) report that the monitor helps them feel more relaxed about their children [9].

The initial physical adjustments and restrictions placed on parents by monitoring, when exacerbated by sleep deprivation, exhaustion, and emotional turmoil, increase irritability and decrease the ability to cope. Trying to maintain a household can be a difficult task for a mother whose time and energy is constantly in demand. A monitored baby can never be left unattended unless he or she is on a monitor, and, even then, a responsible person must be no further than ten seconds away. When not on the electronic monitor, the infant must be carefully observed for breathing and color changes. "We had our spate of false alarms during the early phase, and thought at times we would go crazy if we couldn't get away from our little friend," said one parent. "Ten seconds, even in our little home proved to equate with 'same floor.' Our entire existence revolved around being near the monitor or having Erin in a Snugli carrier so we could watch her. But eventually, we got the hang of it."

Often, it is difficult for the mother as the primary caretaker to accomplish simple chores such as showering, vacuuming, etc., since these have to be done when another person can listen for the alarm. The usual solution is to do "noise" housework when both parents or another adult is present. Support is the key for coping with monitoring. Sharing the work load of household duties, nurturance of the monitored child and the other children, and responding to the alarms at night is essential for positive adjustment to the monitoring experience.

Social (relationship) support offers families information at an interpersonal level that provides emotional, esteem, and network support [16]. Emotional support leads the members of the family unit to believe that they are cared for and loved. Esteem support leads them to believe that they are esteemed and valued. The third type of social support, network support, leads the members of the family unit to believe that they belong to a network involving mutual obligation and mutual understanding [24]. Network support includes extended family, neighbors, friends, medical personnel, other monitoring parents, and social agencies in the form of housekeeping and respite care. As a result of accepting support from these sources, many parents report that the monitoring experience has made them closer to their friends, families, and communities.

Home monitoring will affect all family members, including the infant's siblings. Parents should be encouraged to discuss monitoring with their other children during the time of the infant's hospitalization. In addition to the normal adjustment that any child needs to make when a new sibling arrives, these siblings must be able to accept a "vulnerable" child who, in the words of one brother, is "bionic!" The manner in which this accommodation occurs is a reflection of the child's age, personality, temperament, prior preparation, and perception of his or her parents' feelings about the monitor. Older children may respond by being helpful, or may, like younger children, feel intense sibling rivalry (which can be exacerbated by the jealousy invoked by the rapid response parents make to the infant's calling them via alarms). The monitor should be presented as something that keeps the infant safe and from which the sibling can derive benefit (i.e., "it" can watch the infant while Mommy spends time with him or her). As one parent shares, "From the beginning we included Barbi (age three). We showed her how the monitor worked and even hooked it to her. We also gave her an old cigar box, two sticky electrodes and some old wires to play with. She put them on her doll 'to help her breathe' as she puts it. We made sure to give Barbi special time and told her that the monitor gave us the ability to do that. It seemed to work. We felt more secure with the monitor, and so did she."

The Adjustment Period

When the parents begin to trust the monitor, anxiety in general tends to decrease (it is important to acknowledge that regardless of nights of multiple false alarms, none of the parents in the Black [8] or Wasserman [10] studies had ever considered discontinuing the monitor or ignoring alarms). The ability to adjust to the problems of monitoring appears to be related to the family's premorbid psychic structure, the events before the diagnosis of the apnea, and whether or not the infant has subsequent "spells." If the infant requires resuscitation during monitoring, the psychic costs and tensions in the home increase. Home monitoring has been reported to decrease anxiety in the face of subsequent spells [8]. Parents in the Black study were convinced that their children would have died had the monitor not signaled the distress. Moreover, parents soon become sensitive to their infant and begin to anticipate "bad" nights (nights where there will be alarms) through the observation of color, behavioral changes and/or intercurrent illnesses, thus increasing their sense of control [8].

Learning to live with the physical and social restrictions of monitoring often is difficult. We have found that parents benefit greatly from the support of other monitoring parents who have many concrete suggestions and "tricks of the trade" to share. In addition, the availability of personnel such as respite care and housekeepers, who can be obtained through the Department of Social Services, will give the family greater flexibility and freedom. Medical personnel are a very important source of support during the adjustment period. Telephone calls initiated by the monitoring program staff are viewed as extremely important as is the availability of medical personnel to answer questions, give support, or be available in an emergency. In one study [8], 75 percent of the parents viewed the pulmonary laboratory, its chief physician, and nursing staff as the support on which they relied most heavily.

Short-Term vs. Long-Term Monitoring

There appear to be at least two major groups of infants with apnea. One group is monitored for approximately four months and has no recurrent episodes [25]; the second group has recurrent episodes during sleep requiring significant intervention to terminate [5, 26, 27], with some infants dying during subsequent episodes [5–7]. Approximately 5 percent of infants will continue to need monitoring after twelve months of age. In addition to apneic and bradycardic episodes, we have observed gastrointestinal reflux, seizures, temperature abnormalities, cyclical behavioral abnormalities, appetite disturbances, and episodic color changes in these older children. Families of these infants have a more difficult time coping with the stress of their child's illness. Since many of these abnormalities seen in the older child have not been fully understood medically, the families live with constant uncertainty. Such families usually need more intense support, often with the program psychiatrist or psychologist.

Specific Effects of Monitoring on Family Subsystems

Spouse Subsystem

Factors Affecting Adjustment. The couple's preexisting methods of coping, both as individuals and as a couple, are extremely important in determining how they will adjust to the stresses of monitoring. The broad range of characteristics of individual family members (personal resources) that potentially are available in time of crisis is an important variable in the family's ability to cope with stress. When members have sufficient and appropriate resources, they are less likely to view a crisis situation as problematic. Four basic resources have been identified: (1) financial (economic well-being), (2) cognitive (realistic stress perception and problem-solving skill), (3) physical and emotional "health," and (4) psychological resources (personality characteristics), especially self-esteem and the sense of mastery over one's life. Marital discord, when it occurs during the period of treatment for apnea of infancy, usually is related to the spouses' different attitudes toward monitoring [8]. Moreover, the most effective adjustment appears to occur when families share the burdens and the spouses function through mutual cooperation and support [10]. Fifty percent of the couples in two studies reported that monitoring brought them closer together, and 21.8 percent believed their marriage had improved, with 68.6 percent of the mothers and 91.5 percent of the fathers describing their spouse as offering the most help [9, 10]. In contrast, couples who do not communicate clearly and directly and who either consistently withdraw or turn to others for support rather than to each other (i.e., families of origin, friends, work, alcohol, children, etc.) will experience increased marital stress. In one study, six of thirteen couples who had divorced or were considering divorce, reported that the lack of sharing the responsibility of monitoring was a significant factor in their decision [10], and 10 percent of the mothers in another study reported that they had separated or considered separation because of the monitor [9].

Previous History of Loss. A history of loss, including that of a parent, a sibling, or a previous child, especially the loss of a previous child to SIDS, will affect the spousal relationship. Smialek noted shock, disbelief, denial, negativism, anger, guilt, resurgence of formerly unresolved grief, and recurrent fears of loss as the most common grief reactions of 351 families of SIDS victims [28]. These feelings do not evaporate but rather influence the couple's relationship with each other and the family's perception of the new child. "One cold day in 1974 I awoke to find our 5-month-old daughter had died in her sleep," said one parent. "After the initial shock was over, we started putting the pieces of our lives back together. But, no matter how hard I tried, my husband and I were never able to talk about it. I felt guilty and alone. My husband seemed to hold me responsible for what had happened. We thought that it would take some of the hurt away and bring us closer if we had another child. On September 24, I gave birth to a beautiful, baby boy. When Johnny was born, he was termed a "borderline case." We decided to monitor him, feeling that even if we never had an alarm, it was better than taking a chance we might be wrong. We monitored him for three and one-half years! Every time we'd try to take him off (doctor's orders) we'd find an excuse. My husband kept saying to me 'if anything happens to him, it will be on your shoulders.' Well, eventually I took him off in the face of my husband's anger." Unfortunately, they continued to have problems with him. They were unable to control his behavior—including getting him out of their bed at night. Because of the parents' unresolved grief, anger, and feelings of responsiility surrounding the death of their daughter, Johnny entered a family in which the spouses needed to maintain psychological distance from each other, while at the same time having expectations that he would bring them closer. The relationship between Johnny's parents did not improve with his birth, but Johnny was able to stabilize the system by becoming triangulated between them (Figure 10.2). After monitoring ceased, Johnny continued to be triangulated, with the focus of parental attention being his difficult behavior (also a symptom of his distress). The initial therapeutic focus was in helping his parents to develop mutual support, to have appropriate expectations, and to set appropriate limits on their son's behavior. As would be expected, when Johnny's behavior improved, the couple's issues began to surface. Empowered now as successful parents, they were finally able to express and resolve their feelings about their daughter's death. Mandell recommends that parents who have lost a child to SIDS defer having subsequent children until their grief has resolved and the environment in their homes has become healthier [29].

Exacerbation of Normal Processes. When a child is born, it is common to see a decrease in spousal attention, as each parent's attention becomes focused on the infant. With the development of increasing fatigue and irritability, loneliness and depression can result. In one study, all the mothers and 6 percent of the fathers had signs or symptoms of depression. "During the first week home, we found that we were either having a lot of fights or weren't speaking. Even though we realized that it was just a result of pressure and fatigue, it felt difficult to stop. For John, it was being at work all day, and when he got home, I didn't give him time to unwind. I had taken care of the kids all day, including our monitored daughter, and I wanted him to take over. We weren't talking to each other as we had in the past. There just never seemed to be any time. After the kids were in bed for the night, I was feeling alone and distant. Neither of us felt that our needs were being taken care of. I felt resentful and found myself beginning to get more pleasure from being a mother than a wife. John found little pleasure with me and began seeing me, as he put it, as being either 'unavailable' or 'a critical nag.' John began staying late at work, saying that he 'had to,' but I knew that he felt better there than at home. Understanding didn't help—I still felt resentful and increasingly overburdened." This type of pattern can become self-reinforcing. If the wife is unpleasant or unavailable, the husband is likely to avoid her. The more unavailable the husband is, the more the wife will feel neglected, overburdened, and resentful, and the less available she will be for him, resulting in increased distance be-

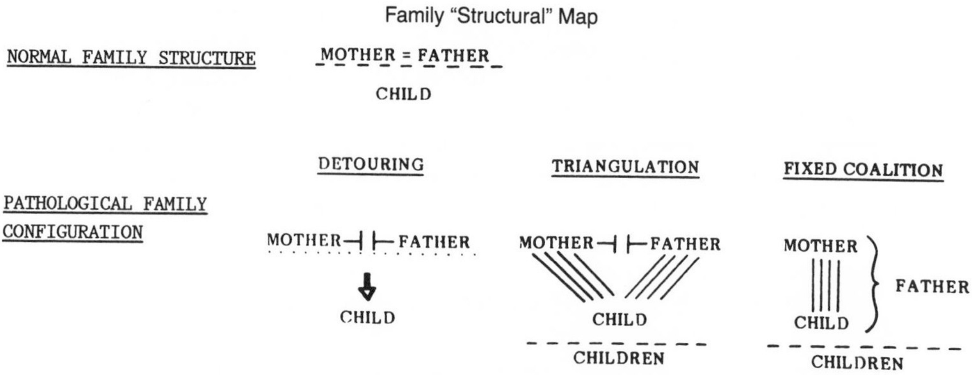

Family "Structural" Map

NORMAL FAMILY STRUCTURE   _MOTHER = FATHER_

                                       CHILD

                     DETOURING   TRIANGULATION   FIXED COALITION

PATHOLOGICAL FAMILY
CONFIGURATION

           MOTHER─┤ ├─FATHER   MOTHER─┤ ├─FATHER   MOTHER ⎞
                  ↓   ╲╲╲ ╱╱╱   ⎟
                CHILD   ╲╲╲╱╱╱   CHILD   ⎬ FATHER
                                        CHILD   ⎠
                                   ─ ─ ─ ─ ─ ─ ─   ─ ─ ─ ─ ─ ─ ─
                                      CHILDREN   CHILDREN

FIGURE 10.2. Alliances/Affiliations—depict the quality of usual transactions between two family members

A) clear (normal)══════   C) weak or unknown ━ ━ ━   E) coalition of several ⎫
B) overinvolved ═══════   D) conflict ──────┤ ├───── members against an- ⎬
                                                     other   ⎭

Detouring: the conflict between two people is deflected through concern for another (i.e., the monitored child).

Triangulation: a husband and wife relate to each other through the inclusion of the child who is asked to side with one parent against the other.

Fixed coalition: a child consistently sides with one parent against the other.

tween the spouses. Fortunately, this couple found a healthy solution (related to their premorbid coping style). "We realized," said the wife, "we had to do what we had always done, and that is if something bothered one of us, we had to talk things out." And talk things out they did. "John has helped me through days I thought would never end. Just having him take our older son and our new baby to the park after dinner so I could spend some time alone made all the difference to me. I could see the difference in John when he had some time alone, too. We began to feel more supportive of each other, and looked forward to spending more time alone together when the kids were alseep. I can't say that the first night or first few weeks were easy, but I can say that all the daily routines did fall into place."

The majority of the families in three studies reported that the monitor had a "significant or drastic effect on their social life" [8–10]. The transition from couple to parent often by its very nature affects the couple's socializing, but monitoring adds an extra dimension. It is difficult to find a CPR-trained sitter and when one is found, many parents are reluctant to leave their infant. Some parents solve this problem by sharing the care of the infant. "For a temporary period of time," states one mother, "we had become married singles. We had found that since we couldn't go out together as frequently as before, we arranged it so that each of us could have time to go out (alone) and be with friends, do errands, etc. The only problem was, we'd meet at the door, with one going out and the other coming in!" Unfortunately, this type of sharing child care usually results in the couple having little time together. In the Cain study [9], seventy-four parents (55.7 percent) noted that the monitor prevented them from going out as much as they would like, whereas in the Black study [8], 10 percent of the families were hesitant to entertain at home because they were reluctant to expose their infants to people who might carry infections. In contrast, many parents do entertain at home while others go out separately but do manage to set aside time for each other. "We haven't gone out alone since Joni was in the hospital, but we go out separately with friends because we need time to get away. In addition we plan a quiet dinner for the two of us alone at home every so often, splurge on a bottle of wine and catch up with each other. God knows, we deserve it!" Other parents resolve this problem by taking the infant out with them. Whatever means of socializing is chosen, spouses need adult time together. With that time, it will become easier for spouses to be parents, inviting the children to become a stable part of their relationship.

Intimacy. Sexual intimacy is related to the couple's continuing affection and shared experiences, as well as their levels of physiologic libido, energy, etc. One study found that a decrease in sleep and sexual interest was common in families who monitored their infant [10]. As one mother stated, "It seems like years have gone by, rather than the mere months it has actually been. Rachael was born in March, we started monitoring in April, and by September, I thought I was the worst mother in the world! Rachael was now six months old and nursing full time. Jack, her brother, was two and one-half years old and as active as any two and one-half year-old could be. I really didn't realize how quick tempered and irritable I had become, and not one person could tell me what was wrong, including my husband, who tried to be supportive and affectionate. Yet, every time he tried to come closer to me—especially if he tried to make love, it felt like an added burden, making me angry—and I'd end up feeling worse about myself! I felt deep down that I was becoming severely depressed. At times my face and whole body were numb and I had no feeling. At other times I would cry at the drop of a hat. The life I had chosen at this point was to be at home with my babies and be 'supermom' (she was a nurse who had intended to return to work part-time, but decided not to because of the need to monitor). All my outside activities revolved around the children and the monitor. Tom, my husband, worked two jobs, and although he is a very supportive husband and daddy, we didn't see much of him at this time. Also, because our insurance didn't cover babysitting, we were not able to get out alone. It started to be more and more of an ordeal to get out alone and to go about my daily routine. Everyday conversations with friends were getting shorter as I was finding less and less to talk about and more and more things to complain about. The worst part was that I was complaining about things that other people did that bothered me, rather than how I was the bothersome one!" While on a routine medical visit with their pediatric pulmonary physician, who includes as an important part of her interview social adjustment questions, this mother began to cry. After talking with her at length, the physician suggested that Mrs. B. and her husband speak with the team psychologist. "Dr. K. told me what the problem was. The simple truth was that I was exhausted, and Tom and I were stressed beyond our limits! Between nursing around the clock and getting up with alarms (real), I wasn't getting nearly enough sleep. I was amazed at what fatigue could do! I wasn't in a depression, I didn't have a deep psychological problem, I was just plain tired! She offered some practical solutions to us and helped us to communicate our needs more clearly. She even gave us the 'assignment' of spending more time together! Within a week I was a new person, and Tom and I were lovers again!"

Sexual intimacy can be affected by having the child sleep in the marital bedroom or bed. Rationalizing that they needed to watch their infant closely, two-thirds of the parents in one study kept the infant in their bedroom for the duration of monitoring, whereas other couples who were able to put the child in his or her own room reported being very aware of the sleeping child and alarms [8]. For those parents who do not practice birth control, the fear of becoming pregnant and either adding to the stresses of monitoring or taking the risk of having to monitor another child can decrease the frequency of sexual relations.

Career and Work. Being a husband or father, wife or mother are but two of the many roles that individuals experience. In addition to these "family roles," the work role is often viewed as important and/or a financial necessity. Because of the need to monitor her infant, a mother who might have planned to continue to work after her child's birth may be unable to do so, resulting in personal disappointment and resentment. In one study, nine of sixteen mothers who wanted to work outside the home felt unable to do so because of their fear of leaving their infant with another caretaker, and only one mother went back to her regular job [10]. Moreover, if the husband becomes the sole provider in a family that had planned their lifestyle around two salaries, there will be increased pressure on him to increase his income. This pressure is intensified by the additional financial burden of monitoring, which has been estimated to cost $1,500 [30]. Some monitoring fathers have assumed longer work hours, a second job, or a job change in order to accommodate the extra burden of monitoring. The potential resentment or hostility that may accompany these "forced" career decisions can affect the spousal relationship, as well as the relationship of parent to child. In contrast, some parents report little or no financial problems related to the cost of monitoring, since for these families, the cost was largely assumed by insurance or assistance programs [9].

There are additional expenses that are not reimbursable and are not addressed by this study. These include transportation (many families live long distances from the medical center), long distance telephone calls, babysitters, and extra expenses related to lifestyle adjustment. As would be anticipated, the longer the infant is monitored, the greater these expenses will be.

The Pathologic Solutions. In those monitoring families who lack mutual support, clear and direct communication, and the skills to resolve disagreements and cope with problems as they arise, one might expect to see a progressive downward spiral of exhaustion, depression, frustration, and tension resulting in either open hostility or increased emotional distance between the spouses. When the spousal distance exceeds the limits of tolerance, one of four family configurations can occur. These include the formation of a stable triangle (triangulation), a coalition, detouring, or divorce [31] (Figure 10.2). These family configurations are not specific to families that monitor, but the monitoring experience can become the catalyst for their development. These processes often begin before monitoring, become "solidified" during monitoring, and continue long after monitoring has ceased. In triangulation, the husband and wife relate to each other through the inclusion of the child, who is pressured by each parent to "take sides." Detouring is the process by which parents deflect the incipient conflict through concern for the child, that is, when they are stressed and begin to argue, they may focus on the child out of concern for alarms, color change, etc. The third configuration is that of a stable coalition. This is a natural outgrowth of the overinvolved parent–child relationship with the complementary underinvolved relationship between the other parent and child, and between the spouses. These family configurations are not considered pathologic when they are transient and, in fact, can occur in normal families. However, they are considered pathologic when they become rigidly fixed and control the functional operations of the family. These patterns can be prevented and, if present, can be reversed. However, the longer they are maintained, the more difficult it is to effect change.

Parental Subsystem

The experience of monitoring exacerbates the emotional and physical stresses that are naturally present when a couple become parents. In one study, 79 of the 105 parents with other children felt that the monitored baby initially had required more time than previous babies [9]. This feeling decreased with time in 42 percent of the parents. Four of the 105 parents reported that they felt irritated with the "demanding" infant, and eleven said that, as a result, they were more irritable with their other children. This maternal irritability will affect the mother–child relationship.

Families who viewed the monitored child as "an irritant" or "a burden" reacted differently to the infant than did the majority of parents who viewed their child as "special" and endowed the illness with positive meaning [32]. When families are able to redefine the stressful situation and give it new meaning (i.e., purpose, value, understanding, etc.), it works to clarify the hardships and tasks so as to render them more manageable and responsive to problem-solving efforts [16]. Redefining monitoring as a "challenge," an "opportunity for growth," etc., or endowing it with special meaning, i.e., "a blessing," "saving our child was God's gift to us," appears to facilitate family coping and adaptation. As one parent of two monitored children stated, "There were many times when I thought God was testing us. But I kept remembering that there were so many worse off than us. At least our children would grow out of their difficulties. God had His own plans for us. He gave us two beautiful, healthy cherubs. He made us stronger and helped us learn the meaning of patience and endurance. He helped us cherish life (through saving our children) and one another. We, the parents of two monitored babies, have been blessed." In contrast some parents perceive their child to be theirs on tenuous loan, and may become hypervigilant and overindulgent. Others are afraid to allow their child to experience any stress, perceiving their child as vulnerable and fearing that frustration might trigger another episode. Still others may perceive their child as so special that they consistently "give" to him. For these parents, if monitoring continues for longer than usual (five to six months), the overprotecting and overindulging may lead to the development of a demanding, "spoiled," vulnerable child. In one study, seven of the sixteen children at a mean age of twenty-one months after discontinuance of monitoring, were characterized as "spoiled" by their parents, and all were viewed as "special because they almost died" [10]. At the time of diagnosis, parents should be reminded that except for having experienced an apneic episode, their child is normal. If parents perceive their child as normal, they will respond normally to each developmental stage, allowing the child to develop appropriate frustration tolerance and autonomy. If this is done early, discipline will be more natural and less traumatic for parent and child.

Spousal tension can affect parenting. Parents must be consistent in their expectations of their children (although they can agree to disagree). They must communicate these expectations to each other and the child in a clear manner. If there is tension in the spouse subsystem, the child is vulnerable to miscommunication, and may be caught in the parental crossfire. Moreover, the child who receives different messages from each parent can learn to manipulate them to his or her advantage. If the child is in a coalition with one parent against the other, he or she may receive inappropriate power from one parent while attracting criticism or punishment from the other.

Other children in the monitoring family will be affected by parental fatigue, irritability, and the "shift" in attention to the new infant. Moreover, the monitored child's siblings have age-appropriate needs as well. If these needs are not appropriately met, the sibling may attempt to get parental attention by becoming "symptomatic," increasing the parental burden [10].

Long-term monitoring parents (monitoring longer than twelve months) have additional burdens. Some of these children develop other medical problems including seizures, "seizurelike" activity, awake apnea, awake and asleep bradycardia, and abnormal appetite, as well as behavioral and temperature control cycles. For these parents, there are many unanswered questions, and anxiety and uncertainty continue to be present. In addition, some families are monitoring simultaneously two and, rarely, three children. We continue to be impressed at how well these families have adjusted and incorporated the monitor into their lives.

Sibling Subsystem

The effect of home monitoring on the siblings of the monitored child is a function of their age, parental relationship, personality, temperament, and fantasies and feelings about the new baby. In addition to the normal adjustment that any child needs to make when a new sibling arrives, this child must accept a baby who is vulnerable and who brings with him a "monitor." Normal reactions seen in an older sibling include anger, jealousy, resentment and a sense of rejection. Moreover, children are perceptive of their parents' feelings about the monitored infant and may act out these feelings (i.e., anger, resentment, fear, etc.) while their parents continue to disown them.

Some siblings may respond favorably to the added responsibilities they might be given and even attempt to cope by becoming "second parents." It is important for parents to set clear limits on how much help is appropriate. Parents must explain about monitoring to the older child in an age-appropriate way. Pam, in talking about her five-year-old son stated, "I am amazed at how quickly our family came to trust and rely on our monitor. My son thought that this instrument with wires and switches and blinking lights resembled "Star Wars" equipment, not surprising since Luke Skywalker and Hans Solo were his current heroes." Another six-year-old boy thought his baby sister was a bionic woman with a power pack! Pam went on to add, "After attaching the leads to his body and allowing him to operate the warning lights (by jumping up and down to increase his heart rate and holding his breath to cause an apnea alarm), he seemed comfortable with his sister's new equipment and understood its function as well as any five-year-old cares to know."

All siblings, especially young children, may experience feelings of jealousy or rejection. As one parent stated, "We had a few problems with our three-year-old, jealousy mostly. Some of it was over just having to share Mommy and Daddy, and some of it was due to the extra attention Sally got from being on a monitor. We solved the problem by making sure that Mary got extra special one-on-one time with each of us. In addition, since we were going to take Sally out anyway, instead of hiring a babysitter, we would take Mary and Sally with us. This seemed to solve her feeling 'left out.' " It is effective to have the parent point out to the sibling that the monitor watches the infant during sleep, enabling them to spend time with the sibling during the baby's naps. As one parent said, "We have been lucky as far as Joseph and jealousy is concerned. There hasn't been any. If Joseph wants me to get him something when I'm busy with John, he tells me 'put John night-night and beep him, Mom!' " Of course with any new baby, siblings should never be left alone with the infant as they have been known to disconnect the monitor. Older siblings, too, can have adjustment problems such as generalized anxiety, decreased attention in school, behavioral problems, enuresis and speech regression [10].

Wanting to "get rid of" a new sibling or "send him back" is quite common. Some siblings have expressed concern that they "caused" the monitored child to have an episode because they hated him, were jealous of him, wanted him to disappear, etc. One child even viewed monitoring her brother as a punishment—she had wanted him gone, and now he was special! Children must be told that they were not responsible for their sibling's illness. In spite of these potential problems, in our clinical experience the majority of the siblings have made a successful adjustment to the monitored infant. It is important for medical personnel to stress the importance of reinforcing the normal sibling relationship between the sibling(s) and the new infant since this relationship definition will persist even after monitoring has ceased.

Individual Subsystem: The Monitored Child

The natural history, including the long-term sequelae of apnea of infancy, is unknown (see Chapter 11). Medical and neurologic symptoms in addition to apnea arise in a small proportion of the children who continue to have apnea after twelve months (approximately 5 percent of the total monitored population). The process of monitoring and the presence of apneic episodes and/or medical sequelae will affect children at each of their developmental stages. In infancy, issues of attachment are important. Usually the monitored infants are watched carefully and have frequent interactions with their parents, although most parents report that they do not treat their monitored infant differently [9]. In one study, one-third of the parents felt they enjoyed their babies more, and were "more attached because of the baby's problem" [8]. In contrast, one-fifth of the infants reportedly were held less, one-third were comforted less, and one-tenth were played with less often. Either "too much" or "too little" can be damaging. Parents must respond appropriately to the child's needs, otherwise the development of a "false self" can occur [33].

Children need to move through their developmental stages with as much parental objectivity and object relatedness as possible. If children are perceived (correctly or incorrectly) as vulnerable and needing extra protection, parents will tend to be hypervigilant and overprotective, and the normal development of the child's autonomy, self-control, and self-confidence will be affected. Parents must be able to trust themselves and the monitor. Babies need progressive freedom to explore their environment, and parents need time to be with their child without the intervention of a mechanical apparatus. A child must have the freedom to crawl, walk, take age-appropriate risks, try and fail, and learn from mistakes. A child also needs the security of appropriate limits for protection, the development of frustration tolerance, and security.

Since most children are not monitored after one year of age, it is the parents' perception of the child (a perception that has been affected by the illness and the monitoring experience) that will affect him or her at each of the subsequent developmental stages. For children who continue to be monitored, it is the parents' perception of them and their continuing medical problems that affect each stage.

As children grow, they become more curious about the monitor. The beeping of the alarm is a curiosity, a powerful means of obtaining the parents' attention, and an excellent vehicle to act out the control struggle. Some children even refuse to be monitored! "Leonard had periods when he decided he no longer needed to be monitored. Refusing to be connected and even trying to break his monitor were hard enough, but we also had to explain to him the seriousness of his problem. Being old enough to shut off all the equipment, he carried the situation a bit too far. One morning we awoke to find him sleeping on the floor next to our bed. At that point we had him see Dr. K., and the appointment was a success! She explained to him that *she* gave him the monitor (which reduced the parent/child control stuggle) and through his recordings she was sure that he still needed it. Now there are nights that he repeats her words of wisdom. 'When you have a problem at night and can't wake up to call Mom and Dad, the monitor calls them for you!' This really made sense to him, and he no longer shuts off his alarm."

The older child who has daytime apnea and bradycardia or other unexplained symptoms during the day cannot be left alone for medical reasons. This will affect his or her sense of autonomy, privacy, and the development of peer relationships. A mother who had three children on monitors stated, "Because Leonard and Erin have problems such as bradycardia, choking, and seizures while awake, they can't go out with friends without Mom or

Dad. Leonard really resents this. If he is doing well, I do allow him to play with friends in a small area of our yard. I then watch constantly but unobtrusively from our window. Their Nana is appropriately trained in CPR and monitor usage, and during a trouble-free period, Len is allowed to go for a visit to her house, or they go for walks. This is a treat for both of them." It has been our experience that the parents (and families) for long-term monitored children are incredibly creative and diligent in fostering normalcy.

Extrafamilial Subsystem: Support Systems

Support is the key ingredient to successful coping for monitoring families. In one study, 68.6 percent of the mothers and 91.5 percent of the fathers described the spouse as offering "much or a great deal" of help [9]. Extended family members such as grandparents, aunts, and uncles were noted to be potential supports especially if they learned CPR. This is in contrast to relatives who were "afraid" of the monitored child or those who questioned the parental anxiety since the child "looked so good." Other important supports include the monitor program staff, local pediatrician, social agencies through which they could get housekeeping and respite care, as well as emergency supports such as police and fire departments. Friends and other monitoring parents also form an important resource for support. Local SIDS chapters and Parents Monitoring Associations maintain support networks through telephone contact, social functions, general meetings, psychological support groups, and periodic newsletters that keep parents abreast of new information concerning monitoring, "helpful hints," and shared parental experiences. In addition, they educate the community about SIDS and monitoring and have pressured for legislative and social services needed for families. As one parent stated when referring to the importance of peer support, "I sometimes become anxious, and during those times, I usually call another parent. It's amazing how helpful a little conversation with someone in the same predicament can be. Just to hear someone say 'I know' and really mean it lifts me right up again!"

The Final Phase

Discontinuing the Monitoring

Most parents view the monitor as a "friend." One monitoring parent commented, "For me the monitor is sanity, a semireasonable night's sleep, nap times with minimum worry, comfort in knowing my baby's distress will not go unnoticed." Mrs. D. added, "It's been two months now that Becky has been on a monitor. We've had our bad days when we've walked around like zombies from lack of sleep and other days when we've gotten cocky because we haven't had an alarm for days. We've been able to get housework done with the help of a homemaker aide and have even hired a neighborhood boy to mow the lawn. We've come to enjoy and respect the monitor—it is very comforting when the baby has slept through the night, and we wake up confident that all is well because the alarm hasn't gone off."

Because most families depend on the monitor and integrate it into normal family life, discontinuing its use can be a difficult task. When the infant has met the general medical guidelines for discontinuing the monitor, his physician makes the recommendation to do so based on the infant's history, recognizing that some parents will need more support than others to follow his recommendation. Some will need to discontinue monitoring gradually, initially stopping for naps and then at night. During discontinuance, the first few nights are difficult for the parents and usually the child is checked frequently. A strong spouse system with husband and wife supporting and comforting each other (in addition to the support of apnea personnel) will make the resolution to discontinue monitoring easier. For some parents, this is relatively easy, especially when monitoring is uneventful. For those whose children experienced additional apneic episodes, it is more difficult. Tommy was monitored for two and one-half years and had two severe episodes of apnea. He had real alarms and "bad" pneumograms. "Taking my child off the monitor sounded so simple," said his mother. "I was sure I could do it with no problems. I sure fooled myself. After several weeks of trying, I decided that I would never take him off. It was as simple as that. I would wait until he was completely grown!" Even though she had described her monitoring experience as one filled with fatigue, she added, "We lived this life for two years and seven months; now Dr. K. was saying we should discontinue monitoring, and it seemed impossible. Every argument was thought up against doing it. We said to each other, 'we didn't mind all the work; better safe than sorry; he wasn't old enough; it hadn't been long enough since his last real alarm; he might be coming down with a cold which had always caused him to have real alarms; we couldn't face life if he died, etc.' Yet there was no doubt about it, Tommy was indeed better. His pneumograms were good, he got through colds without alarms, he had fevers without alarms, he got two new teeth without alarms. One night after many attempts, we shut off the monitor, unsnapped his wires and went to sleep. We forced ourselves to check less often than we wanted to. He slept fine and in a few nights, so did we."

In families for which the monitoring serves as a distance regulator or a conflict diffuser for the spouse subsystem, discontinuing the monitoring usually is more difficult, and even after it has been discontinued it is not uncommon for the child to continue to be a "symptom bearer" [34].

Discontinuing the monitoring will affect all the family's systems, including the sibling subsystem. Older siblings may manifest anxiety and continue to be hypervigilant. It is important to speak with all the children and prepare them for discontinuance. Parents also should consider having them speak with the apnea physician so that they can hear "officially" that the monitor is no longer needed.

Depending on the age of the monitored child and the length of time monitored, the child may perceive its absence. In the rare case in which he or she is old enough, it is very helpful for the child's physician to discuss it with him or her. Once off the monitor, it is extremely important to reinforce the child's normalcy.

We are seeing increasing numbers of parents who monitor more than one child. The majority of these parents report that this is easier for them than the initial monitoring experience because they know what to expect [10]. Moreover, the experience is facilitated because society in general and physicians in particular are more knowledgeable about monitoring, and considerable improvements have been made in the monitoring equipment. In addition, most parents have not seen the subsequent child unresponsive (as in the initial episode for their first child).

Status Post Monitoring

Only one study of fourteen families has commented on the long-term impact of home monitoring [10]. Two studies reported that approximately half of the couples believed monitoring had brought them closer together [9, 10]. One study stated "pre-existing problems appeared to worsen in some families after discontinuance of monitoring," with five of fourteen couples having divorced and a sixth considering divorce [10]. In another study, 14.2 percent felt that monitoring had made things worse, two of seventy-four mothers said they had separated because of the monitor and four others said they seriously considered separation [9]. Moreover, four couples decided not to have other children, reportedly because of this experience.

The Wasserman study noted that nine of thirteen of the monitored children were described by parents as exhibiting neurologic difficulties, specifically exhibiting gross and fine motor problems, decreased attention span, hyperactivity, poor coordination, speech problems, poor balance, and "slowness" [10]. It is important to note that these are subjective data gathered from parental observation. In a study investigating the neurologic, cognitive, and behavioral consequences of nonfatal infant apnea, fifteen formerly apneic-monitored children were compared with age-similar siblings and sex-matched playmates. Significant impairment in gross motor development and mild cognitive deficiencies were observed when apneic children were compared with their siblings but not when they were contrasted with their playmates. The conclusion was that apnea may have a threshold effect on subsequent development [35].

By parents' reports in the Wasserman study, twelve of sixteen older siblings manifested psychological problems, which included anxiety, decreased attention span, general behavioral problems, and regression [10].

Summary amd Recommendations

Having a child who has apnea necessitating home monitoring is a potential stressor affecting each of the subsystems (spouse, parental, sibling, individual) within a family system. The greatest anxiety is experienced during the initial episode and the first month of monitoring. The family then "adjusts" in its own characteristic way. Monitoring can be an exhausting and isolating experience; yet, the majority of families view the monitor as a "friend" giving them security, control, and peace of mind. The key for successful coping with the stresses of home monitoring appears to be open and clear communication, support, education, and prophylactic intervention. Parents need to be encouraged to talk openly with each other, their children, and their physicians.

From the moment of diagnosis, physicians and apnea personnel need to be available to families for medical and psychological support. During routine medical follow-up, physicians should assess the family's psychological coping, quality of family life, and social adjustment. Both fathers and mothers should be encouraged to attend these appointments because involvement of both spouses will support the boundary around the spouse system, and the physician will be able to observe the quality of the spouse interaction. If indicated, older siblings or extended family members should also participate in the medical appointment. Monitoring-related stresses should be anticipated and discussed [25]. It is important to listen to parents' concerns and to reinforce good parenting. In addition, contact with a mental health professional who is considered a routine member of the pediatric pulmonary team should be ongoing if possible. These meetings can be diagnostic, educative, and supportive. If there is concern that a child or family is at risk, more frequent meetings should be established.

In addition to the supports provided by the medical community, parents should be directed toward other psychological and physical support systems. Encouraging parents to have relatives or friends attend monitor and CPR training sessions will encourage empathy and educate individuals who can give the parents free time away from their monitored child, while at the same time providing support and decreasing their sense of isolation. Moreover, parents should be directed immediately (at the time of diagnosis) toward agencies through which they can receive respite care, housekeepers, and financial aid when necessary. Contact with other parents who have monitored an infant (individual parents and/or a monitoring parent organization) should be encouraged.

Psychological Intervention

Combined stresses on basically healthy individuals can create symptoms. By maintaining continuous close contact with each monitoring family, the "family at risk" can be identified, facilitating early intervention that may abort the development of severe emotional problems such as depression, intolerable anxiety, behavioral problems (in children), and marital disruption. Prophylactic knowledge about potential stresses helps parents to perceive them as "normal" when they occur and to ask for help. In addition, parents also are more likely to ask for help if they have a previously positive rapport with the caregiver.

When a family requests help with a particular problem or with "difficulty coping," we work closely with them and their referring physician. We meet with the family in its entirety, and at times the parents and/or children separately. We support and reinforce the family's strengths and are often directive in helping them find solutions to the problem. Occasionally, we broaden our context to include the extended family, medical personnel, schools, and community agencies where necessary. We work therapeutically toward reinforcing the boundaries around the parental and spouse subsystems and help them to integrate the monitored child as a normal son or daughter into the sibling subsystem. Work is often done with the parents and the nonmonitored children. In addition we have found an ongoing, professionally led parents' group to be therapeutically beneficial and are forming a siblings' group. If a parent appears clinically depressed, antidepressant medication may be necessary.

In uncomplicated, short-term monitoring, stress usually is due to the initial episode, adjustment to the monitor, and the changes in the family lifestyle. Our goal is to continue to support the family's positive adaptive style, making suggestions where appropriate and encouraging the family to perceive and respond to the child as a normal infant. For more long-term monitoring families, more intensive psychological support is indicated. For these families, much is still unknown, and everyday life may continue to be difficult and unpredictable.

There is still controversy over the use of home monitoring. Most families in which there is an infant who is considered for monitoring have high levels of anxiety due to the episode of apnea. Monitoring may actually decrease this anxiety [8, 9]. Southall, however, questioned the role of parental anxiety induced by monitoring (and false alarms) in affecting the parent-child relationship and perhaps inducing physical harm [36]. Continuing to make improvements in the monitor and in the treatment of apnea of infancy certainly will help to decrease anxiety. In addition, further controlled, long-term studies must be done to examine the long-term effect of monitoring.

Parents appear to be the staunchest opponents of the monitoring critics.

In all three of the studies done on the psychological stresses of home monitoring, the parents viewed the monitor as helpful [8–10]. Moreover, no study has ever reported a parent voluntarily discontinuing monitoring without a physician's approval. The monitor repeatedly has alerted parents to infants who have required resuscitation and who might have died had they not been monitored [5, 8, 25].

There is no question that home monitoring can be stressful and exhausting and affect the whole family; yet, 72.95 percent of parents in the Cain study reported that the monitor had helped them to feel more comfortable and relaxed about their children [9]. Many of our parents repeatedly expressed that "the end justifies the means," and "as hard as it is, it definitely works."

We conclude this chapter with words from a parent of a monitored infant. "The only thing I can say to new monitoring parents is to accept and trust the monitor as fast as possible. Don't look at the monitor as a burden, just as an inconvenience. And thank God every day, as I do, that your baby is alive and healthy and some day will be off the monitor forever."

References

1. Peterson, D.R., G. vanBelle, and N.W. Chinn. 1979. Epidemiologic comparison of the sudden infant death syndrome with other major components in infant mortality. *Am J Epidemiol* 110:699–707.
2. Guntheroth, W.G. 1982. *Crib Death: The Sudden Infant Death Syndrome.* New York: Futura Publishing.
3. Valdes-Dapena, M.A. 1980. Sudden Infant Death Syndrome: A review of the medical literature 1974–1979. *Pediatrics* 66:597–614.
4. American Academy of Pediatrics Task Force on Prolonged Apnea: Prolonged Apnea. 1978. *Pediatrics* 61 (suppl):651–652.
5. Kelly, D.H., D.C. Shannon, and K. O'Connell. 1978. Care of infants with near miss sudden infant death syndrome. *Pediatrics* 61:511–514.
6. Kelly, D.H., and D.C. Shannon. 1981. Neonatal and infantile apnea. *Advanced Perinatal Medicine* 1:1–44.
7. Duffty, P., and M.H. Bryan. 1982. Home apnea monitoring in near miss sudden infant death syndrome (SIDS) and in siblings of SIDS victims. *Pediatrics* 70:69–74.
8. Black, K., L. Hersher, and A. Steinschneider. 1978. Impact of the apnea monitor on family life. *Pediatrics* 62:681–685.
9. Cain, L.P., D.H. Kelly, and D.C. Shannon. 1980. Parents' perception of the psychological and social impact of home monitoring. *Pediatrics* 66:37–41.
10. Wasserman, A.J. 1984. A prospective study of the impact of home monitoring on the family. *Pediatrics* 74:323–329.
11. Curran, W.J. 1972. An enigma wrapped in swaddling clothes: Congress and "crib death." *N Eng J Med* 287:235–237.
12. Death Investigation. *Synopsis and Analysis of Laws.* Final Report No. HSA 240-80-0027 Dept. H.H.S. 1981.

13. Research planning workshops on the sudden infant death syndrome. 1972–1976. Washington, D.C. Department of Health, Education and Welfare. Nos. 1–12.

14. Brady, J., B. Chir, and J. Gould. 1984. *Sudden Infant Death Syndrome: The Physician's Dilemma.* Chicago: Year Book Medical Publishers.

15. Kelly, D.H., K. O'Connell, and D.C. Shannon. 1979. Electrode belt: A new method for long term monitoring. *Pediatrics* 63:670–673.

16. McCubbin, H., and C. Figley. 1983. *Stress in the Family: Coping with Normative Transitions.* Vol. 1. New York: Brunner Mazel.

17. Bertalanffy, L.V. 1968. *General Systems Theory.* New York: Braziller.

18. Minuchin, S., B.K. Rosman, and L. Baker. 1978. *Psychosomatic Families: Anorexia Nervosa in Context.* Cambridge, Mass.: Harvard University Press.

19. Barr, A. 1975. *At Home with a Monitor: A Guide for New Parents.* Boston: Pediatric Pulmonary Laboratory of the Massachusetts General Hospital.

20. Haight, B.F., D.H. Kelly, and K. McCabe. 1982. *A Manual for Home Monitoring.* Boston: Pediatric Pulmonary Laboratory of the Massachusetts General Hospital and National Sudden Infant Death Syndrome Foundation.

21. Kalis, B.L. 1970. "Crisis theory: Its relevance for community psychology and direction for development." In *Community Psychology and Mental Health,* ed. D. Adelson and B.L. Kalis. Scranton, Pa.: Chandler.

22. Caplan, G. 1964. *Principles of Preventive Psychiatry.* New York: Basic Books, Inc.

23. Lindemann, E. 1944. Symptomatology and management of acute grief. *Am J Psychiatry* 201:144–148.

24. Cobb, S. 1976. Social support as a moderator of life stress. *Psychosom Med* 38:300–314.

25. Spitzer, A., and W. Fox. 1984. Infant apnea—an approach to management. *Clin Pediatr* 23(7):374–380.

26. Keens, T.G., P.C. Dennies, C.D. Low, and A.C. Platzker. 1982. Risk of subsequent apnea in infants surviving near miss sudden infant death syndrome. *Clin Res* 30:151A.

27. Walsh, J.K., O.D. Farrell, W.J. Keenan, M. Lucas, and M. Kramer. 1981. Gastroesophageal reflux in infants: Relations to apnea. *J Pediatr* 99:197–201.

28. Smialek, Z. 1978. Observations on immediate reactions of families to sudden infant death. *Pediatrics* 62:160–165.

29. Mandell, F., and L.C. Wolfe. 1975. Sudden infant death syndrome and subsequent pregnancy. *Pediatrics* 56:774–776.

30. Krous, H.F., and D. Bendell. 1982. What to do about the infant with apnea. *Journal of the Oklahoma State Medical Association* 75:77–78.

31. Minuchin, S. 1974. *Families and Family Therapy.* Cambridge, Mass.: Harvard University Press.

32. Venters, M. 1981. Familial coping with chronic and severe childhood illness: The case of cystic fibrosis. *Social Sciences Medicine* (A) 15:289–297.

33. Winnicott, D.W. 1965. *The Family and Individual Development.* London: Tavistock Publications.

34. Bing Hall, J. 1980. Symptom bearer as a marital distance regulator. *Family Process* 19:355–367.

35. Deykin, E., M. Bauman, D.H. Kelly, M.S. Chungcheng Hsieh, and D.C.

Shannon. 1984. Apnea of infancy and subsequent neurologic, cognitive and behavioral status. *Pediatrics* 73(5):638–645.

36. Southall, D.P. 1983. Home monitoring and its role in the sudden infant death syndrome. *Pediatrics* 72(1):133–137.
37. Umana, R., S. Gross, and M. McConville. 1980. *Crisis in the Family.* New York: Gardner Press.

11

The Apneic Infant: Longitudinal Development

TERRI L. SHELTON, Ph.D. and R. DEBRA BENDELL, Ph.D.

Prolonged, interrupted, infantile apnea initially was viewed as solely a medical problem, but it is now obvious that the effects of apnea extend into areas other than the infant's health. This chapter reviews the available research on the longitudinal cognitive and neurologic development, personality characteristics, and the risk of vulnerability of the apneic infant. Implications for future research are suggested, as well.

Cognitive and Neurologic Status of the Apneic Infant

It has been well documented that anoxia may have adverse effects on the central nervous system and, consequently, on cognitive functioning. Researchers have hypothesized that infants with apnea may experience hypoxic episodes and thus be at risk for cognitive/neurologic deficits. The developmental functioning of apneic children during infancy, preschool, and school-age years has been examined by numerous investigators.

Developmental Functioning during Infancy

Black, Steinschneider, and Sheehe [1] conducted one of the first studies to examine the relationship between neonatal sleep respiratory instability and infant development. Of the 122 infants evaluated in their study, 28 subsequently were placed on home monitors. Approximately 90 percent of these infants were evaluated at seven to eleven months of age (range six to fourteen months) using the Bayley Scales of Infant Development [2]. Among the total sample, infants with high PSA_4 values (i.e., greater respiratory instability) demonstrated significantly poorer mental and psychomotor development during infancy. However, none of the infants demonstrated evidence of serious retardation. When the development of the twenty-eight monitored infants was compared to that of infants not monitored, apneic infants scored higher, on the average, in both mental and psychomotor development although these differences were not statistically significant.

As part of the Sudden Infant Death Research Project at Stanford University, Korobkin and Guilleminault [3] completed neurologic examinations adapted from Amiel-Tison [4] on forty-one near miss infants, seven asymptomatic siblings of SIDS infants, and twenty-one asymptomatic control infants. The infants were examined at various ages, ranging from two weeks to two years of age. Of the thirty-three evaluations of control infants, 94 percent were normal evaluations, whereas of the seventy-six examinations of the near miss group, only 37 percent of the evaluations were normal. (Although a large difference, it is not clear from the article if this difference was statistically significant.) The difficulties of the near miss infants under three months of age were characterized most often by consistent abnormalities of muscle tone, particularly shoulder hypotonia. Many of these problems seemed to resolve with age. Of those near miss infants examined for the first time at more than three months of age, 76 percent were normal. Those having difficulties tended to have problems such as asymmetry of tone, increased adductor tone, or overall developmental delay. Of the nineteen near miss infants who were followed longitudinally, only 58 percent had no developmental delay, with the remaining infants having some type of spasticity, asymmetry of tone, or developmental or language delay. Of the seven siblings of SIDS victims examined between two and sixteen weeks of age (one infant was examined at six months), five or 71 percent had neurologic abnormalities when first examined (e.g., ataxia, developmental delay, hypotonia). The authors speculated that both the hypotonia and the apneic event may be expressions of intrinsic CNS abnormalities; however, another subpopulation of apneic infants may manifest difficulties as a direct result of the apneic episodes. Unfortunately, the scope of this study did not allow the identification of these two subgroups or denote whether the difficulties were associated with severity and/or frequency of apneic episodes.

Preschool and School Age Functioning

A recent longitudinal investigation examining the cognitive and neurologic development of infants with apnea was published by Deykin et al. [5]. This pilot study examined fourteen formerly apneic, home-monitored children, fourteen age-similar siblings, and seven age/sex matched playmates. The children ranged in age from three to six years at the time of the evaluation. Assessment of neurologic status was performed by a pediatric neurologist who evaluated fine and gross motor skills and the establishment of hemispheric dominance, according to a format proposed by Denckla [6], as well as "nonverbal perceptive-expressive abilities" as measured by the Goodenough Draw-a-Person test [7]. Cognitive abilities were assessed using the Peabody Picture Vocabulary Test (PPVT). Behavioral adjustment also was evaluated, and these results are presented later in this chapter.

Comparisons between apneic children and playmates yielded no significant differences with respect to neurologic competence. This was true of the comparisons between apneic children and their siblings with the exception of gross motor skills. When sex, one-minute Apgar scores, birth weight, and medical condition during the first week of life were controlled, subjects with apnea demonstrated a significantly greater risk of gross motor impairment than their siblings. Results from performance on the PPVT indicated that the mean score for the apneic children was lower than that of their siblings (mean = 114.1) or that of the playmates (mean = 105.7) although neither difference was statistically significant. The average paired differences in PPVT scores between apneic children and siblings and between apneic children and playmates were −4.7 and −3.9 points, respectively. Data on the frequency and severity of apneic episodes abstracted from Pediatric Pulmonary Laboratory Charts and from log sheets kept by the families indicated that there was no consistent relationship between the total burden of apnea experienced and developmental deficits.

Wasserman also examined parental perceptions of the developmental status of their formerly apneic children through psychiatric interviews [8]. At the time the target children were to enter kindergarten or first grade, nine of the thirteen children were described as having gross and fine motor problems, decreased attention span, hyperactivity, poor coordination, speech problems, poor balance, and developmental delays. Although the author did not indicate whether or not the relationship between the severity of the apnea and developmental deficits was significant, Wasserman did note that five of these nine children experienced initial apnea episodes severe enough to require resuscitation.

An examination of these studies suggests that the cognitive/neurologic sequelae of infant apnea are unclear. Variations in subject samples, assessment instruments, and the severity of apnea render conclusions across studies tenuous. Nevertheless, with these cautions in mind, one fairly consistent finding was the identification of some type of deficit in motor skills [3, 5, 8]. Other than this finding, the available data suggest that apneic infants as a group generally are not significantly different from other control groups (e.g., playmates, siblings) with respect to cognitive/neurologic abilities. However, an examination of individual cases longitudinally indicates that some children do experience deficits that may not be identifiable early in infancy. Given the well-documented limited predictive validity of infant assessments, it may be that early evaluations at the time of or shortly after discontinuing monitoring are insufficient to answer the questions regarding the ramifications of infantile apnea. As was suggested by the Wasserman study findings [8], some percentage of apneic infants might reflect "soft" neurologic signs and/or learning disabilities later in childhood.

The relationship between the severity of the apnea and later deficits is unclear, as well. Part of the confusion can be attributed to the fact that not all of the early investigations controlled for the variations in the severity of the child's apnea. However, as research in this area becomes more refined, conclusions about the relationship between these variables should be forthcoming.

Finally, if developmental delays are found to be associated with prolonged infantile apnea, the question remains as to the etiology of these deficits. As Korobkin and Guilleminault speculate, in some populations, the delay and the apnea may be expressions of intrinsic CNS abnormalities, whereas in others, the delay may be a function of the apnea itself [3]. In addition, deficits may be a function of maladaptive interaction patterns that result from the early identification of a child as "at risk" [9]. It is important that future investigations attempt to address not only the possible relationship between apnea and development but, if a relationship is found, the etiology of deficits, as well.

Personality and Behavioral Characteristics

A few studies focused on the behavioral characteristics of infants with apnea in the hopes of elucidating differences between apneic and nonapneic populations and/or similarities between SIDS infants and those with prolonged apnea. These studies examined areas such as the characteristics of the infant's cry, the child's temperament, and, to a lesser degree, parental perceptions of the child.

Infant Cry

Perhaps part of the impetus for examining the apneic infant's cry stems from several studies indicating that cries of longer duration and/or abnormal cries are characteristic of neurologically impaired infants [10, 11]. Because some researchers hypothesized a link between apnea and neurologic immaturity and/or SIDS, these studies, as well as those identifying the abnormal cry characteristics of infants who died of SIDS, led a few investigators to examine the characteristics of the cry of the infant with apnea [12–15].

In 1979, Felman et al. used fluoroscopic techniques to examine the relationship between cry patterns and apnea [16]. In their sample of nine infants who exhibited sleep-related upper airway obstruction but were asymptomatic when awake, a particular constriction of the nasopharynx was identified with a corresponding characteristic cry. These results were similar to a cry pattern identified in SIDS and apneic infants by Golub and Corwin [17]. These authors postulated that the infant's cry is a reflection of complex neurophysiologic functions. Thus, analysis of the cry could be used as a diagnostic tool to assess the infant's status. Of the eighty-seven infants examined in their prospective investigation, two infants subsequently died of SIDS, and prolonged infantile apnea was diagnosed in one. This apneic infant was monitored because apnea had been diagnosed in the child's sibling. The computer analysis of the acoustic properties of this group demonstrated significant constriction in the vocal tract consistent with the results reported by Felman et al. [16]. Unfortunately, these studies involved too few subjects, and analysis of the infants' cries has not proven to be a definitive diagnostic tool for differentiating apneic infants from asymptomatic controls.

Temperament

Temperament has been described as an individual's behavioral style. In other words, rather than focusing on what an individual does or why, temperament refers to how an individual responds to the environment. The systematic study of temperament dates back to 1956 when Thomas, Chess, and Birch began the New York Longitudinal Study [18]. The results of this and many other investigations indicated that temperament is a function of both genetic and environmental variables and is an important aspect of an individual's development. As such, the study of temperament in apneic infants has been an important area of research from a physiologic/genetic standpoint as well as from the interactional point of view.

Although Naeye et al. examined parental retrospective observations of SIDS infants and not apneic infants per se, their study served as an impetus for many studies examining temperament characteristics in apneic populations [14]. In that investigation, parents retrospectively rated their infants who had died of SIDS as being less physically active, more breathless and exhausted during feeding, and having less intense reactions to environmental stimuli and more abnormal cries than their siblings. Similar findings were reported from two prospective, longitudinal studies examining temperament in infants who were monitored for apnea. Bendell and McCaffree et al. reported that parents rated apneic infants as more passive in temperament than either their siblings [19] or age/sex-matched controls [20].

Weissbluth et al. extended these studies by not only comparing the temperament characteristics of near miss SIDS infants, asymptomatic siblings of SIDS victims, and normal infants but also examining the relationship between temperament and sleep characteristics in these groups [21]. Twenty asymptomatic infants, eleven symptomatic siblings of SIDS infants, and fifteen infants that had experienced at least one episode of sleep apnea served as subjects. Parents were asked to rate these children on the Infant Temperament Questionnaire [22]. Sleep-related abnormalities and sleep duration also were recorded. No significant group differences were observed on the basis of temperament characteristics. However, the near miss SIDS infants slept less than the other groups. In addition, low activity and low intensity response ratings were correlated significantly with increased apnea and frequency of periodic breathing during sleep among the near miss group. Furthermore, these infants were rated as less sensitive to external stimulation when awake. The authors concluded that the results suggest a relationship between respiratory dysrhythmia during sleep, infant temperament, and sleep duration but with no significant group differences identified.

In 1982, Weissbluth proposed an interesting model for examining the interrelationships among congenital temperament factors, the severity of respiratory control deficits, and progesterone levels [23]. He cited several studies [21, 24, 25] associating not only passivity and high sensory threshold characteristics with sleep dysrhythmia but also infantile colic, difficult temperament pattern (e.g., negative mood, high activity, low rhythmicity), and low sensory thresholds with frequent night awakenings. An examination of these relationships as well as the relationships between progesterone levels and sleep characteristics resulted in the following hypothesis.

In general, plasma progesterone levels rise in response to sleep-related respiratory control deficits. However, in several affected infants, elevated progesterone levels may lead to CNS depression and blunted arousals for sleep. In these children there may be accompanying behavioral changes interacting with congenital temperament characteristics resulting in low activity, low intensity, high sensory thresholds, and the disappearance or absence of colic. Thus, a child with respiratory deficits, atypical progesterone levels, and temperament characteristics of passivity, low intensity, and high sensory thresholds might be at higher risk for death due to SIDS [23]. This hypothesis is consistent with the findings of several studies (e.g., Naeye et al. [14]) associating infants dying of SIDS with temperament characteristics of passivity and lower intensity. However, variations in any one of these variables (e.g., increased activity, increased intensity, lower sensory threshold) might reduce the risk of a death due to SIDS and result in an apneic, near miss event instead. The hypothesized relationships among these variables are depicted in Figure 11.1. This hypothesis would provide a partial explanation for the relationship between infantile apnea and the results of temperament studies. It also suggests a strong relationship between apnea and SIDS that has yet to be proven.

In conclusion, it appears that although studies have indicated that infants dying of SIDS may have a characteristic temperament style, this may not be the case for apneic infants as a group. Rather, there appear to be individual differences that are related to the infant's respiratory and/or sleep difficulties. This individual difference factor and the resultant interaction between temperament and environment has not been addressed specifically in the apneic population. However, other studies examining these variables in "high risk" populations may shed light on the interaction of these variables within apneic infants.

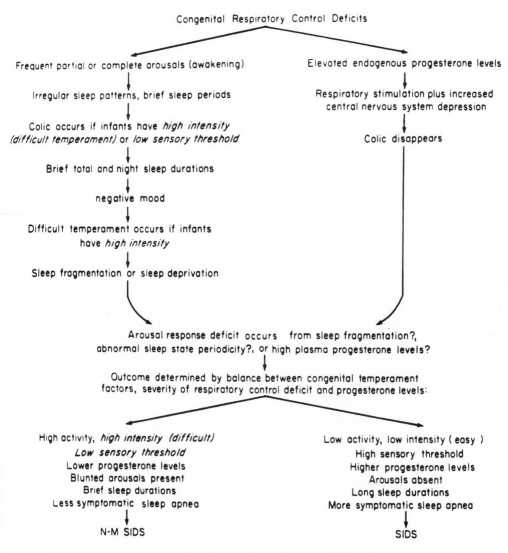

FIGURE 11.1 Progesterone, Sleep Apnea, Sleep Patterns, and Infant Temperament

More specifically, Field [26, 27] and Goldberg, Brachfeld, and DiVitto [28] demonstrated that middle income mothers of preterm infants were extremely active and controlling within the dyadic interaction. In turn, their infants were verbally inactive and gaze averting during these early interactions. It is unclear whether the mothers' behaviors were a reaction to their infants' inactivity or whether the infants' behaviors were attempts to modify the overstimulation from the mother. Nevertheless, this type of interaction pattern set a precedent for later contacts between these parents and their children. In a five-year follow up of these mother-infant dyads, Field suggested that mothers who were overactive during early face-to-face interactions were also overprotective and overcontrolling during later interactions with their children [26, 27]. Similar findings have been reported with other "special" populations (e.g., infants with Down's syndrome [29], hearing impairment [30], or cerebral palsy [31]), suggesting that apneic infants and mothers are at risk for similarly disturbed dyadic interactions. This would be particularly true of those infants rated as more passive and nonresponsive by their parents. Although no current research is available on interaction patterns between mothers/fathers and their apneic infants, a few studies have examined other parental perceptions of infants with prolonged apnea.

Parental Perceptions

In their longitudinal investigation, Deykin et al. evaluated the behavioral status of formerly apneic infants [5]. Using the Behavioral Screening Questionnaire (BSQ), they identified only three of the formerly apneic children as having emotional difficulties. Apneic subjects received slightly lower scores (e.g., fewer behavioral difficulties) than did playmates. However, they received marginally higher BSQ scores than siblings. There were no overall group differences that were significant in this study, but two other investigations provided support that some parents of apneic infants and formerly apneic children perceive these children as somewhat different from others [8, 19].

Bendell, in a study of thirty-eight apneic infants, reported that parents rated these children as more vulnerable [19]. Infants who were considered close to death during the initial apneic episode (e.g., requiring CPR), were perceived by parents as being more difficult to care for. Similarly, Wasserman examined the effects of monitoring on the apneic child by means of longitudinal psychiatric interviews with the parents [8]. At the first follow-up interview (mean of twenty-one months post monitor discontinuation), 50 percent of the children were characterized as "spoiled" by the parents. Like the results of the Bendell study, these children were viewed as special or vulnerable "because they almost died"—even two years after the monitor had been discontinued.

Vulnerability

The available literature on the "vulnerable infant" suggests that the apneic infant is at risk for being perceived as vulnerable by caretakers. The "vulnerable infant" was defined by Green and Solnit as an infant who was expected to die either from real or imagined conditions or illness [32]. This definition is consistent with the circumstances surrounding the diagnosis of prolonged apnea. Although a biologic, one-to-one relationship between SIDS and apnea has not been proven, for the majority of parents, the initial apneic event is equated with near death. Furthermore, research suggests that the initial apneic episode has long-lasting import. The severity of the initial clinical episode has been found to be related to parental stress and the quality of family functioning some six months later [20, 33]. In addition, the coping mechanisms required to stimulate breathing (e.g., ranging from gentle stimulation to CPR), the time elapsed before obtaining medical services, and whether the mother was isolated at the time of the initial incident impact further upon subsequent perceptions of the apneic infant's vulnerability.

Although all infants with apnea are at some risk for being perceived as vulnerable, the vulnerability is most apparent when the apneic infant is also a subsequent sibling of an infant who died of SIDS. Legg and Sherick noted that parents often attempt to assuage the pain and suffering attendant to the loss of a child by quickly conceiving another child [9]. However, literature indicates that an appropriate lapse of time between the SIDS death and birth of the new infant is of utmost importance [9, 34, 35]. The new infant's entry into the family may interrupt, distort, or delay the mourning process, but the infant cannot resolve the grief associated with loss of the SIDS infant. Not only may the birth of an infant disrupt the grieving process, but inadequate time for mourning also may interfere with parental attachment to the new infant and a realistic view of this subsequent child as an individual [36]. Bergman noted that following loss of an infant to SIDS, parents often respond to the new baby with constant "surveillance" [37]. The disruption of the parent–child relationship is accentuated when the "replacement" child is further differentiated as having prolonged apnea. Although it is unclear whether parental perceptions of their child's vulnerability impact on the child's cognitive and behavioral development, one study described the disruptive interactive effect of the loss of an infant to SIDS and the birth of a subsequent infant in whom apnea is diagnosed. Bendell et al. described the adjustment difficulties of a mother of an apneic infant [38]. Prior to the birth of this child, the mother had lost two infants to SIDS. When medical evaluations indicated the necessity of placing the infant on a home monitor following a severe, initial hypoxic event, the mother's resultant anxiety was so great that it interfered with her successful completion of CPR training. The mother refused to practice CPR on a "Resusci-Annie" doll because the doll's face reminded her of her "dead children's faces." Only with behavior therapy techniques such as systematic desensitization and flooding was the mother able to assume the care of her apneic infant at home. Home monitoring should be discontinued once medical criteria for termination have been met. However, Purchit, Ford, and Saylor [39] documented a population who delayed discontinuing monitoring once a medical decision was made. In this population, delayed discontinuation of monitoring appeared related to higher maternal anxiety and past experience with a SIDS death.

Finally, the issue of vulnerability affects not only parental perceptions of the child but also the child's reactions and perceptions. Particularly in the case of a subsequent sibling of a SIDS infant, the profound effect of guilt that may stem from being a "replacement" child must not be discounted. In other words, the child may feel that a predecessor had to die in order for him or her to live. Although cognitively the child may recognize a lack of responsibility for the older sibling's death, it must be recognized that the "psychology of survivorship" may be evident. A child's identification with the SIDS infant is further intensified by a diagnosis of prolonged infantile apnea. Furthermore, as Legg and Sherick postulate, the experience of integration into a grieving family and the assumption of a prefabricated identity may represent a massive insult to early developmental processes [9].

As with the areas of cognitive development and temperament, it is difficult to evaluate fully the ultimate impact of apnea and monitoring on the target children and their resulting relationships with family members without further longitudinal studies. However, the available literature suggests that these children are at risk for being viewed as vulnerable some two years after the monitor has been discontinued. Because vulnerable infants have a narrower range of resources available, further investigations are needed to assess the potential impact on development and, more important, the factors that mitigate the perception of vulnerability.

Implications for Future Research

It appears that with growing attention to early hospital discharge and home care maintenance, monitoring will be increasing. In addition, with greater public education regarding infantile apnea, the diagnosis of prolonged infantile apnea is likely to increase. Continued evaluations of the ramifications of prolonged apnea itself as well as the impact of monitoring are necessary not only to provide information and support to the families but also to allow informed decisions as to the advantages and disadvantages of this treatment regimen. The previously reviewed literature suggests certain trends for future research in terms of methodologic considerations and the specific emphases of such research.

Methodologic Considerations

The variability of instruments and subject characteristics makes comparisons across studies quite difficult. This criticism is valid for many areas of research; nevertheless, the replication of existing studies using similar assessment batteries and subject characteristics would facilitate greatly the understanding of the apneic population and the ramifications of prolonged infantile apnea.

Of particular importance in future investigations is attention to the severity and frequency of apneic events and the length of monitoring, and the subsequent relationship of these variables to cognitive/neurologic deficits, personality characteristics, and parental perceptions. When reported in the past, this information was obtained primarily through initial medical evaluations, periodic diagnostic tests, and parent reports of alarms. While variability in parent reports certainly introduces additional error variance into statistical analyses, use of this information has been beneficial. Nevertheless, other means of obtaining these data, such as the use of trend event recorders, are needed in order to obtain more objective records of the child's apneic episodes during the monitoring period. Parent records are beneficial, particularly when examining their perceptions of the infant, but a more objective means of obtaining information about the child's history of apnea should be used whenever possible.

Typically, previous investigations have used control groups such as asymptomatic siblings or other infants without respiratory or neurologic abnormalities (e.g., playmates). These control groups have been useful in answering some questions, but other populations (e.g., high risk infants, infants with cardiac problems) may be more appropriate comparison groups when evaluating the vulnerability of apneic children or attempting to examine the reason for observed neurologic/cognitive deficits (e.g., whether deficits are the result of hypoxic episodes or lack of developmental opportunities from parental overprotection). Although these "between group" designs are needed, additional information may be obtained only through "within group" designs. For example, it would be of interest to compare those apneic infants or formerly apneic children perceived as vulnerable with those who are not perceived in this way in order to identify personality, developmental, and/or family variables that differentiate these groups. Information obtained from such studies would be particularly useful when attempting to provide more individually tailored support to these families.

Obviously needed are more longitudinal and cross-lag designs. Given the limited predictive validity of infant assessment, developmental evaluations in later childhood are necessary to evaluate fully the sequelae of prolonged apnea. Whereas it is not unexpected for parents to perceive apneic children as "at risk" at the time of monitoring or shortly thereafter, it is of greater interest to examine whether these perceptions persist long after the monitoring is discontinued. These questions can be answered only through longitudinal evaluations.

It has been appropriate to examine unitary relationships such as those between apnea and cognitive deficits or apnea and temperament characteristics, but future research must determine whether more complicated patterns of relationships exist through the use of multivariate statistics and the examination of the interaction of variables. The severity of apneic events may be related significantly to later developmental delays, but parent perceptions of vulnerability and the child's temperament characteristics also provide useful predictive information about this population.

New Directions

Previous research has focused primarily on examining the sequelae of infantile apnea as related to either cognitive/neurologic development or temperament characteristics. More studies are needed to examine parental perceptions of the apneic infant, the quality of the parent-child interaction, and the effects of prolonged apnea and monitoring on the interactional system. In addition, although a few studies have investigated the impact of a SIDS death on siblings, there is little information regarding the adjustment of siblings of apneic children. Information in these areas is needed if professionals are to provide anticipatory guidance as well as identify those children and families who need additional assistance in order to cope more effectively. Infantile apnea is viewed as a temporary medical problem, but inadequate preparation of the family and inattention to the impact of apnea on the monitored child's development may result in long-lasting, negative effects beyond the monitoring period.

Many children are monitored as a function of an initial episode of prolonged apnea, but infants are monitored for other reasons as well (e.g., being a sibling of a SIDS infant, having apnea of prematurity or respiratory diseases, parental anxiety). Results from one study indicate that parental perceptions and subsequent interactions with the monitored infant vary as a function of the initial reason for monitoring [40]. The etiology of the apnea and the reason for monitoring may prove to be an important variable in the study of this population.

Finally, although an inspection of the available literature indicates some identifiable group differences between apneic and non-apneic populations (e.g., gross motor delay), some studies reported nonsignificant group differences. In a few of these studies, significant and important individual differences were identified [1, 21]. It may prove informative for future investigators to examine data not only along group dimensions but also by means of an individual differences model. This approach may not only incorporate new variables (such as the reason for monitoring) along with previously examined variables (e.g., developmental status, severity of apnea, and temperament characteristics), but also may clarify the psychosocial sequelae of prolonged infantile apnea and the directions needed for intervention.

References

1. Black, L., A. Steinschneider, and P. Sheehe. 1979. Neonatal respiratory instability and infant development. *Child Dev* 50:561–564.

2. Bayley, N. 1969. *Manual for the Bayley Scales of Infant Development*. New York: Psychological Corporation.

3. Korobkin, R., and C. Guilleminault. 1979. Neurologic abnormalities in near miss for sudden infant death syndrome infants. *Pediatrics* 64(3):369–374.

4. Amiel-Tison, C. 1976. A method for neurological evaluation within the first year of life. *Curr Prob Pediatr* 7:1–50.

5. Deykin, E., M.L. Bauman, D.H. Kelly, C-C. Hsieh, and D. Shannon. 1984. Apnea of infancy and subsequent neurologic, cognitive, and behavioral status. *Pediatrics* 73(5):638–644.

6. Denckla, M.B. 1974. Development of motor coordination in normal children. *Dev Med Child Neurol* 16:729–741.

7. Goodenough, F.L. 1926. *The Measurement of Intelligence by Drawing*. Yonkers-Hudson, N. Y.: World Book Company.

8. Wasserman, A.L. 1984. A prospective study of the impact of home monitoring on the family. *Pediatrics* 74(3):323–329.

9. Legg, C., and I. Sherick. 1976. The replacement child—a developmental tragedy. *Child Psychiatry Hum Dev* 7(2):113–126.

10. Ostwald, P.F., T. Phibbs, and S. Fox. 1968. Diagnostic use of infant cry. *Biologia Neonatology* 13:68–82.

11. Prechtl, H.F., K. Theorel, A. Gramsbergen, and J. Lind. 1969. A statistical analysis of cry patterns in normal and abnormal newborn infants. *Dev Med Child Neurol* 11:142–152.

12. Colton, R.H., and A. Steinschneider. 1980. "Acoustic characteristics of first week infant cries: Some relationships to the sudden infant death syndrome." In *Infant communication, cry, and early speech,* ed. T. Murry and J. Murry. Houston, Tex.: College Hill Press.

13. Colton, R.H., and A. Steinschneider. 1981. The cry characteristics of an infant who died of the sudden infant death syndrome. *J Speech Hear Disord* 46:359–363.

14. Naeye, R.L., J. Messmer, T. Specht, and T. A. Merritt. 1976. Sudden infant death syndrome temperament before death. *J Pediatr* 88(3):511–515.

15. Stark, R.E., and S.N. Nathanson. 1972. "Unusual features of cry in an infant dying suddenly and unexpectedly." In *Development of upper respiratory anatomy and function: Implication for SIDS,* ed. J.F. Bosma and J. Showacre. Washington, D.C.: U.S. Department of Health, Education, and Welfare.

16. Felman, A. H., G. M. Laughlin, and C. A. Leftridge. 1979. Upper airway obstruction during sleep in children. *AJR* 133:213.

17. Golub, H.L., and M.J. Corwin. 1982. Infant cry: A clue to diagnosis. *Pediatrics* 69(2):197–201.

18. Thomas, A., S. Chess, and H.G. Birch. 1968. *Temperament and behavior disorders in children*. New York: New York University Press.

19. Bendell, D. 1982. The impact of the apnea monitor on parents. Paper presented at SIDS Day, University of Oklahoma Health Sciences Center, Oklahoma City, Okla.

20. McCaffree, M.A., D. Bendell, T.L. Shelton, and C. Mattice. 1983. Longitudinal familial adjustment to infants with interrupted infantile apnea. (abstract) *Clin Res* 17(4):Part 2:100.

21. Weissbluth, M., R.T. Brouillette, K. Liu, and C.E. Hunt. 1982. Sleep apnea,

sleep duration, and infant temperament. *J Pediatr* 101(2):307–310.

22. Carey, W.B., and S.C. McDevitt. 1978. Revision of the Infant Temperament Questionnaire. *Pediatrics* 61:735–739.

23. Weissbluth, M. 1982. Plasma progesterone levels, infant temperament, arousals from sleep, and the Sudden Infant Death Syndrome. *Medical Hypotheses* 9:215–222.

24. Carey, W.B. 1972. Clinical applications of infant temperament measurements. *J Pediatr* 81:823–828.

25. Carey, W.B. 1974. Night waking and temperament in infancy. *J Pediatr* 84:756–758.

26. Field, T. 1977. Effects of early separation, interactive deficits, and experimental manipulations on infant–mother face-to-face interactions. *Child Dev* 48:763–771.

27. Field, T. 1983. "Social interactions between infants and adults." In *Advances in Clinical Child Psychology*, ed. B. Lahey and A. Kazdin. New York: Plenum Press.

28. Goldberg, S., S. Brachfeld, and B. DiVitto. 1980. "Feeding, fussing, and playing with parent-infant interaction in the first year as a function of prematurity and perinatal problems." In *High risk infants and children: Adult and peer interactions,* ed. T. Field, S. Goldberg, D. Stern, and A. Sostek. New York: Academic Press.

29. Jones, O. 1980. Mother–child communication in very young Down's syndrome and normal children. In *High risk infants and children: Adult and peer interactions,* ed. T. Field, S. Goldberg, D. Stern, and A. Sostek. New York: Academic Press.

30. Wedell-Monig, J., and J. Lumley. 1980. Child deafness and mother–child interaction. *Child Dev* 51:766–774.

31. Kogan, K. 1980. Interaction systems between preschool aged, handicapped or developmentally delayed children and their parents. In *High risk infants: Adult and peer interactions,* ed. T. Field, S. Goldberg, D. Stern, and A. Sostek. New York: Academic Press.

32. Green, M., and A. Solnit. 1964. Reactions to the threatened loss of a child: A vulnerable child syndrome. Pediatric management of the dying child. Part III. *Pediatrics* 34(1):58–66.

33. Cain, L.P., D.H. Kelly, and D.C. Shannon. 1980. Parents' perception of the psychological and social impact of home monitoring. *Pediatrics* 66:37–41.

34. Cain, A.C., and B. Cain. 1964. On replacing a child. *J Am Child Psychiatry* 3:443–456.

35. Poznanski, E.D. 1972. "The replacement child." A saga of unresolved parental grief. *J Pediatr* 81(6):1190–1193.

36. Berezin, N. 1982. *After a pregnancy fails: Help for families affected by a miscarriage, a still birth or the loss of a newborn.* New York: Simon and Shuster.

37. Bergman, A. 1972. Sudden infant death. *Nursing Outlook* 20(12):775–778.

38. Bendell, B., T.L. Shelton, H. Krous, and M. Shirley. 1984. Behavioral treatment of CPR anxiety: A case study. *Children's Health Care* 13(2):77–81.

39. Purchit, D.F.M., and C. Saylor. 1986. Maternal delay in discontinuation of

home monitors. Paper presented at the Fourth Conference on Infantile Apnea and Home Monitoring. Rancho Mirage, Calif.

40. Shelton, T.L., and D. Bamrick-Konarske. 1985. Parental evaluation of support services and familial adjustment to monitoring. Paper presented at the Third Conference on Infantile Apnea and Home Monitoring: Managing Apnea from Prematurity to Puberty, Rancho Mirage, Calif.

12

The Parents of SIDS Victims Fight Back: The Story of the National SIDS Foundation

ABRAHAM B. BERGMAN, M.D.

Several days before I began studying at Western Reserve University Medical School in 1954, I attended a talk sponsored by a medical fraternity seeking to attract new members. The talk, presented by the colorful and brilliant Cleveland forensic pathologist, Lester Adelson, was about a mysterious entity called "crib death." It was the first and last time I heard of crib death throughout my medical school and pediatric residency training. I vaguely recall during my residency being called to the emergency room to lay my stethoscope on the chests of several lifeless infants who had been rushed to the hospital in order to fulfill the legal requirement of pronouncing them dead. I do not recall their faces or names, however, because I had no involvement with the infants or their families. They were, after all, not my patients. I had no idea what happened to the dead bodies, let alone to the grieving parents. They were not my responsibility.

It was a full ten years later when I again heard about crib death, this time in a lecture by my friend and colleague, J. Bruce Beckwith, pathologist at Children's Orthopedic Hospital and Medical Center in Seattle. I then learned who was taking responsibility for the dead bodies and grieving parents. Nobody! My lack of knowledge about crib death was typical for physicians of my generation. It wasn't written about in pediatric textbooks or talked about in hospital conferences.

Why the "knowledge black-out" about sudden infant death syndrome (SIDS), as it later came to be known, among health professionals? Certainly not because of any conspiracy of silence. The reason is that SIDS victims were not seen in doctors' offices or hospitals. If they came to hospitals at all, it was only to an emergency room to be pronounced dead, and thence to the morgue. Thus the individual clinician would have little occasion to come in contact with SIDS. Those who were very much aware of SIDS were coroners, medical examiners, and morticians. These individuals, however, tended to have little interaction with physicians practicing clinical medicine, and virtually no influence on medical education.

For similar reasons, organized research on infants dying suddenly and unexpectedly was virtually nonexistent. An investigator usually is stimulated to embark on a research path when his curiosity is piqued by a perplexing clinical problem with which he comes in contact. Individuals who perform scientific research, however, usually inhabit teaching hospitals or research institutes. Therefore, capable research scientists didn't even know of the existence of SIDS. The miniscule amount of research work that was conducted on crib death took place in understaffed and underfunded county morgues. Tribute must be paid to pioneers such as Jacob Werne and Irene Garrow, of New York, Clara Raven, of Detroit, and Lester Adelson for dispelling the centuries-held belief that crib death was the result of mechanical suffocation. These pathologists carried out their studies without research grants amidst heavy volumes of service work.

In 1958, only a handful of pathologists were interested in the problem of sudden, unexpected infant death; there was no organized research effort and no prospect of same was in sight. Although these pathologists were aware that crib death was a large problem, they had no idea of its prevalence. They also did not know whether infants dying suddenly and unexpectedly were succumbing to a single, unknown disease entity, or coincidently to a variety of known diseases. If these pathologists knew so little about crib death, obviously the state of knowledge among the general medical community was less, and among the lay public, totally absent.

Picture the agony of parents losing a child to crib death. No one could tell them why their baby had died, and there was no organized research trying to find answers. This appalling state of ignorance would still be with us today were it not for the efforts of a small group of aggrieved parents who were unwilling to accept the status quo. These parents and their allies succeeded in raising the consciousness of the medical establishment as well as federal, state, and local government agencies to address the problem of sudden infant death syndrome.

Death of Mark Addison Roe

In 1958, Mark Addison Roe died in Greenwich, Connecticut. It was on an October morning that the six-month-old boy was found dead in his crib. At the insistence of his pediatrician, an autopsy was performed. Cause of death: acute bronchial pneumonia. Case closed. However, for Mark's parents the case was only beginning. Jed and Louise Roe had no reason to expect the tragedy to occur as they settled into a life of privilege in the summer of 1958. Jed worked in an investment house in New York City, and Louise spent her days tending their two sons in the affluent Connecticut suburb. Everything was just as they had hoped it would be.

Two weeks before his death, Mark had been pronounced normal by his pediatrician on a well-baby check up. He had been a full-term baby and received the best of care. There was no indication of future "problems." Why, then, did he die?

It was this question that occupied the Roes for the next three years. For Louise, there was also the fear that Mark would be a small memory to her, alone. For Jed, there was the desire to try to prevent other deaths such as Mark's. The first few months after Mark's death were spent trying to sort out the isolation and guilt. It was all so inexplicable and no one could even begin to give them an answer. What had they done wrong?

During these months, they began to hear of others who had lost babies in the same mysterious way. Friends and acquaintances told them of their own losses, newspaper obituaries listed case after case of infants found dead in their cribs. Slowly, the isolation lifted and the sense that Mark's death was not a solitary incident led Jed to begin the search for a foundation or a research project to which he might contribute a substantial insurance policy given to Mark by his grandfather at birth. He was persistent, and not dissuaded by the often-barbed suggestions of some physicians that laymen should not meddle in scientific matters.

By early 1962, Jed's quest had led him to every physician who had done any scientific research into sudden, unexpected infant deaths. They were few, they were scattered, and there were but a few minor facts on which they all agreed. But he did not find any foundation or project in which he and Louise could participate or establish a memorial to Mark. He then began to investigate the possibilities of forming a foundation himself, one that would serve as a clearinghouse for physicians and families, and organize and support research.

At the same time, a comprehensive epidemiologic study on crib death was being carried out in the office of Dr. Milton Helpern, chief medical examiner of New York City. Under the direction of Dr. Renate Dische, the investigators hoped to investigate every case of sudden, unexpected, and unexplained infant death occurring in New York City with home visits, parent–physician interviews, and thorough postmortem examinations. After talking to Dr. Dische, Jed was convinced of the importance of his "cause" as well as the necessity of forming a foundation to further research and understanding.

In August of 1962, the Mark Addison Roe Foundation was incorporated in the state of Connecticut. Its trustees were Jed and Louise, Dr. Dische, Mark Roe's pediatrician, Dr. J. Frederick Lee, and a young Greenwich attorney, Lowell Weicker, Jr., a close friend of the Roes, who is now a U.S. senator. Doctors Rustin McIntosh and William Silverman of Columbia University were its medical advisors. The most important recruit, however, was Dr. Marie A. Valdes-Dapena, a pediatric pathologist who then worked at St. Christophers Hospital in Philadelphia. Dr. Dapena had started her work on crib death studying infants brought to the medical examiner's office in Philadelphia. There was no office and no staff for the Roe Foundation. It was funded by the insurance policy, contributions from friends and relatives, and the Roes themselves.

Early Years of the Foundation

For the first five years of its existence, the foundation remained much as it had been envisioned. The primary concentration was on the "grants to research program" through which funds were channeled to assist ongoing research projects. In late 1966, the first chapter of the Roe Foundation was chartered covering Nassau and Suffolk counties on Long Island in New York. Special emphasis was placed on the role of public education. During this same period, the foundation and its medical advisors, led by Dr. Dapena, developed a common reporting form for sudden infant death that would aid research in finding new clues as to the cause. The forms provided for a relatively complete pre- and postnatal history of the victim and a simple family medical history, as well as a socio-economic record. They were to be completed by the attending physician or medical examiner in consultation with the parents as soon as possible after the death. Although the form had excellent therapeutic value for the families and could have elicited some good results, the foundation could not prepare a plan for acceptable distribution and analysis. It was a project that required far greater financial resources than the Mark Addison Roe Foundation possessed at the time.

While the foundation continued to operate under the guidance of the Roes, others volunteered their time and resources and began to play a role in the growth and direction of the fledgling organization. Some were parents who had suffered similar tragedies and others were friends who were moved by the suffering they saw. Chapters continued to develop and soon the foundation was pulled into a more national role.

In 1967, the Roes moved to Denver. They had arranged for office space in the basement of a Greenwich law firm, but Ann and Arthur Siegal offered office space in their advertising agency in New York City. Their offer was accepted and the foundation moved to New York City, changing its name to the National Foundation for Sudden Infant Death, Inc. This was done at the urging of the Roes, who felt that the organization could no longer serve just as a memorial to Mark but should be a memorial to all victims of SIDS. (In 1976 the name changed again to the National SIDS Foundation.)

The move to New York and the change of name did not alter the fact that the foundation was a volunteer operation. The office, equipment, and telephone were donated by the Siegals; volunteers staffed the office on a rotating basis; and stationers and printers donated their products and services. The emphasis placed on public education took its toll on the volunteers.

The lay and medical press began to write more frequently about the "mystery killer." More and more families reached the foundation's door and telephone. The poignant question was always the same: "Why did my baby die?"

In 1968, the first full-time salaried employee, Judie Choate, was hired to function as the Executive Secretary and to direct the volunteers in the day-to-day operation. She had lost a baby to SIDS, and had spent most of her time counseling other families on the telephone and in person. The direction of the foundation remained primarily the concern of its Board of Trustees and President, Ralph Colin, Jr., a former Air Force colleague of Jed Roe.

In the fall of 1970, the foundation again changed gears. Less attention was given to the research grant program, mostly because little money had been raised. It was apparent that a single office in New York, staffed by one paid employee and a group of volunteers, could not serve as the sole source of information about SIDS or provide solace to all the grieving families. More emphasis was placed on organizing local chapters and getting other organizations to help. This national perspective was provided primarily by Judie Choate. Meanwhile, important developments were occurring 3,000 miles away from New York in the state of Washington.

Mary Dore

Not until 1975 was there any semblance of an organized research effort to find the cause of and seek possible preventive measures against SIDS. It would have been 1995 before research was underway if it had not been for the efforts of Mary Dore. Fred and Mary Dore of Seattle lost their fourth child, a three-month-old daughter, on September 8, 1961.

Fred and Mary had heard vaguely of crib death before, but were shocked to learn of its prevalence in their own community. They worried about the term "pneumonia" on the death certificate. Pneumonia, of course, is a recognizable illness for which treatment should be sought. How could conscientious parents neglect signs of pneumonia in their baby? The local coroner, Leo Sowers, explained that the baby really didn't have pneumonia, but, for lack of a better term, that was the term that many physicians and coroners chose to apply.

As the months passed, Mary read the newspaper obituary columns every day and learned of about eight other families who had lost their babies in a similar manner. She wrote or called the mothers and began collecting newspapers and magazine articles, as well as names and addresses of other parents. She became a one-person support group for the parents of crib death victims.

Two features set the Dores apart from other SIDS parents. Fred was a veteran state senator who served as chairman of the Appropriations Committee (he now is a justice of the Washington State Supreme Court). Mary is smart, dedicated, and tenacious when she has a goal in mind.

Like most parents, they asked their pediatrician, Dr. Robert Polley, about the cause of crib death. "It's just one of those things," he responded. "We don't know the answer." The Dores, like the Roes in Connecticut, took it one step further. "If you don't know," they said, "is there any research going on anywhere to find the answer?" Fortunately, Dr. Polley took their inquiry seriously.

At the behest of Dr. Polley and the Dores, the Washington State Medical Association set up a special committee to study the problem of sudden and unexpected death in infancy. After several months they reported back to the Dores that, just as Jed Roe had learned, no organized research was taking place in the United States or anywhere else. The committee proposed that if research were to be undertaken, the first step should be to have all victims autopsied in one central location. That was no small issue. Death investigation throughout the United States is carried out under the jurisdiction of counties. Practices vary enormously. The costs of performing autopsies and transporting bodies were also barriers. The figure of $20,000 a year was projected by the committee for initiation of a pilot study in the state. The Dores went to work.

Washington State Law. Senate Bill 180 was introduced in 1963 into the Washington State Legislature by Senator Dore. It provided that all cases of sudden and unexpected death in children under the age of three years be studied at the University of Washington Medical School. The lobbying was done by Mary Dore, a Democrat, assisted by the wife of Coroner Sowers, a Republican. The Sowers also had lost a baby to crib death several years earlier.

Mary went immediately to the wives of the other legislators. On March 11, 1963, the day before the Dores' next child was born, SB-180 passed the Washington State Legislature. The bill as originally passed directed that "all babies under three years of age dying suddenly when in apparent good health, without medical attendance, within 36 hours preceding death be autopsied through the facilities of the University of Washington School of Medicine." A $20,000 appropriation to carry out the new law also passed.

Mary Dore did not confine her lobbying to legislators. Even before the bill was introduced, she descended upon the medical school. Her pleas fell upon receptive ears. Dr. Warren Guntheroth, a pediatric cardiologist and Dr. Donald Peterson, the epidemiologist for the Seattle/King County Health Department, who also taught at the school, began studies. Her most important convert, however, was the chairman of the Pediatric Department, Dr. Robert Aldrich. Early in 1963, Aldrich was tapped by President John F. Kennedy to be the first director of the newly created National Institute of Child Health and Human Development (NICHD). When Aldrich moved to Washington, D.C., he took with him another Seattle pediatrician, Dr. Gerald LaVeck, who was to succeed him as institute director.

One of Aldrich's first actions in 1963 was to award a contract to the University of Washington to conduct the "First International Conference on the Causes of Sudden Death in Infancy." This was the seminal event for SIDS research.

In 1965 Mary Dore founded the Washington Association for Sudden Infant Death Study, which in 1971 became a chapter of the National SIDS Foundation. Working in concert with the research team at Children's Orthopedic Hospital and Medical Center, consisting of J. Bruce Beckwith, C. George Ray and Abraham B. Bergman, the chapter established the prototype community management program for the families of SIDS victims, which has been replicated throughout the country.

Senator Warren G. Magnuson

Washington State had another important connection to the SIDS saga in the person of Warren G. Magnuson, who served in the United States Senate from 1944 to 1980. In 1968 he became chairman of the Appropriations Subcommittee that controlled the budget of the Department of Health, Education and Welfare (HEW). Through a high school classmate who worked on his staff, I had become an unofficial advisor on health matters to the senator. Aided by Mary Dore and other SIDS parents in Washington State, it was not difficult to interest the senator in the SIDS problem. Even in the face of opposition from the House of Representatives and a presidential veto of the HEW Appropriations Bill in 1973, Magnuson was able to earmark $4 million for the NICHD to embark on an expanded SIDS research program. In the previous year, the institute had funded but a single research grant on SIDS for $72,000. It was a big jump forward.

Judie Choate

Back on the East Coast, Jed and Louise Roe established the SIDS Foundation; and Mary Dore initiated the organized research effort by making dollars available for interested scientists. Judie Choate, who was named executive director of the foundation in 1970, however, was most responsible for the national campaign to "humanize" the handling of crib death. She described how she became involved in the book, *Why Did My Baby Die?* [1].

I was a young, rather inexperienced New York housewife with little interest in medicine except as it ensured the well-being of my two sons, Michael, 3 years, and Robert, 5 months. On a March morning in 1965 my life changed with a jolt and part of medicine became an all-consuming interest. My five month old son was discovered lifeless in his crib. No warning sickness, no struggle, no cry. Another tiny victim of "crib death." Like all cases of sudden, unexpected and unattended deaths in our city, Robbie was a Medical Examiner's case. His body was left in the apartment, in a closed bedroom with a policeman in attendance until mid-afternoon when a medical investigator (from the Medical Examiner's office) observed the body and interviewed us. Questions such as, "How many times did you hit the baby?" and "Did your other child choke or in any way abuse the baby?" provoked a commitment to see that no family would ever have to endure the agony of responsibility for their child's death. I can remember thinking, as they took the baby to the morgue, what happens to families who don't speak English, who have never heard of crib death, who don't have private medical care. I suppose it was, in part, easier to think about abstracts than to face my own terror. I spent a manic day trying to track down a foundation concerned with crib deaths. I had read about it; I knew it was in Connecticut. I knew it was a child's name and I knew I had to help. I called every medical school, library and hospital in New York with no results. No one knew what I was talking about. I finally started calling the major women's magazines. At the moment they took the baby's body from the apartment, I was given the name of the Mark Addison Roe Foundation by the editor of a national magazine.

I had enough knowledge about crib death to know that the Foundation could not tell me why Robbie died, but that was not my need. I just wanted to help in any way I could; thus, one week later when I began to correspond with other parents across the country, I had no idea that my involvement would be long-term nor did I suspect the horror stories I would come to know well. I guess I have kept going with the thought that although I could never save a baby's life, I could help ensure that someone would try. That I could, however, save families from the anguish and misery of holding themselves responsible for the death of their child.

A Tall Order

In 1972, I became president of the foundation. It was the last thing in the world I wanted to do. Judie Choate, among others, convinced me, however, that in order to get national recognition, a health organization is more apt to be heeded if a person with an M.D. degree is the spokesperson. Also, by then I was thoroughly outraged by how families were being treated and felt that it should not be left to SIDS parents alone to redress their grievances.

In putting together a "battle plan" it was apparent that there were two separate but related aspects of the SIDS problem. First and foremost, a research effort had to be launched. Research support had been the exclusive interest of the tiny Roe Foundation. A few small grants were awarded, but the foundation lacked the capacity for any sort of substantial campaign. Money was not all that was lacking. Few scientists with potential talent even knew of the existence of crib death; they had to be recruited to work in the field.

The other dimension was the fate of families losing children to SIDS. The veil of mystery covering both health professionals and the lay public had to be dispelled. We thus were required to put together a multifaceted campaign consisting of promoting research, professional and public education, and support services for bereaved families. It was a tall order for an organization with only one paid employee!

Where Were the Troops?

What about health professional organizations? In response to prodding by Mary Dore, the Washington State Medical Association formed a special committee to study the problem of SIDS. Their example was not emulated elsewhere. Logically, pediatricians would be expected to take the lead in addressing child health problems. My own "union," the American Academy of Pediatrics, was supportive, but unwilling to take any initiative. Groups like the American Medical Association and the American Public Health Association were silent, as were the professional societies of pathologists. Interest within the Department of Health, Education and Welfare was totally absent. It was left, then, to SIDS parents and their supporters to mount the barricades. For practical purposes in 1971, this meant two organizations, the National SIDS Foundation and the Guild for Infant Survival.

The Guild for Infant Survival was founded by Saul and Sylvia Goldberg of Baltimore in November, 1964. The Goldbergs' two-month-old daughter Suzanne died of SIDS in December of 1963. Their story is similar to that of the Roes and Dores. They were insistent that something be done about the malady that had taken their child. There were abortive attempts to get together with the Roes, but the styles did not mix, and the Goldbergs formed their own organization. By design, the guild never had a strong central organization; they believed in confederacy with individual guilds setting their policies for operation. At the time of this writing, they have virtually ceased to function as a national organization. In the 1970s, however, there were several chapters centered in Baltimore, Philadelphia, Washington, D.C., and Northern Virginia.

In addition to a decentralized structure, there were two other major differences between the foundation and the guild. All foundation policies and pronouncements about SIDS were reviewed by a Medical Board, made up of knowledgeable scientists. The guild eschewed "professional direction." Also, although not unsympathetic, the Goldbergs did not share our zeal for organizing health professionals like public health nurses to assist families of SIDS victims. They believed more in parent-to-parent assistance, and in raising funds for research. Although the styles and philosophies differed, the guild and foundation were reasonably successful in avoiding public disputes. (For more information on the philosophy of the Guild for Infant Survival, see Richard Raring's book, *Crib Death* [2].)

"No Longer Can We Accept"

In the fall of 1971, the foundation launched a national campaign to achieve the twin goals of promoting research and "humanizing" the management of SIDS. The occasion was the first parent-medical conference held in Chicago. The "marching orders" are recounted in detail to provide perspective on what has been achieved since 1971 to the present time. They were entitled "No Longer Can We Accept":

1. . . . a death certificate diagnosis, in SIDS cases, of "interstitial pneumonitis," "tracheal bronchitis," "suffocation," or any other meaningless diagnosis. Physicians must know that SIDS is a disease, readily diagnosed during the course of a simple autopsy. More important, parents must know that their babies have died of a specific entity.

2. . . . callous coroners' or medical examiners' administrative procedures whereby families are kept waiting months for autopsy results or subjected to cruel inquests in SIDS cases.

3. . . . physicians confusing all sudden, unexpected infant deaths with true SIDS. The condition can be diagnosed and must be for the sake of statistical identification and the emotional health of the family.

4. . . . suspicion of neglect on the part of firemen, policemen, morticians, newspapermen, and even clergymen with the unexpected death of an infant. These people are most often the first in contact with the stricken family; their lack of information can only further add to the feelings of guilt, grief and frustration in the family.

5. . . . the fact that some families are denied autopsies because of lack of funds or that low income families, not receiving private medical care, rarely receive any information about the syndrome.

6. . . . the lack of instruction about SIDS in medical and other health professional schools. Without knowledge, there will be no impetus for new research nor will young physicians and nurses be prepared to deal with the syndrome should it occur in the course of their professional careers.

7. . . . the existence of only a handful of research projects into the cause (or causes) of SIDS.

8. . . . the lack of knowledge of the syndrome on the part of pediatricians and family physicians. Every doctor should be prepared to offer the family more than the small consolation of "these things happen."

9. . . . newspaper articles of syndicated doctors' columns discussing suffocation, allergy or countless other unsubstantiated theories as the cause of SIDS. This kind of misinformation has done in the past, and continues to do, incalculable harm.

10. . . . the fact that volunteer families have been asked to alone form local parent groups. This is a monumental undertaking which has, in the past, been directed by mail and telephone from the NSIDSF in New York.

We Therefore Propose . . .

1. . . . a standardized procedure in every community for handling cases of infants who die suddenly and unexpectedly that is both compassionate and medically sound. Autopsies must be performed and parents promptly informed of the results.

2. . . . that the criteria for the diagnosis of SIDS be disseminated to coroners and medical examiners throughout the United States, and that the term, "sudden infant death syndrome" be utilized on the death certificates.

3. . . . that every SIDS family receive authoritative information about SIDS from a physician, nurse, or other health professional who is both knowledgeable about the disease and skilled in dealing with characteristic grief reactions.

4. . . . that a major effort be undertaken to increase the amount of research being conducted on SIDS through solicitation of the scientific community by the National Institute of Child Health and Human Development.

5. . . . that parent volunteer groups be available in every state or large community to promote the aims of the Foundation on a local level. Close ties should be maintained with local physicians, particularly pediatricians and pathologists.

The strategy for achieving the above goals would be:

1. Strengthening of the national office of NSIDSF to provide:
    a. Authoritative public information,
    b. A speaker's bureau,
    c. Consultants to assist in formation of local chapters, and
    d. Liaison with other organizations.

2. Alliance with professional medical and health organizations (e.g., pediatricians, pathologists, nurses, social workers, etc.) so that they can educate their own members about SIDS.

3. Involvement of national, state and local government to:
    a. Promote SIDS research,
    b. Upgrade autopsy procedures, and
    c. Disseminate authoritative information through health department, coroner's and medical examiner's office and law enforcement agencies by means of literature, seminars, consultants, etc.

4. A dignified public relations campaign to educate the public about SIDS without producing undue anxiety. Educational efforts will be specifically directed toward those most apt to come into contact with SIDS, such as morticians, clergy, police and firemen, and media representatives.

Campaigning in Local Communities

A measure of the Foundation's enormous success is that we now take for granted most of the parents' rights spelled out above. Yet, in 1972 when a group of graduate students working under my direction surveyed SIDS management practices in 148 U.S. cities, a dismal picture emerged [3]. In only 25 percent of communities were autopsies routinely performed. An incredible variety of terms were used on death certificates. Information and counseling was the exception rather than the rule. Every year a number of grieving parents were jailed for suspected child abuse when their infants died of SIDS. The situation, though not optimal, is far different today. Why? Mostly because of strenuous campaigning by dedicated chapter members at local and state levels.

The campaign invariably involved convincing the local coroner/medical examiner and health department director to join forces in establishing a compassionate program for handling all cases of sudden, unexpected death. When these individuals were sensitive, as was the case in such areas as New Orleans, San Francisco, Minneapolis-St. Paul, St. Louis County, Vermont, Oregon, and Oklahoma, the job was relatively easy. When they were less receptive, as in Houston, New York City, Los Angeles, Chicago, and Milwaukee, consciousness-raising had to take place. This process was aided by sympathetic newspaper or television reporters depicting how families were treated.

SIDS parents didn't do the job alone. Each chapter had a medical advisor, invariably a warm-hearted practitioner who was already 150 percent committed, to help run interference with other health professionals. Sympathetic individuals who had not lost babies joined the cause.

My personal pantheon of heroines contains the women who considered themselves "only SIDS mothers," yet assumed leadership positions in the local chapters and succeeded in moving mountains. One example is Carolyn Szybist, who organized the Chicago chapter in 1969, and later succeeded Judie Choate as national executive director in 1976. Few could rival Szybist's moving manner of speaking and skill in comforting newly-bereaved parents.

Federal Legislation

In January 1972, spurred by numerous letters written by guild and foundation members, the Senate Subcommittee on Children and Youth, chaired by Senator Walter Mondale, held a hearing on SIDS. Technically, all the hearing accomplished was a nonbinding Senate resolution calling for increased research on SIDS, and assistance to families. Actually, however, the publicity generated by the hearing lent respectability to the efforts of our chapters in local communities and gave them a big boost. To SIDS parents, the mysterious disease entity was at last being recognized.

The management study [3] concluded that community management programs could not develop without some source of public funding. In 1973, the foundation raised funds to establish a prototype regional center at Loyola University Medical School in Chicago, but that was the lone example. In particular, the costs of autopsies, and public health nurses' visits could not be expected to be borne solely by local governments. After hearings in the House and Senate, I worked with Steve Lawton, aide to Congressman Paul Rogers, who chaired the House Health Subcommittee, to draft what was to become the SIDS Act of 1974. The legislation, which was adopted despite the opposition of HEW, authorized funds to establish regional centers to perform autopsies, and provide information and counseling to SIDS families.

In 1975, twenty-two federally funded regional SIDS centers were established in twenty-one states and grew to forty-two centers in thirty-seven states in 1981, at which time responsibility for SIDS activities were turned over to the states under the Maternal and Child Health Block Grant. A description and evaluation of the regional centers is beyond the scope of this chapter. Suffice it to say that most of the centers were responsible for materially improving the standard of SIDS management in the areas they served. Others were ineffective. The degree of success seemed to correlate with the extent with which center professionals and community chapter volunteers respected each other and worked cooperatively.

Technical Assistance

With great effort the foundation managed to carry out basic functions such as printing and distributing literature, arranging for speakers, and above all, answering the mail and telephone. In communities with strong chapters, such as Seattle, Oakland, San Diego, Omaha, New Orleans, and Long Island, it was possible to organize appropriate management programs. In most of the rest of the country, however, we were stymied. Such an effort required sending out trained community organizers, which we could not afford. Recognizing that proper handling of SIDS survivors could prevent mental illness, the National Institute of Mental Health (NIMH) came to our assistance. In 1974, NIMH awarded a three-year contract to the foundation for $163,513 to establish such services. Two public health nurses were hired who performed yeoman service. Fifteen of the first twenty-two project grants awarded under the new law in 1975 were a direct result of the foundation's technical assistance provided under the NIMH contract.

In 1976, a somewhat similar contract was awarded to the foundation by the Office of Maternal and Child Health (OMCH) to organize community resources in areas not served by the projects. Eight "community organizers" were employed at various times over three years, seven of them being SIDS parents. All had originally been active in local foundation chapters, with the exception of one, who was active in the guild. The program was amazingly successful; tangible improvements in SIDS management took place all over the country. Unfortunately, there were constant disputes between officials of the foundation and OMCH over program direction. In 1979, the "mobilization contract" was withdrawn from the foundation and awarded to Lawrence Johnson and Associates, a Washington, D.C., for-profit social science consulting firm.

Foundation Moves

In 1976, after being "on call" twenty-four hours a day for ten years, Judie Choate stepped down as executive director. To my knowledge, no one at either the national or chapter level ever volunteered for a job; everyone had to be drafted. Such was the case with Carolyn Szybist who replaced Choate only after she correctly perceived that if she did not, the foundation would dissolve. This required moving the national office from New York to Chicago. In 1977, Stanford Friedman, a professor of pediatrics and psychiatry at the University of Maryland, was induced to succeed me as foundation president. When Szybist stepped down as director in 1981, the office moved to its current location in Landover, Maryland, a Washington suburb. (Address: National SIDS Foundation, Two Metro Plaza, Suite 205, 8240 Professional Place, Landover, MD 20785. Toll-free phone: 1-800-221-SIDS.) Marie Valdes-Dapena took over as president in 1984.

State of the Chapters

Although we knew that the development of strong local chapters was imperative to achieve our objectives, the variation between them was enormous. Some wanted to be exclusively involved in raising money for research, and others preferred to serve as a support group for other parents. The philosophical orientation usually depended on the composition of the group. There were three general categories: (1) "new parents" who had recently lost children and were still in the throes of their grief-guilt reactions, (2) "old parents" who had not lost children within two years, and tended to have a more global perspective, and (3) volunteers, many of them nurses, who had not lost children to SIDS, and who were drawn to the cause for idealistic reasons.

There was no such thing as a typical chapter. Some, like the ones in Seattle, Long Island, and on Northern California's East Bay were relatively large and contained a mixture of all three groups. A chapter on Chicago's North Shore was made up of mostly suburban housewives, none of whom were SIDS parents. The Alaska chapter centered in Anchorage was organized by public health nurses who perceived a need for a community program after making home visits to SIDS families. Some chapters were in fact energetic couples like the Salzsteins in San Diego and the Greenes in Maine, who did the work of ten people.

Burnout

In our chapters, there could be any number of members listed on the rolls, but only a few could be relied on to do the work. This situation, of course, pertains to all organizations, but in the NSIDSF there was an important difference, in that the work engendered such intense emotions. This was true not only in SIDS parents, for obvious reasons, but also in the rest of us. We always seemed to be unappreciated underdogs staging guerilla warfare; very few positive strokes were ever given for foundation work.

The set-up was an obvious one for rapid burnout. With very few exceptions, it was difficult to continue in active chapter work for more than a few years. SIDS parents could hurl themselves into the fray partly as a means to resolve their own grief. As the normal healing process occurred, however, it was only natural, and indeed healthy, to disengage. Leadership necessarily had to be transitory. This meant a waxing and waning of chapter activities based in large measure on the attributes of the current SIDS parents.

The phenomenon that never ceased to fascinate and inspire me was the emergence of strong, grass-roots leaders, who before their children died, never thought of themselves as especially accomplished. Suzie Behr in Omaha, Maria Orr in Honolulu, Sherryl Collins in Kewaskum near Milwaukee, Lynn Runfola in Buffalo, Judy Roth in Detroit, Ann Barr in Marblehead near Boston, Donna Musslewhite in Atlanta, Linda Hash in Oakland, Jane Adams in New Orleans, Glenda Rowe in Oklahoma City, and many, many others were "ordinary" housewives who were drawn into leadership roles only when their lives were touched by tragedy. Although, of course, they would have preferred alternate means, their work with the foundation chapters opened new vistas in their lives.

Conclusion

The inspiring saga of the National SIDS Foundation should stand as a lesson. A small band of volunteers, most of them suffering from personal grief, caused an enormous health problem to be "discovered" by the scientific establishment, the government, and the general public. The movement was successful when health professionals and volunteers joined forces and worked cooperatively.

Until the cause or causes of SIDS are discovered and means of prevention found, the need for a broad-based organization like the foundation will continue. A source of unbiased and authoritative information about SIDS is needed. Funds for research, both public and private, have to be obtained. This work cannot be left solely to the government. Grieving families still must be assisted to prevent disabling guilt reactions. The National SIDS Foundation will continue to speak for the children who have died and the families who survive with the hope that every child shall live.

Note: *More details about the events described in this chapter are contained in a book written by Dr. Bergman entitled* The "Discovery" of Sudden Infant Death Syndrome: Lessons in the Practice of Political Medicine, *published in 1988 by the University of Washington Press.*

References

1. Bergman, A.B., and J.A. Choate. 1975. *Why Did My Baby Die?* New York: The Third Press.
2. Raring, R.H. 1975. *Crib Death.* Hicksville, N.Y.: Exposition Press.
3. Bergman, A.B. September 20, 1973. "The management of SIDS in the United States." In *Hearings of the Senate Committee on Labor and Public Welfare on S. 1745.* Washington, D.C.: U.S. Government Printing Office.

Author Index

Subject Index

Adrenal medullary hyperplasia/hypoplasia, 25, 30. *See also* Hypoxic tissue markers
Airway Muscle Relaxation Theory, 62–63, 71–78
Airway Muscle Spasm Theory, 62, 65, 66–71, 78
Airway Obstruction theories, 62–83
Anesthesia reaction, as cause of SIDS or apnea, 12, 67–68, 74, 77
Apnea: 22, 33–34, 63–64, 66, 122, 126, 130–31, 133, 147–49, 151–52; central, 66, 78, 81, 96–97, 100–103, 107–8, 110, 112, 140, 142, 145–46; feeding, 105–6, 142; idiopathic, 69, 77, 133, 151–52; of Infancy (AOI), 140, 142, 144, 146, 151–52; Interrupted Infantile, 11–12, 22, 227–38; mixed, 66, 69, 78–81, 96, 99–103, 107–10, 113–15; obstructive, 64–66, 69, 71, 73–82, 94, 96, 98–103, 105, 107–11, 113–15, 143, 152; Obstructive Sleep Apnea Syndrome, 24–25, 59, 64, 109, 113, 152; of Prematurity, 69–71, 77–80, 105, 152; prolonged, 64, 139–42, 145–46, 151–52, 198; short, 139; sleep, 22, 30, 59, 69, 73–76, 80–82, 94–96, 98, 101, 105, 107–10, 112–13, 140–42, 151–52, 198
Apneic infants: behavioral and personality characteristics, 230–36; longitudinal development, 221, 227–30; neurologic functioning, 221, 228–31
Arcuccio, 19, 182–83
Arcutio, 182–83
Attachment, parent-infant: in parents of SIDS infant, 161–63; related to intensity of grieving, 165–66, 188–90
Autonomic Nervous System, 124–25

Bereavement, 157–58, 163, 166, 171. *See also* Grief; Mourning

Botulism, infant, as cause of SIDS, 11–12, 22, 141
Bradycardia, 63, 71, 76, 79, 98–99, 105–6, 108–10, 113, 139–40, 142–43, 145–48, 151–52, 198
Brainstem gliosis, 25, 30–32. *See also* Hypoxic tissue markers; SIDS, Neuropathology
Breathholding, 70–71, 80

Cardiac arrhythmia, 33–34, 80, 108, 110, 112–13, 121–28, 131, 141, 147
Cardiac lesions, 33–35
Cardiac sympathetic innervation, 122–27
Cardiac Theory (in SIDS), 121–34
Cardiopulmonary monitoring, 141. *See also* Electronic monitoring; Home monitoring
Cardiopulmonary resuscitation (CPR), 12, 77, 80, 95, 139–42, 147–49, 151–52, 203
Carotid body abnormalities, 25, 27–28, 94. *See also* Hypoxic tissue markers
Central Congenital Alveolar Hypoventilation Syndrome (CCHS), 107, 110
Clostridia botulinum, 22. *See also* Botulism, infant
Cot death, 3, 19
Crib death, 3, 242–43
Crouzon's Syndrome, 65, 100, 107
Cry, characteristics in apneic infants, 230–31
Cyanosis, 63–64, 70–71, 77, 80, 82, 105, 130, 139, 146, 198

Ear oximeter, 96–98, 108, 145
Education of caregiver, regarding Home Monitoring, 147–49, 152
Electronic monitoring, 139–40, 149, 198. *See also* Cardiopulmonary monitoring; Home Monitoring

Fulminant infection, as cause of SIDS, 6, 18, 21–22

Sudden Infant Death Syndrome

Designed by Ann Walston.

Composed by Brushwood Graphics, Inc.
in Times Roman text and Helvetica display type.

Printed by The Maple Press Company
on 50-lb. S. D. Warren's Sebago Eggshell Cream offset,
and bound in Joanna Arrestox cloth.